I0131959

Frontiers in Clinical Drug Research
Anti-Infectives
(Volume 2)

Editor

Atta-ur-Rahman, FRS

Kings College
University of Cambridge
Cambridge
UK

CONTENTS

CHAPTERS

The designed cover image is created by Bentham Science and Bentham Science holds the copyrights for the image.

PREFACE

The second volume of **Frontiers in Clinical Drug Research – Anti Infectives** comprises of seven chapters in various important fields including utilization of analytical techniques for identifying the nosocomial pathogens and antimicrobials, topical antimicrobials, anti-infective drug safety at global level, antimicrobial resistance and others.

In the first chapter, García-Contreras and colleagues discuss the current advancement in novel bacterial anti-infective drug development. They also discuss the *in vitro* and *in vivo* activity of anti-infective agents by analyzing their mechanisms of action and other recent advances in this field.

In the second chapter, Totapally and Raszynski have discussed the threat of antibiotic resistance at the global level, the causes involved in the development of antibiotic resistance and some solutions to overcome this huge problem.

Castro-Pastrana *et al.*, in the third chapter discuss certain aspects of chemoinformatics, predictive clinical pharmacology and systems biology. They also discuss the utilization of preclinical models, *in silico* methods, translational biomarkers, genomics and the strategies of postmarketing surveillance during the development of anti-infective drugs for safety evaluation and risk management.

In chapter 4, Paulson discusses the topical antimicrobial products and describes their classification, mechanism of action, indications and the information regarding the products available in the market. Horka and colleagues mainly focus on nosocomial infections in chapter 5 and the analytical techniques helpful in the identification and estimation of levels of antibiotics and microorganisms in real samples.

In chapter 6, Fernández and Camacho present an overview of the use of natural product extracts, compounds and fractions that are known for their antimalarial activity. They also highlighted the strategies and challenges linked with contemporary antimalarial natural drug research, in the light of recent literature. In the last chapter, Teixera *et al.* discuss the antimicrobial agents that can be used for therapy in vaginal infections, different dosage forms and the risks and benefit associated with them. They also explain the new strategies and approaches applied in the vaginal drug delivery.

I would like to thank all the authors for their excellent contributions. I am grateful to the outstanding efforts of the team of Bentham Science Publishers, comprising Dr. Faryal Sami and Mr. Shehzad Naqvi led by Mr. Mahmood Alam, Director Bentham Science Publishers.

Prof. Atta-ur-Rahman, FRS

Kings College
University of Cambridge
Cambridge
UK

CONTRIBUTORS

Alberto J. Martín-Rodríguez	Institute for Bioorganic Chemistry "Antonio González", Center for Biomedical Research of the Canary Islands (CIBICAN), Department of Organic Chemistry, University of La Laguna, Tenerife, Spain and Oceanic Platform of the Canary Islands (PLOCAN), Gran Canaria, Spain
Andre Raszynski	Nicklaus Children's Hospital, Miami, FL 33155. Herbert Wertheim College of Medicine, Florida International University, Miami, FL, USA
Anna Kubesová	Institute of Analytical Chemistry of the Czech Academy of Sciences, v. v. i., Veveří 97, 602 00 Brno, Czech Republic
Balagangadhar R. Totapally	Nicklaus Children's Hospital, Miami, FL 33155, USA & Herbert Wertheim College of Medicine, Florida International University, Miami, FL, USA
César de la Fuente-Nuñez	Synthetic Biology Group, MIT Synthetic Biology Center, Research Laboratory of Electronics, Department of Biological Engineering, Department of Electrical Engineering and Computer Science, Massachusetts Institute of Technology, Cambridge, Massachusetts, USA and Broad Institute of MIT and Harvard University, Cambridge, Massachusetts, USA
Dana Moravcová	Institute of Analytical Chemistry of the Czech Academy of Sciences, v. v. i., Veveří 97, 602 00 Brno, Czech Republic
Daryl S. Paulson	BioScience Laboratories, Inc., Bozeman, Montana, USA
Filip Růžička	The Department of Microbiology, Faculty of Medicine, Masaryk University, Brno, Czech Republic and St. Anne's University Hospital, Brno, Pekařská 53, 65691 Brno, Czech Republic
Gabriel Becerril Aragón	Department of Physicochemical Biology, Faculty of Biology and Soil Studies, Irkutsk State University, K. Marx St.1 Irkutsk, 664003, Russia
Héctor Quezada	Laboratorio de Investigación en Inmunología y Proteómica, Hospital Infantil de México Federico Gómez, Mexico City, Mexico
Israel Castillo-Juarez	Colegio de Postgraduados, Campus Montecillo, Texcoco, Mexico
Jiří Šalplachta	Institute of Analytical Chemistry of the Czech Academy of Sciences, v. v. i., Veveří 97, 602 00 Brno, Czech Republic
Joana Barbosa	CBQF-Centro de Biotecnologia e Química Fina – Laboratório Associado, Escola Superior de Biotecnologia, Universidade Católica Portuguesa/Porto, Rua Arquiteto Lobão Vital, Apartado 2511, 4202-401 Porto, Portugal
Jozef Šesták	Institute of Analytical Chemistry of the Czech Academy of Sciences, v. v. i., Veveří 97, 602 00 Brno, Czech Republic
Lenin Domínguez-	Department of Chemical and Biological Sciences, School of Sciences,

Ramírez	Universidad de las Américas Puebla, Cholula, México
Lucila I. Castro-Pastrana	Department of Chemical and Biological Sciences, School of Sciences, Universidad de las Américas Puebla, Cholula, México
Marie Horká	Institute of Analytical Chemistry of the Czech Academy of Sciences, v. v. i., Veveří 97, 602 00 Brno, Czech Republic
Marie Tesařová	Institute of Analytical Chemistry of the Czech Academy of Sciences, v. v. i., Veveří 97, 602 00 Brno, Czech Republic
Norma Rivera Fernández	Laboratory of Malariology, Department of Microbiology and Parasitology, Faculty of Medicine, National Autonomous University of Mexico. Mexico City, 04510, Mexico
Paola Serrano-Martínez	Department of Cell Biology, University Medical Center Groningen, University of Groningen, Groningen, The Netherlands.
Paula Teixeira	CBQF-Centro de Biotecnologia e Química Fina – Laboratório Associado, Escola Superior de Biotecnologia, Universidade Católica Portuguesa/Porto, Rua Arquiteto Lobão Vital, Apartado 2511, 4202-401 Porto, Portugal
Perla Y. López Camacho	Department of Natural Sciences, Metropolitan Autonomous University, Cuajimalpa, Mexico City, 11850, Mexico
Rodolfo García-Contreras	Department of Microbiology and Parasitology, Faculty of Medicine, UNAM, Mexico City, Mexico
Sandra Borges	CBQF-Centro de Biotecnologia e Química Fina – Laboratório Associado, Escola Superior de Biotecnologia, Universidade Católica Portuguesa/Porto, Rua Arquiteto Lobão Vital, Apartado 2511, 4202-401 Porto, Portugal
Thomas K. Wood	Department of Biochemistry and Molecular Biology, Pennsylvania State University, Pensylvania, USA and Department of Chemical Engineering, Pennsylvania State University, USA
Toshinari Maeda	Department of Biological Functions Engineering, Kyushu Institute of Technology, Kitakyushu, Japan
Valentina P. Salovarova	Department of Physicochemical Biology, Faculty of Biology and Soil Studies, Irkutsk State University, K. Marx St.1 Irkutsk, 664003, Russia

Frontiers in Clinical Drug Research
Anti-Infectives
(Volume 2)

Frontiers in Clinical Drug Research
Anti-Infectives
(Volume 2)

2

Frontiers in Clinical Drug Research – Anti Infectives

Volume **2**

Editor: **Prof. Atta-ur-Rahman**

ISSN (Online): **2352-3212**

ISSN: Print: **2452-3208**

ISBN (eBook): 978-1-68108-153-3

ISBN (Print): 978-1-68108-154-0

© [2016}, Bentham eBooks imprint.

Published by Bentham Science Publishers – Sharjah, UAE. All Rights Reserved.

© Bentham Science Publishers – Sharjah, UAE. All Rights Reserved.

BENTHAM SCIENCE Bentham *e* Books

CHAPTER 1

Recent Advances in Novel Antibacterial Development

Alberto J. Martín-Rodríguez[1,2,£]**, Héctor Quezada**[3,£]**, Gabriel Becerril Aragón**[4,£]**, César de la Fuente-Nuñez**[5,6]**, Israel Castillo-Juarez**[7]**, Toshinari Maeda**[8]**, Valentina P. Salovarova**[4]**, Thomas K. Wood**[9,10]**, and Rodolfo García-Contreras**[11,*]

[1]*Institute for Bioorganic Chemistry "Antonio González", Center for Biomedical Research of the Canary Islands (CIBICAN), Department of Organic Chemistry, University of La Laguna, Tenerife, Spain;* [2]*Oceanic Platform of the Canary Islands (PLOCAN), Gran Canaria, Spain;* [3]*Laboratorio de Investigación en Inmunología y Proteómica, Hospital Infantil de México Federico Gómez, Mexico City, Mexico;* [4]*Dept. of Physicochemical Biology, Faculty of Biology and Soil Studies, Irkutsk State University, K. Marx St.1 Irkutsk, 664003, Russia;* [5]*Synthetic Biology Group, MIT Synthetic Biology Center, Research Laboratory of Electronics, Department of Biological Engineering, Department of Electrical Engineering and Computer Science, Massachusetts Institute of Technology, Cambridge, Massachusetts, USA;* [6]*Broad Institute of MIT and Harvard University, Cambridge, Massachusetts, USA;* [7]*Colegio de Postgraduados, Campus Montecillo, Texcoco, Mexico;* [8]*Department of Biological Functions Engineering, Kyushu Institute of Technology, Kitakyushu, Japan;* [9]*Department of Biochemistry and Molecular Biology, Pennsylvania State University, Pensylvania, USA;* [10]*Department of Chemical Engineering, Pennsylvania State University, Pensylvania, USA and* [11]*Department of Microbiology and Parasitology, Faculty of Medicine, UNAM, Mexico City, Mexico*

Abstract: Bacterial infections remain one of the leading causes of death worldwide, and the options for treating such infections are decreasing, due to the rise of antibiotic-resistant bacteria. In fact, the continuing rise of antibiotic resistance is such a major global health concern that the World Health Organization has warned that we may enter a "post-antibiotic era" within this century, and they propose that urgent actions should be taken. Nevertheless, since the pharmaceutical industry has not produced a new class of antibiotics for more than a decade, researchers are taking several approaches towards developing new classes of bacterial anti-infectives, including focusing on new targets and processes, such as bacterial biofilm formation, that is related to approximately 65% of human infections. Moreover, significant advances have been made in the development of therapies aimed to attenuate the damage produced by bacterial infections by the downregulation of bacterial virulence instead of directly targeting bacterial growth, in contrast to conventional antibiotics. Furthermore, other active research areas are the utilization of molecules produced by commensal and mutualist bacteria as antibacterials to inhibit the growth of pathogenic species, and to boost the immune system in order to promote the elimination of infections. Other alternative treatments are focused on

*****Corresponding author Rodolfo García Contreras:** Department of Microbliology and Parasitology, Faculty of Medicine, UNAM, Av Universidad 3000, Coyoacán, Copilco Universidad, 04510, Mexico City, Mexico; Tel: + 52 55 56232300, Ext. 32356; E-mail: rgarc@bq.unam.mx
[£]These authors contributed equally to this work

Atta-ur-Rahman (Ed)
All rights reserved-© 2016 Bentham Science Publishers

inhibiting bacterial multidrug resistance mechanisms, such as the active efflux of antibiotics by multidrug efflux pumps. In this chapter, we discuss the recent advances in the development of novel bacterial anti-infectives, analyzing their anti-infective mechanisms, their activity *in vitro* and *in vivo,* and the advances toward their clinical implementation.

Keywords: Bacterial anti-infectives, biofilm inhibitors, host defense peptides, silver nanoparticles, gallium, quorum sensing inhibitors, quorum quenching, probiotics, prebiotics, eubiotics, bacteriocins, vaccines, immunomodulation.

INTRODUCTION

Although antibiotics probably saved more lives than any other kind of drugs during the course of human history, bacterial infections remain one of the main mortality causes, and the options for treating such infections are decreasing, due to the dramatic rise of antibiotic-resistant bacteria. In fact, currently several bacterial strains from different species are resistant to virtually all known antibiotics, therefore producing virtually untreatable infections; hence, there is a pressing need to develop new antimicrobial therapies due to the steady rise of antibiotic resistant bacteria coupled with the lack of novel drugs capable of killing these pathogens. Indeed, it has been estimated that, if no new antibiotics are discovered by 2050, 10 million people will die worldwide each year as a direct result of drug-resistant infections. The situation is so alarming that the World Health Organization has warned that we may enter a "post-antibiotic era" within this century, and they propose that urgent actions should be taken, including the development of new antimicrobial classes, effective to treat the already multi and pan resistant strains. In this regard, antibiotics with new suitable targets sometimes obtained from yet unexploited sources are under research. In addition, several new classes of antibacterials are being designed under the premise of not inhibiting growth *per se* but instead to decrease bacterial tolerance against normal antimicrobials or to target bacterial virulence which could attenuate the damage produced to hosts, allowing the immune system to get rid of the infection. Another novel approach to fight bacterial infections is to selectively boost the immune system so it can clear the infection at a faster rate. In this chapter, the recent developments in all the mentioned fields are summarized, with an emphasis on the discovery of new antibacterials, their mechanisms, their activities *in vitro* and *in vivo,* the current progress in their implementation, and their efficacy for treating antibiotic resistant strains. We also review the possible ways bacteria may adapt and develop resistance against these treatments, which are all crucial aspects that should be taken into account before these new drugs can be utilized in the clinic.

Current Antibacterial Therapies

Essentially, current antibiotics are designed to inhibit a limited set of important physiological processes directly linked to bacterial survival, such as protein, DNA, RNA, and cell wall synthesis; others are also designed to alter bacterial permeability or to disrupt specific essential metabolic processes such as the folic acid biosynthetic pathway (Table **1**). The limited amount of suitable targets for the generation of new antibiotics, the lack of investment for the discovery of new antibiotics, as well as other several factors had hampered the discovery and implementation of new antimicrobials in the clinic; in fact, the pharmaceutical industry has not produced a new class of antibiotics for more than decade [1]. However significant advances in the discovery of new antibiotics with novel action targets and mechanisms have been produced by several researchers around the world and some of these compounds exhibit several interesting properties that make them suitable and potential candidates for their clinical implementation.

Table 1: Current antibacterial targets.

Target	Antibacterials	Examples
Cell wall		
	β- lactams	penicillins, cephalosporins, carbapenems
	glycopeptides	vancomycin
Protein synthesis		
	Aminoglycosides	gentamicin, kanamycin, tobramycin
	Macrolides	azithromycin, erythromycin
	Others	tetracyclines, chloramphenicol, clindamycin
Cell membrane		
	Cationic peptides	polymyxins
Folate metabolism		
	Sulphonamides	Trimethoprim/sulfamethoxazole
DNA/RNA synthesis		
	Quinolones	ciprofloxacin, ofloxacin
	Others	rifampicin

EXPLOITING NOVEL TARGETS FOR THE DEVELOPMENT OF NEW ANTIBACTERIALS

Inhibitors of Biofilm Formation

Bacterial establishment and survival during infections are complex phenomena that involve multiple factors from the bacterial and host physiology; hence, often the *in vitro* models used for evaluating the potential of new antimicrobials do not take into account several aspects of such a complex relationship. In fact it was recognized not long ago that both in the environment and in clinical settings, bacteria are not often free-floating planktonic organisms but instead tend to organize in multi-cellular communities known as biofilms. Bacteria living within biofilms are physically protected from their surroundings by a matrix composed of sugars, proteins, extracellular DNA, lipids and water [2-4]. Biofilms exhibit an increased resistance to a myriad of environmental stresses that would be lethal to their free-swimming counterparts, including antibiotics, UV damage, metal toxicity, anaerobic conditions, acid exposure, salinity, pH gradients, desiccation, bacteriophages, amoebae, *etc*. [2-4]. Indeed, bacteria in biofilms are estimated to be between 10 and 1000-fold more resistant to antibiotic treatment compared to their free-swimming counterparts, thus resulting in treatment failure in the clinic [2-4]. In addition, biofilms cause at least 65% of all infections in humans. These biofilm infections are particularly prevalent in devices, on body surfaces, and are a leading cause of chronic infections [2-4]. Despite the importance of biofilms to human health, no antibiotics are currently available that effectively eradicate these recalcitrant structures [5]. Hence, a very active research field is the search for suitable anti-biofilm compounds that are designed to kill bacteria in biofilms, to prevent *de novo* biofilm formation or to promote the detachment of already formed biofilms. To achieve those goals, one of the first steps is to study the genetic and environmental determinants that influence in the different steps of biofilm formation to aid in understanding this complex phenomenon. Basically, biofilm formation is a developmental process consisting of least 4 different steps. Attachment is the first step, mediated by electrostatic interactions such as van der Waals forces, and involves the participation of several bacterial determinants such as surface proteins, as well as appendages such as fimbria and flagella [6, 7], Irreversible attachment: is the second step mediated also by type 1 fimbriae, curli, conjugative pili and specific surface proteins [8, 9], Next is maturation, the three-dimensional growth of the biofilm, including bacteria and matrix components, expression of autotransporter adhesins and the synthesis of multiple matrix components such as diverse exopolysaccharides, amyloid fibers, extracellular DNA (e-DNA) [8, 10, 11]. The last step is biofilm dispersal which consists of the detachment of cells from the biofilm mediated by either external forces like fluid shear or abrasion or by active bacterial processes such as the enzymatic degradation of the biofilm matrix or the biofilm substrate [12].

Based on these different stages in biofilm formation, several antibiofilm compounds have been discovered [13], among them are those designed to prevent initial cell attachment and biofilm development by several different strategies, including interfering with bacterial appendages such as fimbriae and pili. Among this kind of compounds that target type I pili are mannocides that compete for binding in the mannose binding pocket present in the FimH pilus lectin of type I pili, blocking its binding with their mannose rich receptors in eukaryotic cells. To date, compounds like biphenylmannosides have proved effective *in vitro* to prevent biofilm formation of the uropathogenic *Escherichia coli* (UPEC) and also to disrupt preformed biofilms; their oral administration was effective in clearing chronic urinary tract infections in mice and in potentiating the activity of the antibiotic trimethoprim sulfamethoxazole [14]. Similarly, compounds termed pilicides inhibit the assembly of type 1 pili [15], while curlicides inhibit curli biogenesis in UPEC and prevent the polymerization of CsgA, the major curli subunit protein. Interestingly, some of the curlicides also prevent the formation of pili and thus exhibit dual pilicide-curlicide activity [16]. Both pilicides and curlicides also inhibit UPEC biofilm formation and curlicides attenuate bacterial virulence during experimental infections [16, 17].

In addition to curli and fimbriae, flagella also play a pivotal role in the initial phases of biofilm formation, and hence they may be a suitable target for the development of antibiofilm compounds. To date, a proof of this principle was done by generating monoclonal anti-flagellin single-domain antibodies (VHHs) that were successfully used to inhibit swimming and biofilm formation by *Pseudomonas aeruginosa in vitro* [18]. Interestingly, although inhibition of flagellar motility is suitable to inhibit biofilm formation, motility is also a suitable way to inhibit this process, likely by interfering with the initial attachment. The fact that the enhancement of swimming motility is able to prevent biofilm formation was first realized in 2005 when, after screening the ability of 13,000 plant compounds to inhibit the formation of *P. aeruginosa* PAO1 biofilms, Ren and collaborators found that ursolic acid was a suitable candidate, further demonstrating that 10 µg/mL of this compound also inhibited biofilm formation of *E. coli* and *Vibrio campbellii* (previously *Vibrio harveyi*), and that this biofilm inhibition was not related to compound toxicity since at similar concentrations, it was innocuous for the growth of the 3 bacterial species used and to hepatocytes [19]. Although the mechanism by which ursolic acid is able to decrease bacterial biofilms is likely complex and multifactorial, global gene expression analysis in *E. coli* showed that it increases the expression of several genes that codify proteins involved in swimming motility (including *cheA*, and *motAB*), while deleting *motAB* counteracts the ursolic acid effect [19]. Other effects of urosolic acid in biofilm inhibition analysis are quorum sensing independent and related to sulfur metabolism [19]. Further studies demonstrated that ursolic acid is also effective in inhibiting biofilm formation by the main bacterium involved in dental caries, Gram-positive *Streptococcus mutans*, grown in composite resins [20], inhibits methicillin-resistant *Staphylococcus aureus* (MRSA) biofilm formation by interfering with amino acid metabolism and with the expression of adhesins [21], interferes with the growth of other important oral pathogens such as *Actinomyces viscosus* [22], and inhibits the biofilm formation, virulence and viability of *Listeria monocytogenes* [23]. Therefore, ursolic acid has a broad spectrum of activity as an antibiofilm and antimicrobial compound.

Another class of compounds that inhibit biofilm formation by decreasing attachment is diverse exopolysaccharides (EPS). Paradoxically, although EPS are one of the main constituents of the biofilm matrix, it was recently found that often the EPS produced by one bacterial species is able to inhibit the biofilm formation of other species and to promote the destabilization of preformed biofilms. Among the EPS with antibiofilm properties reported are Pel and Psl from *P. aeruginosa*, that have the ability to disrupt preformed *S. aureus* and *S. epidermidis* biofilms [24, 25]. Furthermore, the PAM galactan EPS, isolated from *Kingella kingae*, has a broad spectrum of biofilm inhibition, including the producer species itself and also *K. pneumoniae*, *S. epidermidis*, and *C. albicans* [26]. Also, the group II capsule EPS from *E. coli* inhibits the biofilm formation of a wide range of Gram-positive and Gram-negative bacteria including *S. aureus, S. epidermidis, P. aeruginosa, Klebsiella pneumoniae,* and *Enterococcus faecalis* [27]. Several other EPS compounds from several bacterial sources also inhibit biofilm formation [28]. One attractive feature of the group II capsule EPS from *E. coli* is that acquiring resistance against this anti-biofilm agent, at least by inactivation of single genes, is relative rare, since single inactivation of genes in *E. coli* only provide partial resistance that can increase, but not to very high levels when some of those individual mutations are combined. As expected, the general effects of such mutations were the induction of changes in the physicochemical properties of the bacterial surface that counteract the changes induced by group II capsule EPS [29]. Nevertheless, it would be interesting to design experiments to evaluate the rate of spontaneous resistance development against this and other anti-biofilm compounds not only in *E. coli* but in other susceptible bacterial species, as well as the frequency of resistance among clinical isolates, before going forward with its implementation in the clinic.

Antibiofilm Agents Derived from Host Defense Peptides (HDPs)

Another complementary way to combat biofilm formation, besides interfering with the biofilm process itself, is to target biofilm-growing cells with novel drugs. This is important since currently there are no antimicrobial agents available that can effectively eradicate bacterial biofilms [5]. Host defense (antimicrobial) peptides (HDPs) are evolutionarily-conserved molecules of the innate immune system that defend virtually all organisms on Earth against microbial infections [30]. These peptides are typically small (12-50 amino acids in length) and amphipathic, as they possess both positively charged and hydrophobic amino acid residues [30]. Their amphipathic nature allows these peptides to interact with membranes and penetrate into negatively-charged bacterial and host cells, which constitutes the basis for their broad biological properties. Among their biological functions, the peptides are able to directly kill microorganisms by means of their antimicrobial activity, and can modulate the immune system to control infections *via* their immunomodulatory properties [30, 31].

Recently, the HDP human cathelicidin LL-37 was shown to inhibit *P. aeruginosa* biofilms [32]. This initial observation encouraged subsequent studies aimed at investigating the antibiofilm properties of HDPs as well as the design and synthesis of optimized synthetic peptide variants derived from natural HDP templates. Since then, antibiofilm agents have been identified with improved, clinically relevant properties such as the ability to: i) disperse biofilms at low concentrations and to induce cell death at higher levels ii) act in combination with different classes of antibiotics to eradicate biofilms, iii) protect against lethal infections in animal models.

Small molecules derived from peptides naturally-produced by the innate immune system have also recently emerged as potential therapies against biofilms. These anti-biofilm peptides are capable of eradicating both Gram-negative and Gram-positive bacterial biofilms, synergize with different classes of conventional antibiotics, and be effective in animal models. Recent efforts have allowed the synthesis of potent antibiofilm peptides inspired by the amino acid sequence of known HDPs with antibiofilm activity, which include the human cathelicidin peptide LL-37 and the bovine neutrophil peptide indolicidin [32]. These synthetic peptides were subsequently screened for increased antibiofilm activity while preserving their size (smaller peptides cost less to produce) and low cytotoxicity towards mammalian cells.

One of the first agents identified was 1037, a very small peptide (9-amino acids long) that lacked relevant antimicrobial activity [minimum inhibitory concentration (MIC) of 304 µg/ml *vs P. aeruginosa*] but inhibited biofilms formed by Gram-negative bacteria and the Gram-positive organism *Listeria monocytogenes* [33]. This study and others [34, 35] revealed that it was possible to optimize naturally-occurring peptide templates to obtain improved antibiofilm peptides while reducing the synthesis cost as many of these peptides were of smaller size than their predecessors.

The HDP bactenecin from cow neutrophils has also been exploited for the production of peptides with enhanced antibiofilm activity. One example is peptide 1018, which exhibited potent broad-spectrum anti-biofilm activity against some of the most relevant pathogens in our society, including *P. aeruginosa*, *E. coli*, *Acinetobacter baumannii*, *Klebsiella pneumoniae* and methicillin-resistant *S. aureus* at concentrations well below their MIC [36]. The activity of this peptide was shown to be concentration-dependent in experiments using *P. aeruginosa* biofilms grown in a flow cell device, as very low peptide concentrations (0.8 µg/ml) dispersed cells from biofilms, whereas higher concentrations (10 µg/ml) led to biofilm cell death [36] (Fig. **1**). This peptide may constitute a useful tool to modulate biofilm formation in the model organism *P. aeruginosa* and potentially in other bacterial species as well.

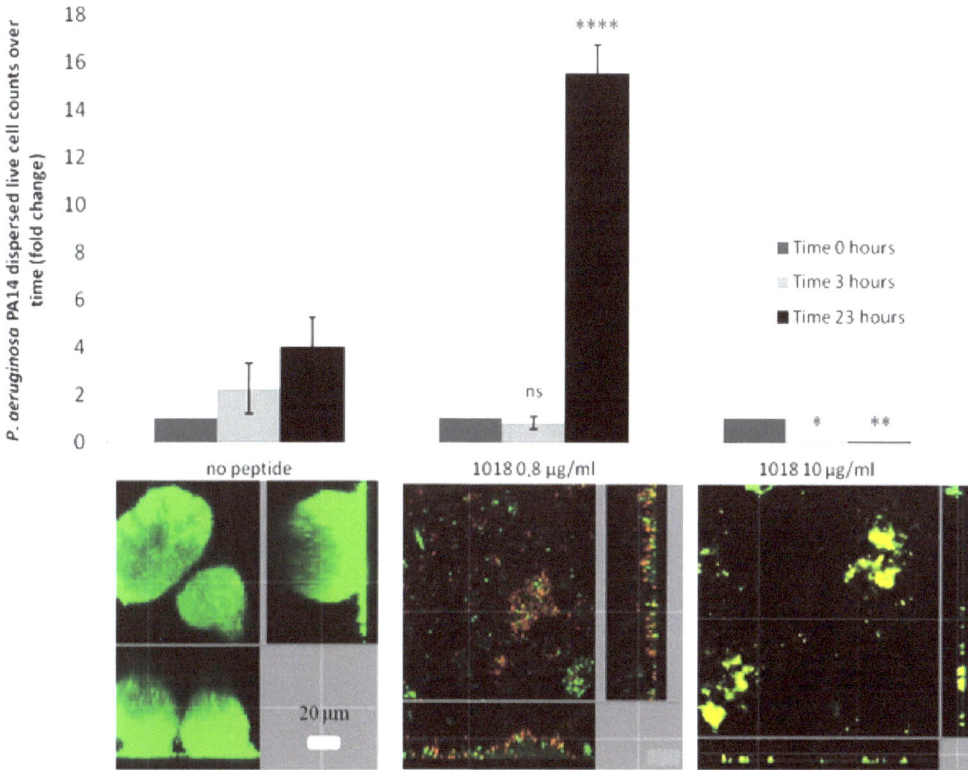

Figure 1: Concentration-dependent modulation of biofilm development by antibiofilm peptide 1018. *P. aeruginosa* PA14 cells dispersed from biofilms (grown in flow cells) upon treatment with the peptide were collected and quantified by performing CFU counts. The panel below shows confocal microscopy images of bacteria that remain attached to the flow cell chambers after peptide treatment. At 0.8 µg/ml, the peptide triggers biofilm dispersal, whereas at 10 µg/ml it stimulates biofilm cell death and therefore no detectable levels of viable dispersed bacteria. This image is published under the Creative Commons Attribution (CC BY) license.

Another clinically relevant characteristic of some antibiofilm peptides described in the literature is their ability to enhance antibiotic action to eradicate biofilms [37, 38]. For example, peptide 1018 was highly synergistic with different classes of antibiotics, including ceftazidime, ciprofloxacin, and imipenem, in eradicating pre-formed bacterial biofilms formed by *P. aeruginosa, E. coli, A. baumannii, K. pneumoniae, Salmonella enterica* and methicillin-resistant *S. aureus* [38].

One of the main limitations of HDPs and their derivatives is that they are susceptible to enzymatic degradation by proteases that can be produced by bacteria [39] or by the host [40]. Recent studies [41] have overcome this by designing peptides composed entirely of D-enantiomeric amino acid residues, which are not recognized by proteases and are therefore resistant to their effect. These D-enantiomeric peptides were very effective at eradicating biofilms formed by both wild-type and multidrug resistant bacterial pathogens, enhanced antibiotic action against biofilms, and protected the invertebrates *Caenorhabditis elegans* and *Galleria mellonella* from otherwise lethal *P. aeruginosa* infections [41].

Mechanistic insights have been obtained for some of these peptides. In particular, peptide 1018 binds *in vitro* to the second messenger nucleotide guanosine tetraphosphate (ppGpp) subsequently leading to its disappearance in experiments using bacterial cultures [36]. D-enantiomeric peptides were also capable of preventing ppGpp accumulation [41]. This is important as ppGpp is produced by bacteria in response to different stresses, binds to RNA polymerase and acts as a transcriptional modulator in order to allow cell survival [42]. In addition, ppGpp has been shown to be important in biofilm development and is a key regulator for the formation of persister cells [43], a subpopulation of cells that inhabits the inner layers of biofilms [44].

Metals with Anti-Biofilm Properties

The following section will summarize another important category of anti-biofilm compounds, bioactive metals. Among them are metal containing nanoparticles, which are generally smaller than 100 nm with potent biocidal effects due the combination of their small size and high surface-to-volume ratio, which allow close interactions with the microbial membranes [13]. So far, silver containing nanoparticles are the most studied ones, since silver has been used as an antimicrobial for decades. The antibacterial effects of silver are at least partially due its reactivity towards thiol-groups which enable the inactivation of several thiol containing enzymes involved in DNA replication, the electron transport chain and protein synthesis [45, 46], therefore providing a wide antibacterial effect against planktonic and biofilm cells. Silver-containing nanoparticles are able to inhibit *in vitro* biofilm formation of *P. aeruginosa* and *Staphylococcus epidermidis* [47]. Moreover, they are also effective against *in vitro* biofilms produced by multidrug resistant (MDR) *P. aeruginosa* strains [48], and *in vivo* against *S. aureus* biofilms developed in coated titanium implants in rabbits [49].

In addition to silver nanoparticles, other metals such as Zn are remarkably potent biofilm and virulence inhibitors in *P. aeruginosa* laboratory and clinical strains, including MDR [50, 51]. Another metal with remarkable antibacterial properties is gallium; importantly gallium nitrate was used in the clinic to treat hypercalcemia of malignancy and it is currently used in cancer diagnosis [1]. Gallium is a non-redox iron analogue that is internalized to the bacterial cells and interferes with several iron-dependent processes by displacing iron, such as in iron transport by siderophores and in iron-containing enzymes including some complexes of the respiratory chain, ribonucleotide reductase, and some antioxidant enzymes such as catalase [1]. The broad effects of gallium are understandable since iron is an essential metal cofactor for most living organisms including most pathogenic bacteria, and is often required for growth, virulence and biofilm formation. In fact, the importance of iron acquisition by pathogens is so pivotal that the human host has evolved a set of primary mechanisms that maintain very low free iron concentrations in the bodily fluids and tissues. These mechanisms include the utilization of high affinity iron chelating proteins such as transferrin and lactoferrin. Concomitantly, pathogenic bacteria have also evolved several interesting mechanisms to obtain iron from their hosts, including the utilization of siderophores that capture iron with high affinity and then deliver it back to bacteria, hemophores that bind and transport heme groups from host proteins and proteases that degrade the iron carrier proteins of the hosts [52]. Accordingly, several gallium compounds have potent bactericidal and bacteriostatic activities against a wide range of pathogenic bacteria *including P. aeruginosa, A. baumannii, Mycobacterium tuberculosis*, laboratory and clinical strains, including MDR [53]. Gallium is also effective in alleviating several infections in animal models and has synergy with some conventional antibiotics and anti-virulence compounds that inhibit the biofilm formation of *P. aeruginosa*

[54-58]. Active research toward the implementation of gallium as an antibacterial includes clinical trials in humans, the development of bacterial resistance, and remarkably, the role of gallium in the production of virulence factors at sub lethal concentrations [59-61].

Anti-Infectives that Target Bacterial Virulence

Beyond targeting bacterial growth, there is a trend to find new suitable targets to fight bacterial infections, among them, interfering with bacterial virulence is one of the best studied ones. Several Gram negative and positive pathogenic bacteria, including *P. aeruginosa*, *A. baumannii*, *Vibrio cholerae* and *S. aureus* coordinate the expression of multiple virulence factors like toxins, redox active compounds, siderophores, exoproteases, lipases and biofilm formation by a mechanism known as quorum sensing, that allows the simultaneous expression of such factors once a certain threshold cell density is reached. This coordination of the bacterial attack maximizes the chances of establishing an infection and allows bacterial dissemination [62, 63]. Hence, interfering with this process is useful for decreasing virulence factor production and consequently the damage to the host, presumably without affecting bacterial growth *per se*, thus decreasing the emerging of bacterial resistance [64]. There are several sources of quorum sensing inhibitors (or quorum quenchers), but by far the more diverse and abundant are those derived from natural sources such as algae and plants.

Quorum Quenching Compounds from Plants and Other Natural Products

Natural products represent the major source of approved drugs and still play an important role in supplying chemical diversity as well as new structures for designing more efficient antimicrobials [65]. They are also the basis for the discovery of new and novel mechanisms of antibacterial action [66]. However, research in antibiotics and natural products has declined significantly during the last decades as a consequence of diverse factors, such as a loss of interest from industrial corporations and the preference for the synthesis and modification of chemical structures derived from well-known natural sources [67, 68]. Nevertheless, natural products remain the most promising source of new antibacterial compounds and in recent years an increase in the study of antibacterial natural product derivatives is occurring [69, 70]. In this regard, a large number of substances, mainly extracts from various natural sources, have been obtained in order to identify their quorum quenching (QQ) activity [71].

To date, plants constitute the main natural source of novel QQ molecules reported in the current literature (Fig. **2**). To overcome their lack of immune systems, plants have evolved an immense arsenal of chemical defenses towards grazers and pathogens that has been exploited by humankind since the dawn of its existence. The pharmacoactive repertoire of plant secondary metabolites is huge and covers a very broad range of scaffolds, molecular targets and modes of action. It is not surprising then that in recent years, great interest in finding QS disruptors from plant sources has occurred. The search has been successful, as evidenced by the abundant literature on this topic. Similarly, sessile organisms such as algae have faced the evolutionary need to combat epibiosis in seawater, a very harsh environment prone to biofouling, thus constituting novel sources of QQ molecules. In response, microbes developed their own chemical warfare. From the study of bacterial-bacterial and bacterial-fungal interactions, knowledge on bacterial and fungal metabolites specifically targeting bacterial QS-regulated behaviors and other downstream physiological processes have begun to emerge. Thus, the most recent advances in the characterization of QQ molecules from natural sources are discussed in the following sections.

Quorum Quenchers Derived from Plants

As introduced above, plants lack immune cells able to be mobilized to the sites of infection, or the sophisticated adaptive immune systems of vertebrates [72]. Instead, they rely on i) their pre-formed defenses, of a physical nature, such as the plant cell wall and cuticule, and ii) their innate immune system, which is organized in two branches, the first recognizing and responding to molecular patterns specific to microbes, pathogenic or not (*e.g.*, flagellin), and the second, reacting specifically towards virulence factors or their effects on the plant host [73, 74]. The role of QS signals as modulating agents of plant-microbe interactions has been recently reviewed by Hartmann and co-workers [75]. Remarkably, QS signals do not only trigger immune responses in plants, but conversely, plants also produce compounds that mimic or interfere with bacterial QS.

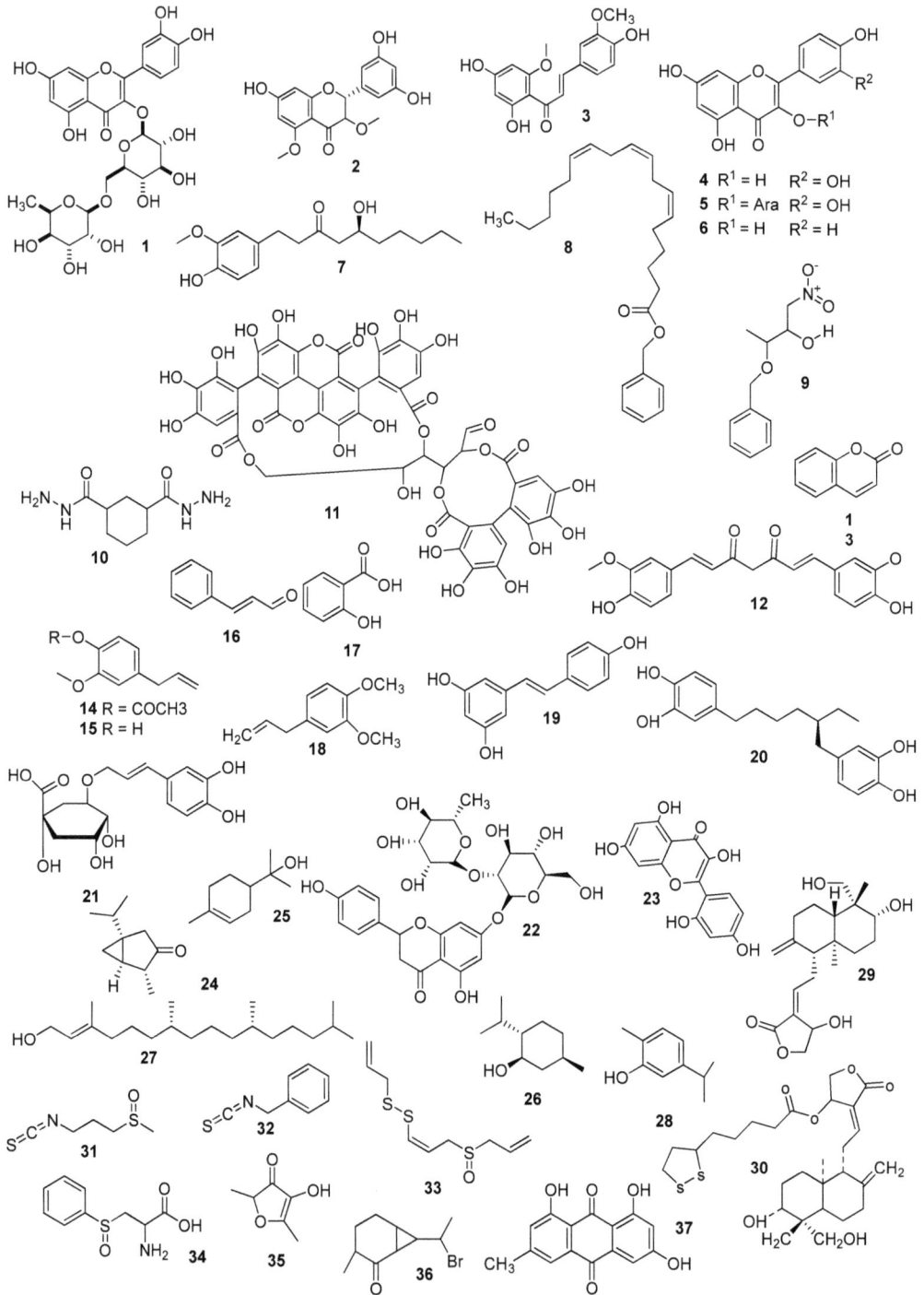

Figure 2: Plant natural products reported with QQ activity.

Flavonoids are widespread plant secondary metabolites with an extraordinary chemical diversity. More than 10,000 flavonoids have been identified thus far [76]. Several glycosylated flavonoids from *Cecropia pachystachya* are inhibitors of acyl homoserine lactone (AHL) mediated QS, with rutin (1, numbers in parenthesis in this and the following section correspond to chemical structures in Figs. **2** and **3**), the only *O*-diglycosylated flavonoid isolated, the most active compound [77]. Recently, Martín-Rodríguez and co-workers reported a series of flavonoids from *Piper delineatum,* two of which (**2-3**) were able to modulate bioluminescence and biofilm formation in *Vibrio campbellii* in a non-toxic fashion, most efficiently at high micromolar concentrations (250-500 μM) [78]. Phenotypic analyses with *V. campbellii* QS knockout mutants suggested a molecular target downstream LuxO for these compounds; however, subsequent testing of these flavonoids in a *V. campbellii* strain displaying luminescence independent of QS suggested that there could be targets outside the QS signaling circuit contributing to the phenotypic output, and further research is required to elucidate their precise mode of action (Martín-Rodríguez *et al.*, unpublished data). Flavonoid-rich fractions of *Psidium guajava* leaves also exhibited QQ activity in *C. violaceum* and *P. aeruginosa* [79]. The activity was attributed to quercetin (4) and quercetin-3-*O*-arabinoside (5), the major constituents of the active extracts [79]. Recently Gopuet and colleagues, using a molecular docking and molecular dynamics simulation analysis, suggested that the mechanism of action of quercetin is related to competition for binding with LasR receptor protein, so the QQ activity occurs through the conformational changes between the receptor and quercetin complexes [80]. Similarly, flavonoid-rich extracts from *Centella asiatica* inhibit QS-regulated phenotypes in *C. violaceum* and *P. aeruginosa* [81]; the main activity was attributed to kaempferol (6).

Other plant phenolics have been widely reported as QS disruptors. In a detailed study, 6-gingerol (7), the active constituent of ginger (*Zingiber officinale*), was found to repress biofilm formation and virulence gene expression in *P. aeruginosa* [82]. Interestingly, treatment with 6-gingerol significantly reduced animal mortality in a mouse model at low micromolar concentrations (10-100 μM). The authors postulated that 6-gingerol elicits its activity by antagonism with *P. aeruginosa* QS receptors LasR and possibly RhlR; these inferences are supported by *in silico* simulations [82]. The structural simplicity of 6-gingerol encourages the preparation of improved synthetic derivatives, as assessed by Kumar and co-workers [83]. In this regard, knowledge on the potential biological targets of the compound is an asset. Other phenolic QQ compounds include those of *Salvadora persica*; organic extracts from this strain show QQ activity in the *C. violaceum* system. By GC-MS analysis, three phenolic compounds were identified (benzyl (6Z,9Z,12Z)-6,9,12-octadecatrienoate(8),3-benzyloxy-1-nitro-butan-2-ol (9) and 1,3-cyclohexane dicarbohydrazide(10)). Molecular docking suggested that the activity of these compounds could be derived from efficient binding to the QS DNA-binding response regulators of *Streptococcus mutans* and *S. aureus* [84].

Another careful evaluation provided by Li and colleagues [85] showed that sub-MIC concentrations of punicalagin (11), a polyphenolic compound abundant in pomegranates, acts at the transcriptional level in *Salmonella thypimurium* by repressing genes involved in bacterial motility and virulence. Although *S. thyphimurium* adhesion to HT29 cells was not affected by punicalagin, bacterial virulence was notably reduced. Curcumin (12), the well-known pigment of *Curcuma longa,* attenuates several QS-dependent phenotypes such as biofilm formation, alginate production, swimming and swarming motility in an array of uropathogens [86]. Similarly, coumarin (13), a characteristic plant benzopyrone, inhibits AHL-mediated QS in several bacterial models [86]; however, the effective doses were high (>1 mM).

Eugenyl acetate (14) from clove buds (*Syzygium aromaticum*) represses virulence factor production in *P. aeruginosa* and *S. aureus*, as well as violacein production in *C. violaceum* [87]. Such a broad-spectrum activity, including both Gram-negatives and Gram-positives, clearly deserves further investigation. From the evaluation of cinnamon bark oil, eugenol (15) and cinnamaldehyde (16) were identified as inhibitors of biofilm formation and pyocyanin production in *P. aeruginosa* at non-toxic concentrations [88]. In addition, cinnamon bark oil significantly inhibited the expression of the *csgAB* operon involved in curli biogenesis. In a different study, cinnamaldehyde was the most potent hit in a screening program searching for AHL-synthase inhibitors together with other plant natural products tested at millimolar concentrations [89]. Remarkably, in spite of its non-lactonic nature, cinnamic acid was successfully docked to the SAM binding pocket of LasI, but not to that of EsaI. Experimental evidence supports the hypothesis that cinnamaldehyde targets short-chain AHL synthases specifically. In that study, salicylic acid (17) was also identified as a hit in the screening project. Subsequently, the activity of both cinnamic and salicylic acid was thoroughly evaluated in *Pectobacterium* spp., expanding the knowledge on their activity as QQ compounds [90]. Similarly, the methanolic extract of *Cuminum cyminum* strongly interferes with violacein production, bioluminescence, biofilm formation, flagellar motility and exopolysaccharide production [91]. Using molecular docking analysis, methyl eugenol (18) was suggested as the main active metabolite, which interacts antagonistically with the LasR protein [91].

Resveratrol (19) is abundant in grapes and other foods. To overcome its poor solubility in aqueous media, Duarte and co-workers prepared resveratrol-hydroxypropyl-γ-cyclodextrin inclusion complexes that inhibited the biofilm formation in *Campylobacter* spp. and *Arcobacter butzleri*, as well as violacein production in *C. violaceum* [92]. The activity of the complex was attributed to resveratrol, although the precise mode of action of this compound remains to be elucidated. In a screening of 1,920 natural products using molecular docking analysis against LasR and RhIR receptor proteins, two derivatives of caffeic acid (rosmarinic acids (20) and chlorogenic acid (21)) and two flavonoids (naringin (22) and morin (23)) were identified as suitable QS receptor antagonists. These metabolites significantly inhibited the production of several virulence factors of *P. aeruginosa*, such as protease activity, elastase and hemolysin; in addition, they also disrupted the biofilm architecture [93].

Terpenoids are the largest class of natural products, include one or several units of isoprene, and are present in all living organisms [94]. Low-molecular weight terpenoids are volatile, and regulate numerous interactions with the plant and its environment [95]. In a study with plant volatiles, thujone (24) and α-terpineol (25) exhibited the most potent activities in the *P. aeruginosa* PQS and *C. violaceum* QS systems, respectively [96]. Menthol (26), a major constituent of *Mentha piperina,* exhibited a broad-spectrum QQ activity in several Gram-negative models, and increased the survival of *Caenoharbditis elegans* infected with *P. aeruginosa* PAO1 [97]. The activity of menthol was attributed to its interaction with the LasR receptor [97]. Phytol (27), an acyclic diterpenoid, was also reported to interfere with *P. aeruginosa* QS-regulated processes [98]. The monoterpenoid carvacrol (28) inhibited *cviI* expression in *C. violaceum*, along with several QS-regulated processes such as biofilm formation, violacein biosynthesis and chitinase activity, at concentrations below 500 μM. Remarkably, it also reduced biofilm formation in *C. violaceum, S. thypimurium* and *S. aureus* [99]. Andrographolide (29), an important constituent of *Andrographis paniculata*, significantly reduced cell damage in chicken type II pneumocytes exposed to *E. coli* APEC-O78 by interfering with the AI-2 signal transduction pathway, repressing the expression of virulence genes [100]. A previous study showed that 14-alpha-lipoyl andrographolide (30) can also inhibit LasR-homoserine lactone interactions and repress the transcription of the QS-regulated genes *lasR, lasI, rhlR*, and *rhlI* in a dose-dependent manner [101].

The mode of action of iberin (31), an organosulfur compound from *Armoracia rusticana*, was unraveled by a powerful 'omic' approach that combined RNA sequencing and proteomic analyses [102]. Iberin was shown to inhibit the expression of three small regulatory RNAs (srRNAs) RsmY, RsmZ and PhrS. Beautifully, iberin acts at the post-transcriptional level on LadS, a sensor kinase that phosphorylates GacS, which is responsible for activating GacA and the subsequent expression of *rsmY* and *rsmZ* [102]. As expected, *P. aeruginosa* biofilm formation was dramatically reduced in the presence of 500 μM of iberin, highlighting srRNAs as targets for antimicrobial drug development. In a different study, other isothiocyanates such as benzyl isothiocyanate (32) interfered with the QS system of *C. violaceum* [103]. (Z)-ajoene (33) from garlic (*Allium sativum*) thwarts *P. aeruginosa* QS, although a more detailed evaluation is required [104]. Supporting the screening of natural-product-like small molecules for the discovery of novel QQ, Kasper and colleagues synthesized and evaluated a collection of analogues of naturally-occurring compounds produced by *Petiveria alliacea*, among which compound 25 (34) exhibited the best profile as a biofilm inhibitor against oral bacteria and, potentially, as an AI-2 QS disruptor [105]. Further studies are required to determine whether the observed activities are indeed due to interference with QS signaling. Furaneol (35), a furanone abundant in strawberries, has potent activity on QS-regulated phenotypes in *P. aeruginosa* at very low concentrations (0.1-1 μM), that were attributed to interference with AHL-mediated QS, consistent with the mode of action described for other furanones [106, 107]. Anther halogenated compound, the 7-(1-bromoethyl)-3-3-dimethyl-bicyclo [4.1.0] heptan-2-one (36), which was identified in extracts of *Melia dubia* by GC/MS analysis, suppresses hemolysis, swarming and biofilm formation in *E. coli*. Docking studies indicate that this molecule interferes with SdiA, which is homologous to LuxR [108].

Emodin (37) an anthraquinone isolated from *Rheum palmatum* and widely distributed in other plant species inhibits the biofilm formation of *P. aeruginosa* and *Stenotrophomonas maltophilia*. By employing an assay of TraR degradation in *E. coli*, it was determined that the mechanism involves the induction of proteolysis of the quorum-sensing signal [109].

Numerous studies have addressed the search for novel QQ from plant extracts and essential oils. Table **2** summarizes the main findings reported over the last four years, and reinforces the potential of plant secondary metabolites as a source of naturally or naturally-inspired chemical probes targeting bacterial QS.

Table 2: Extracts from plants and other natural sources reported to inhibit bacterial QS.

Source	Major Constituents	Concentration	Target	Refs.
Plants				
Achyranthes aspera	3,12-oleandione, betulin	125 μg/mL	*Streptococcus mutans*	[201]
Adenanthera pavonina	Not provided	0.25-1.0 mg/ml	*C. violaceum, P. aeruginosa*	[202]
Allium cepa	pantolactone and myristic acid	50, 100 μM	*P. aeruginosa*	[203]
Amphipterygium adstringens	Anacardic acid mixture	166-500 μg/mL	*C. violaceum P. aeruginosa*	[204]
Andrographis paniculata	flavonoids, phenolics, saponins, and tannins	No available	*C. violaceum P. aeruginosa*	[205]
Arctium lappa	Arctiin, *o*-hydrobenzoic acid, luteolin, quercetin, chlorogenic acid, caffeic acid, cynarin, benzoic acid	2.5 mg/ml	*S. aureus L. monocytogenes*	[206]
bitter orange (ccitrus)	*o*-glycosylated flavanones	200 μg/mL	*C. violaceum Y. enterocolitica*	[207]
Centratherum punctatum	Sesquiterpene lactones of the goyazensolide and isogoyazensolide-type	200 μg/ml	*P. aeruginosa*	[208]
Citrus spp.	Not provided	97.50-243.75 μg/ml	*V. campbellii C. jejuni*	[209]

Table 2: contd....

Emblica officinalis	Not provided	39-78 µg/ml	Streptococcus mutans	[210]
Hydrastis canadensis	Not provided	40-80 µg/ml	S. aureus	[211]
Ferula asafetida, Dorema aucheri	Not provided	25 µg/ml	C. violaceum, P. aeruginosa	[212]
Hyptis suaveolens	Undecanoic acid, phenanthrenemethanol	50-400 µg/ml	C. violaceum, E. coli Proteus spp. S. marcescens	[213]
Kigelia africana	Not provided	0.31–8.2 mg/mL 2 mg/mL	C. violaceum A. tumefaciens	[214]
Lavandula angustifolia	linalyl anthranilate, linalool,β-caryophyllene, isoborneol, cis-β-farnesene, trans-β-ocimene, 3-octanone, hexyl butyrate, caryophylleneoxide	0.01-0.05 % (v/v)	E. coli	[215]
Leptospermum spp. Manuka,propiolis	Isoprenyl caffeate	450 µg/ml	C. violaceum	[216]
Lippia alba	limonene, neral, carvone, geraniol,bicyclosesquitelandrene,geranial, piperitenone, β-bourbonene, trans-β-caryophyllene	0.6-67 µg/ml (IC$_{50}$)	C. violaceum	[217]
Lippia graveolens	Not provided	0.015-0.12 5mg/ml	C. violaceum	[218]
Essential oils of Lippia alba and Ocotea sp.	Citral	P. putida E. coli		[219]
Melaleuca alternifolia and Rosmarinus officinalis	Not provided	0.5 µL/mL	C. violaceum	[220]
Melicope lunuankenda	Not provided	4 mg/mL 20 µL 3 mg/mL	C. violaceum E. coli P. aeruginosa	[221]
Minthostachys mollis	Pulegone, D-menthene, caryophyllene, limonene, isomenthone	0.02 % (v/v)	C. violaceum	[222]
Murraya koenigii	Caryophyllene, caryophyllene oxide,cinnamaldehyde, α and β-phellandrene, eugenol	0.02 % (v/v)	C. violaceum, P. aeruginosa	[223]
Nymphaea tetragona	Methyl gallate, pyrogallol	600 µg/disc	C. violaceum	[224]
Piper nigrum, Piper betle and Gnetum gnemon	Not provided	250 µL, 20 µL50% v/v	P. aeruginosa E. coli C. violaceum	[225]
Psidium guajava	Not provided	100-1000 µg/ml	C. violaceum	[226]
Rhizophora annamalayana	1H-purin-6-amine,cycloheptasiloxane,cycloocta siloxane,cyclononasiloxane,	1000 µg/mL	C. violaceum V. campbellii	[227]

Table 2: contd....

	cyclononasiloxane,octadecamethyl,cyclodecasiloxane eicosamethyl and1,1,1,5,7,7,7-heptamethyl3,3-bis (trimethylsiloxy) tetrasiloxane.			
Rosa rugosa	Several polyphenols and flavonoids	80-1200 µg/ml	*C. violaceum* *E. coli* *P. aeruginosa*	[228]
Sclerocarya birrea	Quercetin	25-200 µg/ml	*P. aeruginosa*	[229]
Scutellaria baicalensis	Not provided	Not provided	*C. violaceum* *P.Carotovorum*	[230]
Syzygium aromaticum	Not provided	3 mg/mL	*C. violaceum* *E. coli* *P. aeruginosa*	[231]
Terminalia chebula	3-*O*-methyl-4-*O*-(β-*D*-xylo pyranosyl) ellagic acid,*S*-flavogallonic acid,methyl *S*-flavogallonic acid,3,4,8,9,10pentahydroxyldibenzo (β,δ) pyran-6-one AND Ellagic acid	0.5-1.0 mg/ml	*P. aeruginosa* *P. aeruginosa* *C. violaceum A. tumefaciens*	[232, 233]
Trigonella foenum-graecum	Caffeine, methyl 14methylpentadecanoate, palmitic acid, pyrogallol,linoleic acid methyl ester, capric acid	125-1000 µg/ml	*A. hydrophila, P. aeruginosa*	[234]
Triticum sp.	Not provided	0.016-0.5 % (v/v)	*S. aureus*	[235]
Zingiber officinale	Not provided	1, 5 and 10%	*P. aeruginosa*	[236]
Several *Meliaceae, Melastomataceae, Lepidobotryaceae, Sapindaceae,* and *Simaroubaceae* species	Not provided	45-266 µg/ml (IC$_{50}$)	*C. violaceum, P. aeruginosa*	[237]
Bacteria				
Endophytic bacteria from *Pterocarpus santalinus: Bacillus firmus*PT18 and *Enterobacter asburiae* PT39	Not provided	Not provided	*C. violaceum, P. aeruginosa*	[238]
Bacteria from fish farms:*Pseudomonas* sp. FF16 and *Raoultella planticola* R5B1	Not provided	400 µg/disc	*A. tumefacienes* *C. violaceum*	[239]
Endophytic bacteria from *Phaseolus vulgaris*, mainly *Microbacterium testaceum* strains	Not provided	Not provided	*C. violaceumE. coli* *V. campbellii*	[240]
Marine bacteria, particularly *Pseudoalteromonas* sp. K1 and B2	Not provided	Not provided	*C. violaceum, S. marcescens, V. campbellii*	[241]
Paenibacillus sp.139SI from*agricultural soil	Not provided	1.0-4.5 mg/ml	*P. aeruginosa*	[242]
Alcaligenes faecalis	Not provided	Not provided	*Vibrio*	[243]

Table 2: contd....

			alginolyticus	
Nocardiopsis dassonvillei subsp. *dassonvillei*	nocapyrones	100 mg/mL	*C. violaceum* *P. aeruginosa*	[244]
Stenotrophomonas maltophilia BJ01	*Cis*-9-octadecenoic acid	3.6 mg/mL	*C. violaceum* *P. aeruginosa*	[245]
Fungi				
Agaricus blazei	Not provided	0.025-0.10 mg/ml	*P. aeruginosa*	[246]
Marine endophytic strains: *Sarocladium strictum* LAEE06, *Fusarium* sp. LAEE13, *Khuskia* sp. LAEE21, *Epiccocum nigrum* LAEE14	Sespendole, fusaric acid, emericellamide A, variecolorin N and other secondary metabolites	50-500 µg/ml	*C. violaceum*	[247]
Agaricus spp.	Mainly γ-tocopherol		*P. aeruginosa*	[248]
Algae				
Asparagopsis taxiformis	Not provided	5 µLextract	*C. violaceum* *S. liquefaciens*	[249]
Several macroalgal species	Not provided	0.1-10X tissue level	*C. violaceum, P. aeruginosa*	[250]
Lichens				
Unsea longissima (extract-Aucolloidal nano-formulation)	Orcinol, arabitol,apigenin, usnic acid	5-15 %	*C. violaceum, S. mutans*	[245, 251]
Animals				
Eunicea knighti	cembranoid diterpenes	50, 100 µM	*C. violaceum* *P. aeruginosa* *V. campbellii*	[252]

Quorum Quenchers from Bacteria, Fungi, and other Natural Sources

Even though literature shows a clear dominance of plant-derived natural products, there is an increasing number of QS inhibitors from alternative sources being reported (Fig. **3**). Thus, 2,4-bis(1,1-dimethylethyl) phenol (38) produced by the marine bacterium *Vibrio alginolyticus* G16, an epiphytic strain of the red alga *Gracilaria gracilis*, disrupted QS in *Serratia marcescens* at 250-500 µg/ml [110]. Over the last few years, indole (39) has gained increased attention as a signaling molecule in bacteria [111-114]. Indole was characterized as a QQ in *C. violaceum*, *P. chloroaphis* and *S. marcescens* at 0.5-1.0 mM, and contributed to *C. elegans* survival in infection tests [115]. Anthraquinones (40) from the exudates of *Penicillium restrictum* displayed very potent activities towards the *agr* QS system of *S. aureus*, the most potent of which had an IC_{50} of 8.1 μM *in vitro* [116]. Furanone F202 (41) originated from the red alga *Delisea pulchra* and a tiophenone analogue named TF101 (42) elicited potent activities at 10 μM against *E. coli* and *V. campbellii* QS-regulated phenotypes [117]. Both compounds interfered with AI-2 QS, and modulated *E. coli* O103:H2 biofilm formation and virulence. The synthetic compound exhibited better activity than the natural one, reinforcing previous findings [118, 119] and providing support to the development of novel thiophenones with improved performance. In that regard, further toxicity tests are certainly needed. Finally, horse colostrum hexapolysaccharide (43) was characterized as a QQ in *S. aureus* [120]. An interesting finding of that study was the ability of the hexapolysaccharide to interfere with Gram-negative QS as well, by degrading both short- and long-chain AHLs, therefore quenching QS. Protoanemonin (44) is a metabolite that has been reported to be present in plants of the Ranunculaceae family, but has recently been identified in *Pseudomonas* (B13 and *reinekei* MT1) with QQ activity. As elucidated by transcriptomics and proteomics studies, it significantly reduces gene expression and secretion of proteins controlled by QS in *P. aeruginosa* [121].

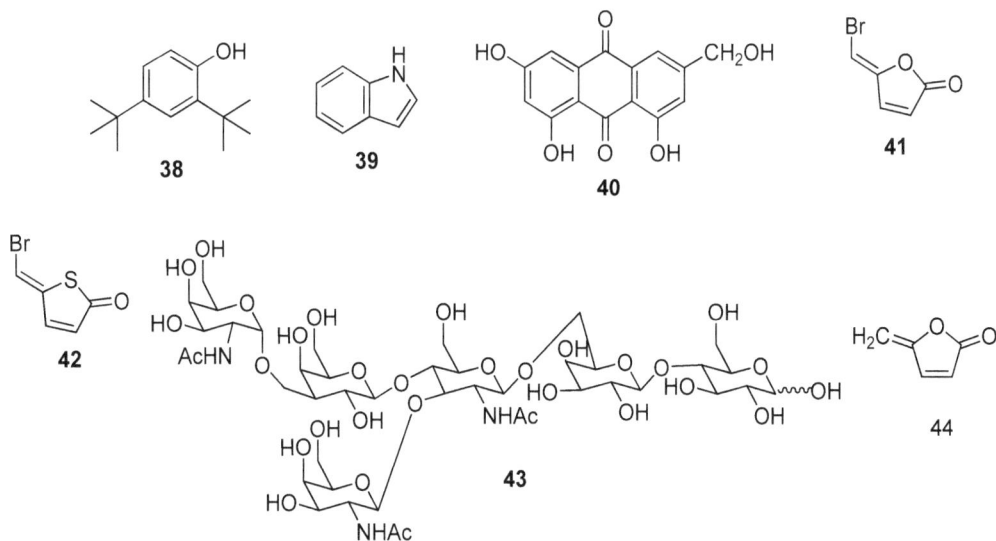

Figure 3: Compounds from non-plant sources reported with QQ activity.

Quorum Quenching Enzymes

To date, there are several quorum quenching enzymes which can degrade or modify AHL autoinducers; the catalytic reactions have been summarized in Fig. (**4**).

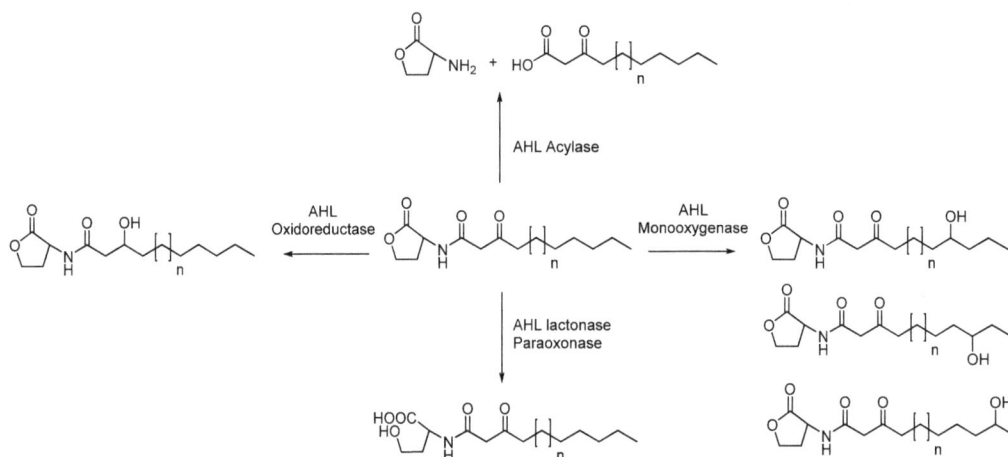

Figure 4: Mechanisms of acyl homoserine lactone quorum quenching enzymes.

Lactonases

These enzymes cleave the lactone ring of AHL autoinducers; thereby, QS systems can be disturbed through the degradation of AHL molecules. A variety of lactonase enzymes have been found in many bacteria, for example, the halotolerant and thermally-stable lactonases [122, 123]. The enzymes are metalloenzymes having two zinc ions for catalysis and stability [124, 125]. In addition, paraoxonases, which hydrolyze paraoxon, are QQ enzymes which can inactivate AHLs [126]. The enzymes were originally found in mammalian cells [127]; hence, mammalian tissues potentially have QQ activity.

Acylases

These enzymes hydrolyze AHL autoinducers into carboxylate and amino acids. The resulting products do not work anymore as autoinducers. Acylase of *P. aeruginosa* is a member of the N-terminal nucleophile hydrolase superfamily [128]. In addition, acylase derived from *Acinetobacter* sp. Ooi24 is a member of the amidase family [129], and is a zinc metalloenzyme [130].

Oxidoreductases

These enzymes catalyze the reduction of AHL autoinducers to produce hydroxyl-AHLs. As a result, a QS system can be disturbed by the modification of AHLs. For example, several AHL oxidoreducatases convert 3-oxo-C(8-14)-AHLs into 3-hydroxy-AHLs [131] and 3-oxo-C12-AHL into 3-hydroxy-C12-AHL [132]. Basically, the enzymes have been characterized as a member of the short-chain dehydro-genase/reductase (SDR) family which probably uses NADPH as a co-substrate. Monooxygenases also catalyze the hydroxylation of AHLs at the ω-1, ω-2, and ω-3 carbons of the acyl chain. The oxidized AHLs showed smaller effect than the original AHLs as an autoinducer signal [133].

PROBIOTICS AND COMPOUNDS ISOLATED FROM BACTERIA

From prehistorical times, antimicrobials of natural origin have been used for food preservation and human health purposes. However, the extensive use of antibiotics in the recent decades has induced resistance to antimicrobial compounds in many bacteria. Antibiotics usually prescribed for humans are also administered to animals and plants involved in the food chain, and therefore reduce their effectiveness in patients even before being submitted to treatment [134]. The search and implementation of alternatives to antibiotics, has become a crucial task for public health institutions and the food industry, who aim to avoid opportunistic infections in living resources (livestock, poultry, fish and others) [135]. In the recent years, the abundant research in probiotic microorganisms, prebiotics and substances produced by bacteria, such as bacteriocins and organic acids, is leading to potential solutions for these problems.

Probiotics

Growing individually or in co-culture, a large number of bacteria produce compounds with antimicrobial action, such as hydrogen peroxide, benzoic acid, diacetyl, reuterin, volatile fatty acids (VFA) and bacteriocins. *Probiotic microorganisms* are bacteria, fungi (yeast and molds), and Archaea [136] whose regular consumption benefits the health of the host (human or animal) by stimulating the growth and function of indigenous intestinal flora, inhibiting colonization by enteropathogens, and improving food utilization. In order to accomplish their functions, probiotics should withstand the acidity of the stomach, resist the action of hydrolytic enzymes, and, at least partially, avoid absorption in gastrointestinal tract [137].

In 1907, the Russian zoologist I. Mechinikov first reported health benefits upon long-term consumption of yoghurt containing *Lactobacillus bulgaricus*, although for centuries the diet of people of the Near East had included lacto-fermented beverages. The positive effects of probiotic lactic acid bacteria (LAB) include:

- Improvements in digestion by the production of short- and medium chain VFA and vitamins.

- Generation of low pH and a low redox potential, what allows normal flora to outcompete gut pathogens such as pathogenic *E. coli*, *Salmonella* spp. *(enterica, arizonae)* and *Yersenia* spp. for attachment sites on entherocytes [134].

- Inhibition of the growth of competing species by the production of antimicrobial peptides (bacteriocins).

- Enhancement of intestinal flora composition.

- Regulation of cholesterol levels.

- Mitigation of lactose intolerance.

- Modulation of immune response, including prevention of neoplastic disorders [138].

Recent definitions of probiotics include not only live microorganisms, but also products of their metabolism, like those of milk fermentation [139]. *L. bulgaricus*, for instance, is unable to survive in the gut, but it produces the enzyme lactase which causes alleviation of lactose intolerance [140].

Probiotic Preparations

Probiotic preparations can consist of single strains or mixtures of microbes. LAB (*lactobacilli, bifidobacteria* and *enterococci*) are used alone or together with non-pathogenic enteric microorganisms such as the fungi *Saccharomyces* ssp., *Aspergillusoryzae* and/or the anaerobic genera: *Bacteroides, Clostridium* and *Veillonella*. Three variants of mixtures of probiotic strains are prepared [141]:

- Defined: strains are mixed after individual cultivation and the numbers of cells are controlled.

- Semi-defined: Strains of the same genus are co-cultured and no cell number control is possible.

- Undefined: The inoculum is taken directly from the biological source (*e.g.*, caecal content, mucosal scraping) and then cultivated in conditions that do not equally favor all strains.

Horizontal gene transfer between bacterial strains with optimal functioning in distinct environments and differences in resistance to reactants and phages open many possibilities. Although, when a probiotic strain is isolated from a different source than the environment in which it is utilized, then inter-strain antagonistic interactions can appear [142]. Paradoxical results of clinical tests show that the application of genetically-modified probiotics is still a challenge, and calls for a ban of their human use have been issued worldwide [143]. Concern arose over the outcome of the 2008 trial of the Dutch Acute Pancreatitis Group with a mixture of *Lactobacillus acidophilus, L. casei, L. salivarius, Lactococcus lactis, Bifidobacterium bifidum* and *B. lactis*. Individually, the strains inhibited pathogen growth, but after 28 days, administration of the 'probiotic drink' to a group of patients caused opportunistic infections and mortality to increase significantly compared to those of the placebo group [144].

Prebiotics and Eubiotics

Prebiotics are nonliving, non-digestible edible resources with health promoting effects on intestinal flora [145]. The most abundant prebiotics are fibers and oligosaccharides formed by 2 to 20 hexose residues. The list of prebiotics for human consumption includesfructo-, galacto-, soy-, isomalto- and xylooligosaccharides, inulin, pyrodextrins and lactulose. Prebiotic compounds should meet the following criteria:

- Resistance to the low pH level in the stomach.

- Ability to withstand enzymatic hydrolysis.

- Should not be totally absorbed along the gastrointestinal tract of the host.

- Capable of undergoing fermentation by endogenous gut flora.

The research into prebiotics has been aimed mainly at human use because ruminants and other animals degrade oligosaccharides. A fraction of the consumed prebiotics passes to the large intestine providing nutrients to the intestinal mucosa and giving competitive advantage to *Bifidobacteria*, *Butyrivibrio* and other beneficial strains. Long term administration of inulin and oligofructans to people has been proven to modulate immune system's activity and to reduce the incidence of inflammatory bowel disease, colitis and atopic dermatitis [137, 146].

The term "eubiotics" stands for a more general concept that includes food supplements and feed additives such as probiotics, prebiotics, essential oils, organic acids (VFA), and compounds of Zn and Cu [147].

Mechanism of Action of Probiotics

After birth, microbes from the mother and the environment colonize the gut protecting the child from pathogens and contribute to the digestion of fermented dietary substrates, VFA define and B-vitamins [141]. When the intestinal flora matures, all its ecological niches are occupied so that no nutrients are left for invading microbes. Nevertheless, such a homeostatic system is affected by stress to the host, diet changes and physical conditions. Probiotic LAB act upon gut flora by a mechanism composed of multiple functional elements:

- Competitive exclusion (CE) is the interference of probiotics with pathogenic strains for colonization sites and nutrients [139]. This occurs according to the principle stated by the Russian biologist G. Gauss in 1932: "two species that compete for the same resources cannot stably coexist in a constant environment".

- Production of antimicrobial VFA, which reduce the competitive fitness of enteropathogens (VFA are also synthesized by gut-indigenous bacteria).

- Production of antimicrobial peptides (bacteriocins, defensins, colicins and others), that inhibit or eliminate pathogenic competitors within the same niche in the ecosystem,

- Modulation of the immune system activity of the host [141].

The structural and functional elements of multimicrobial environments, such as the intestinal tract and skin, can be harnessed in order to improve the health of the host [148]. Symbiotic, the combined use of probiotics and prebiotics, is aimed at achieving a synergistic reduction of pathogens and other benefits. The effects are obtained by varying the competitive pressures on the species by coupling CE and the other functions of probiotics with prebiotic-induced changes in the gut environment [149]. The yeast *Saccaromyces*, for instance, consume oxygen in the gut, which improves conditions for anaerobic bacteria [150]. In several countries, symbiotic approaches have been used in the strategy to eliminate from cattle antibiotic resistant *E. coli O175:H7* and *Salmonella* [151], because this method has low economic and labor costs and is considered eco-friendly [139].

Bacteriocins

Peptides with antimicrobial properties (AMP) are synthesized by many organisms as part of their normal metabolism. Unicellular archaea, bacteria and fungi produce archaeocins, bacteriocins and defensins, respectively; multicellular arachnids synthesise defensine-like toxins; plants, insects and mammals produce defensins, while in the human body, antimicrobial lysozymes are produced [134, 152]. This section, however, is focused on bacteriocins synthesized by probiotic LAB.

Bacteriocins are heat-stable, arginine/lysine-rich cationic AMP with massed less that 10 kDa. These molecules fold into amphiphilic structures, which allows them to cross the phospholipid bilayer forming pores on it [152]. This ability of bacteriocins to kill bacteria is restricted to strains that are closely related to the producing species, which reduces the risk of damage to native gut flora [153]. Bacteriocins are synthesized by ribosomes, undergo post-translational modification, and are easily degraded by digestive proteases, so that they are safe for human consumption.

Bacteriocins are usually sorted into three major classes [154]. The peptide members of each class share sequence homology, particularly on the *N*-terminal leader region. The proteins associated with the secretion and processing of bacteriocins of the same class, also share conservative structural features.

Class I. Lantibiotics

Lantibiotics are peptides containing 18-39 amino acids that undergo extensive post-translational modification. In a first stage, serine and threonine residues are enzymatically transformed into dehydroalanine, dehydrobutyrine and 2-aminoisobutyric acid. Then these dehydrated amino acids form intramolecular covalent bridges with neighboring cysteines leading to the synthesis of the polycyclic thioether amino acids typical for this class: lanthionine and methyllanthionine. There are two types of lantibiotics:

- Type A. Amphiphilic, cationic, screw-shaped, flexible peptide molecules of mass 2-4 kDa, such as nisin and lacticin 3147. These lantibiotics depolarize the membrane of the target species before forming pores on it.

- Type B. Globular peptide molecules of mass 2 to 3 kDa with either neutral or negative charge that interfere with cellular enzymatic reactions of the target microbial species.

Class II. Non-Lantibiotics

Non lantibiotics is a class of diverse, relatively heat-stable, membrane-active peptides of mass less than 10 kDa.

- Subclass IIa. Pediocin-like antimicrobial peptides with N-terminal consensus sequence Tyr-Gly-Asn-Gly-Val-Xaa-Cys. They can reach a 40-60% degree of sequence homology if during their synthesis the leader peptide is removed by proteolytic processing after a double glycine residue, like in the case of pediocin PA-1 and sakacin A. This subclass also includes *Listeria*-active bacteriocins, such as salivaricin.

- Subclass IIb. Refers to bacteriocins formed by 2 peptides, which work synergistically in order to exert antimicrobial activity, what occurs, for example, with lactacin F and lactococcin G.

Class III. Bacteriocins

This class includes heat-labile polipeptides of mass than 30 kDa.

- Subclass IIIa. Bacteriolysins that catalise the hydrolysis of cell walls resulting in autolysis of the targeted bacteria. Some members of this subclass are lysostaphin, that hydrolizes *Staphylococcus* species, helveticin-I derived from *Lactobacillus helveticus*, and enterolysin produced by *Enterococcus faecium*.

- Subclass IIIb, Non-lyltic peptides that inhibit metabolic processes dependent upon electron transport, disrupt the membrane potential and cause ATP efflux. This class includes non-pore forming colicins E3, E4, E5 and E6 that inhibit protein synthesis, colicins E2, E7, E8 and E9 that degrade chromosomal DNA and others.

Mechanisms of Action of Bacteriocins

- Membrane disruption. The most general antimicrobial mechanism of bacteriocins is the formation of pores in the membrane of the infective agent. The pore-formation process occurs in three steps: attachment of bacteriocin molecule to the membrane, insertion and permeabilization. At initial stages, bacteriocins align parallel to the plane of the membrane, but when the quantity of built-in peptides exceeds peptide/lipid ratio threshold of the membrane, then the peptide assembling process turns perpendicular to the plane and goes on forming transmembrane pores. Such is the action of defensisn, epidermins, cathelicidins, colistins and many other bacteriocins [155]. The highest levels of bacteriocin's adsorption to the cell surface and antibacterial activity are reached at pH values below 5. Lantibiotic and non-lantibiotic bacteriocins are extremely active against Gram-(+) bacteria, which allow passage of large molecules, but also against Gram-(-) *Enterobactiaceae*, whose inhibition is reached already at nanomolar concentrations of the peptides.

- Inhibition of cell wall synthesis and cellular targets. Several lantibiotic peptides cannot span the lipid bilayer. Instead they kill Gram-positive bacteria by removing lipid II from the cell division site and, consequently, by blocking cell wall synthesis. Mersacidin produced by *Bacillus sp.* acts according to this mechanism. Bacteriocins can attack cellular targets: microcin J25, produced by *E. coli*, inhibits bacterial RNA synthesis; duramycin C, produced by *Streptomyces* and *Streptococcus spp.* inhibits phospholipase A2.

- Double action. Nisin uses both mechanisms: membrane pore formation and disruption of cell wall synthesis. In the case of two-peptide bacteriocins, like lacticin 3147 (Class I) and lactacin F (Class II), the joint activity of both monomers is required to induce ion leakage and/or interfere with cellular ATP production.

In bacterial cells, specific sensing or immune proteins regulate the synthesis and transport of bacteriocins for avoiding potential self-damage. In the case of mutualistic microbe-host associations, antimicrobial peptides play an immunoregulatory role. In commensal bacterial relationships, like that of *S. aureus* with LAB *Streptoccous mutans*, the former develops resistance to antimicrobial peptides produced by the latter. In some cases the resistance is developed against a whole class of antimicrobial peptides.

Medical Uses of Bacteriocins

The use of LAB-produced bacteriocins as industrial food preservatives has been the main motivation for their intensive study. Bacteriocin-producing LAB are inoculated directly to the food system and, as more recently, are also dispensed in food packaging films [156]. Lantibiotics meet as antimicrobials the requirements for food preservation and impede the growth of food-borne pathogens such as *Listeria monocytogenes* and others.

Bacteriocins as immunoregulators and bactericidal agents cause pleiotropic effects, but the affinities to their multiple targets are different. Hence, for pathogens, it is practically impossible to develop full insensitivity to bacterioicins, which makes them a promising object for pharmaceutical industry. The most promising anti-infective drugs are those produced by the LAB genera *Lactobacillus, Lactococcus, Leucnostoc, Pediococcus* and *Streptococcus*. Nisin produced by *Lactococcus lactis* is used as a drug for bovine mastitis [152].

The development of bacteriocin-based drugs faces serious challenges: the high cost of peptide synthesis and the indispensable testing of the multiple mechanisms of resistance that can appear in the target pathogens. AMP-based anti-infective drug studies rarely proceed from preclinical to clinical trials. The knowledge obtained by the study of natural AMP has allowed developing drugs with improved antimicrobial properties by means of introduction of non natural D-amino acids, amidation of the C-terminal residue, and cyclic formations.

The gene-encoded nature of bacteriocins also makes them responsive to bioengineering approaches [153]. Research groups are constructing and testing recombinant probiotic strains with strong adherence to the intestine and engineered genes for enhanced production of becteriocins [157]. Furthermore, *in silico* studies allow predicting the dynamics of the interaction of natural and genetically modified bacteriocin-producing strains, and their competitive capabilities and fitness in concrete environments [158].

NEW ANTI-INFECTIVE TECHNOLOGIES INVOLVING THE IMMUNE SYSTEM

Recent advances in genomics, cellular and molecular biology have resulted in promising technologies which enable the engineering of immune responses against pathogens, cancer cells and some autoimmune and chronic diseases [159]. In the following paragraphs, we briefly elaborate on these technologies emphasizing their anti-bacterial perspective. Most of this section is dedicated to vaccination which has been one of the most successful procedures in medicine. Recent vaccine research includes DNA vaccines transfected to host cells, identification of the best antigens through analysis of pathogen's genomes, structure-based epitope design and recombinant live cellular vaccines in which vectors like dendritic cells (DC), non-infective pathogenic or commensal bacteria, carry selected heterologous antigens to elicit immunity against pathogens for which traditional vaccination procedures have failed [159-161]. Some of these vectors efficiently elicit mucosal and systemic immunity or can improve immunogenicity against intracellular pathogenic bacteria [160-162]. The use of viruses as vectors carrying DNA or heterologous antigens is also under active development [163, 164]. Furthermore, the study of the molecular basis of bacterial cell recognition, led to the development of new adjuvants mimicking bacterial molecular patterns [165]. Besides vaccines, the recent discovery of neutrophil extracellular traps (NETs), in which the antibacterial properties of histones and DNA contribute to infection clearance [166, 167] and the use of drugs with immunostimulatory effects, demonstrate that modulation of the immune system is a potent tool to fight against challenging bacteria.

Anti-Bacterial Immune Response

Clearance of a bacterial infection by the immune system is a complex process involving the coordinated action of many cell types. The oversimplified description below is intended to highlight the recent anti-infective technologies in the general picture of events that take place during infection and vaccination.

During the early steps of infection macrophages and neutrophils that are part of the innate immune system are in charge of the phagocytosis and lysis of bacterial cells [168]. Their non-specific recognition of the infectious agents is mediated by the binding of pathogen-associated molecular patterns to specialized receptors. This is the basis for development of a new class of adjuvants that mimic such patterns [165]. Recently it was discovered that neutrophils play a dual role at this stage, besides phagocytosis and lysis, these cells excrete a bactericidal net of DNA, histones, proteases and peptides known as NETs [166]. If the action of macrophages and neutrophils is not enough to clear the infection, the adaptive immune system is activated which results in a specific response targeting small structures like peptides or carbohydrates (antigens) present exclusively on the infectious agent. The main players in this response are the various types of lymphocytes whose functions include orchestration of the response (T helper cells), destruction of infected host-cells (CD8$^+$ cytotoxic T lymphocytes), production of antibodies which inactivate and tag bacterial cells for destruction (B lymphocytes), and to stay vigilant after the infection, to rapidly react when the same pathogen invades again (memory T cells) [168]. The link between innate and adaptive immune systems is the action of antigen presenting cells, mainly DC and macrophages. They phagocytose and lyse pathogens to display the resulting antigens in the external face of their characteristic plasma membrane protrusions [161, 168]. Some of the presented antigens result complementary to regions in the variable region of T-cell receptors in naïve T helper or CD8$^+$ T lymphocytes. Such complementary activates these lymphocytes which initiates a specific immune response targeting the recognized antigen [168]. Vaccination mimics the whole process by administering the hosts attenuated or killed pathogens, protein subunits, polysaccharides, or glycoconjugates, which are recognized and processed as infectious agents eliciting, with the aid of adjuvants, efficient, specific and long-lasting immune responses [168]. Since antigen immunogenicity is the basis of vaccination, recent vaccine research has focused on selection, design, delivery and presentation of antigens from pathogens and cancer cells for which no effective vaccines are available [159, 160].

New Technologies in Vaccine Research

Vaccination has been one of the most successful anti-infective practices in medicine; every year immunization programs save millions of lives. Effective vaccines have been licensed for many pathogens, most of which show low antigenic variation and a predominantly antibody-mediated control of infection. Nonetheless, traditional vaccination methods have failed in developing effective vaccines for some highly variable or intracellular pathogens like HIV, tuberculosis or malaria [159, 160]. New technologies in recombinant vaccine development join the power and specificity of the immune system with the recent advances in genomics, molecular biology, bacteriology and virology; combining engineered antigens with new adjuvants in heterologous prime-boost combinations. These technologies are paving the way for the development of new effective vaccines not only for prophylactic pediatric use, but also to target nosocomial infections by antibiotic-resistant bacteria, persistent chronic infections and pathogens relevant for specific groups like pregnant women or elderly people [159].

DNA Vaccines

Introduction of plasmid DNA, naked or coated with fine gold particles, into the host cells results in the transient expression of the selected DNA-coded antigen which is recognized as a foreign protein. Subsequent fragmentation and presentation of the resulting peptides by the MHC class I, results in a specific cytotoxic CD8+ T cell-mediated immune response. If the antigen is also excreted, it may be recognized and processed by antigen presenting cells like DCs and elicit a specific antibody-mediated response [159, 160, 169]. The main advantages of these vaccines are the safety of a vector and pathogen-free administration, cheap production, lack of pre-existing anti-vector immunity and lack of the inherent drawbacks of recombinant proteins like wrong folding or contamination. DNA vaccines are effective in eliciting humoral and cellular long term responses in pre-clinical studies and some are in commercial veterinary use [159]. Antigens from different pathogens including bacteria and cancer cells have been expressed in pre-clinical studies [160]. However, in humans, they show low immunogenicity apparently due to low transfection efficiency, low antigen expression and low production of cytokines and other immunostimulatory molecules [160]. Other possible drawbacks include DNA integration into the host genome and development of anti-DNA antibodies [159]. The strategies currently under investigation to improve this technology include the co-expression of proteins that enhance immunogenicity, delivery by harmless vectors like virus or live bacteria and the combination of different ways to administer the same antigen (heterologous prime-boost vaccination) combining protein-based and DNA-based vaccines [159, 160].

Reverse Vaccinology

Whole genome sequencing of pathogenic bacteria allows the *in silico* identification of surface exposed proteins well conserved among different relevant serotypes but not among closely related species or commensal bacteria. These proteins represent new potential antigens for vaccine production. After identification, they are expressed in heterologous hosts, purified as recombinant proteins and used for immunization of animal models. The antigens that elicit good immunogenicity, intense humoral and cellular responses and long-term protection are then chosen for safety and immunogenicity trials in humans. This process is known as sequence based reverse-vaccinology [159, 160, 170]. The first commercial product obtained by this approach is Bexsero®, the recently approved vaccine for serogroup B *Neisseria meningitides* [159, 170, 171]. Vaccines for several other pathogenic bacteria and eukaryotic pathogens are ongoing in pre-clinical and clinical studies [171].

Structural Vaccinology

X-ray crystallography and molecular dynamics studies of antigens bound to antibodies offer the possibility to identify the molecular determinants of effective binding. These studies have been done using viral epitopes and monoclonal antibodies. Based on this information, researchers modify epitopes to increase their binding capacity to the corresponding monoclonal antibodies [172]. This has been done by chemical modification, stabilization of certain conformations, amino acid substitutions or inserting/deleting short sequences. This could be the basis for the structure-based design of effective vaccines through stabilization and efficient display of conserved epitopes [159]. This approach has increased the immunogenicity of an engineered viral epitope [172].

Live Attenuated Vectors

If genetically attenuated bacteria or viruses expressing heterologous antigens are administered as vaccines, their natural adjuvant properties and invasiveness promote a specific immune response targeting the vector´s proteins as well as the carried antigen which may come from bacteria, virus, parasites or cancer cells [160, 173]. A key feature of these live vectors is that they can be administered *via* mucosal surfaces eliciting both mucosal and systemic immunity [160, 173]. Recombinant live bacterial vaccines must show stable or inducible expression of single or multiple heterologous antigens maintaining their invasiveness and infecting long enough to elicit an effective immune response; they however, should not proliferate into the host and must be antibiotic sensitive [173]. The most studied bacterial vectors are pathogenic bacteria unable to revert to the virulent form like recombinant *Salmonella enterica* (*S. typhi* and *S. tiphimurium*) or *Listeria monocytogenes*. Commensal or probiotic bacteria like *Lactococcus lactis* or *Lactobacillus casei* have also been used although their immunogenicity has been lower than that of recombinant pathogenic bacteria. Some of these vaccines have reached phase I clinical trials [160]. Since approximately 90% of human infections initiate at mucosal membranes [174], protection at these sites is desirable. In addition, live recombinant vaccines are easily administered (by nose or mouth) and have a low production cost.

Specific localization signals can be fused to the heterologous antigens so that they are displayed on the external cell surface, excreted to the media or secreted by the type III secretion system into the cytosol of host cells; all these properties have been shown to increase the effectiveness of recombinant vaccines [160]. Furthermore, live bacterial vectors can also carry genes for co-expression of cytokines and other stimulatory molecules to increase immunogenicity and to elicit efficient immunity. However the use of these vaccines has raised some concerns about the administration of genetically modified bacteria, pre-existing immunity to the vector and pathogenic reversion [173].

Dendritic Cells as Cellular Vaccines

A special type of cellular vaccine is the use of DC cells as antigen carriers. If a selected antigen is introduced into DC, they recognize and process it as a foreign protein and present the resultant peptides to naïve T helper and B cells, if displayed on the MHC II, or to naïve $CD8^+T$ cells if displayed on MHC I. Activation of T helper or B cells results in antibody-mediated immune response, while activation of $CD8^+$ T cells results on cytotoxic T lymphocytes-mediated response; in any case, the selected antigen is specifically targeted. This ability of DC of triggering both branches of adaptive immune response makes them good candidates to develop cellular vaccines. Furthermore, depending on the selected type of DC, one branch can be favored over the other [161]. So far, this approach has been used mainly for cancer antigens [161] although some studies have used it to target intracellular bacterial pathogens like *Listeria monocytogenes* and *Mycobacterium tuberculosis* [175].

Activation of DC, by targeting some surface proteins with specific antibodies, promotes capture and processing of the administered antigen if proper maturation signals are also present. This has been done *ex-vivo* and *in vivo* resulting in the expansion of antigen-specific $CD4^+$ and $CD8^+T$ lymphocytes. Some encouraging results in clinical trials of antitumor vaccines keep this technology as a promising vaccination method [161].

New Adjuvants

Adjuvants are compounds that boost immune response against the administered antigens. In the absence of adjuvants, vaccines are not effective. Currently, the most used adjuvants are based on aluminum compounds although the exact mechanism of immune stimulation is not known. Recent research on bacterial recognition through pathogen-associated molecular patterns and specifically by the Toll-like receptors (TLRs) has broadened the list of compounds that can be used as adjuvants [165]. In cells of the innate immune system, TLR stimulation by lipopolysaccharides, flagellin, lipoproteins, and others results in induction of immune and inflammatory responses. The licensed adjuvant monophosphoryl lipid A (MPL) is a partial TLR4 agonist, and the promising adjuvant flagellin is recognized by TLR5 [165]. Research on these types of adjuvants may result in the ability to enhance and modulate immune response in the most appropriate manner for every particular vaccine [165].

Engineered Antibodies

The new vaccine technologies described above are associated with antigen engineering and active immunization. Passive immunization of engineered antibodies represents an alternative to prevent and treat infectious diseases [176]. Recent advances in identification and characterization of broadly neutralizing antibodies, cloning of monoclonal antibody-producing cells, and directed mutagenesis of antibody-coding genes have resulted in engineered antibodies with enhanced potency and breadth [176]. Molecular basis of affinity and specificity in the variable regions have been explored by library-based selection of broadly neutralizing antibodies from infected patients and their subsequent structural and bioinformatics characterization. This information is the base for rational design of improved antibodies. This technology however, can result in polyreactivity, autoreactivity, reduced solubility or shorter *in vivo* half-lives [176]. So far, this approach has been used mainly for HIV antigens although it has the potential to be used in antigens from other pathogens like bacteria. Furthermore, selected or engineered antibodies can be passively administrated or can be expressed by the host cells by vector-mediated gene transfer [177] which results in stable long-term endogenous expression of the selected antibody.

Neutrophil Extracellular Traps

As part of the innate immune system, neutrophils produce an extracellular net of DNA, histones, proteases and antimicrobial peptides which efficiently entraps and kill bacteria during infection [166]. Although the underlying mechanism of the capacity of DNA and histones to kill bacteria is not well understood, it involves the permeabilization of the bacterial cell membrane and the chelating activity of DNA [166, 167]. NETs kill between 40 to 90 % of the entrapped bacteria, and this activity varies for different species and sites of infection [167, 178]. Due to the recent discovery of NETs, this process has not yet been used as an anti-infective tool. However, further studies will clarify unknown aspects of the innate immune system which may be useful to fight against infections.

Drugs with Immunostimulatory Effects

Non-specific boosting of the immune system has been achieved with the use of immunostimulatory cytokines [179, 180], TLR agonists [180, 181] and inhibitors of TNF-α secretion [180, 182]. Although these effects have been mainly used in anti-cancer immunotherapy [180], some studies have addressed their potential use for the control of pathogenic bacteria, for example, IFN-γ has been considered beneficial for protection against *M. tuberculosis* [183], interleukin-6 (IL-6) shows tuberculostatic activity in infected murine bone marrow-derived macrophages [184], interleukin 1 alpha (IL-1α) and IL-6 stimulated the innate immune response in human keratinocytes, improving control of bacterial infections in cultured composite keratinocyte grafts [185] and several human chemokines have shown antibacterial activity [186]. Modulation of intracellular signals in the host cells using tyrosine protein kinase inhibitors has also been beneficial for the control of intracellular pathogens [187-189] and the use of thalidomide, an inhibitor of TNF-α secretion, stimulated the immune response against *E. coli* and *P. aeruginosa*

[190, 191]. The use of adjuvants like recombinant cytokines or chemokines and immunomodulatory drugs may contribute to treating antibiotic-resistant or intracellular pathogenic bacteria. The immunomodulatory properties of host peptides with antimicrobial activity have been discussed in the section Antibiofilm Agents Derived from Host Defense Peptides (HDPs) [30, 31]. Remarkably, anti-infective technologies involving the immune system can impact positively on treatments of pathologies involving bacteria, virus, parasites and cancer cells.

PERSPECTIVES AND CONCLUDING REMARKS

According to the OMS, 10 million people are predicted to die by 2050, from antibiotic-resistant infections, if no new antimicrobials are developed. The majority of these infections are biofilm-related and it is therefore imperative to effectively target bacterial biofilms. Hence, biofilm inhibitors are one of the more suitable anti-infectives with ample possibilities to be soon implemented in the clinic; for example, bacterial EPS, pilicides, curlicides, metal containing compounds and HDPs are excellent scaffolds for the design of potent antibiofilm molecules. These synthetic derivatives eradicate biofilms in a broad-spectrum manner, synergize with otherwise ineffective antibiotics, and are active in different animal models. Nevertheless, more work is needed, particularly extensive pharmacokinetics and formulation studies will be required to definitely establish antibiofilm peptides as an alternative to currently available antibiotics in the treatment of persistent biofilm infections. In addition, studies to determine the development of bacterial resistance against anti-biofilm compounds as well as strategies to combat resistance selection are highly recommended. Besides biofilm inhibitors, QQ metabolites isolated from natural products are excellent resources for developing potent anti-virulence drugs insofar as they may provide novel scaffolds for drug design [64]. However, to date most of these studies were done *in vitro*, and the active metabolite and the target which they operate are unknown, so, it is necessary to structurally identify the active molecules.

Using assays to evaluate the inhibition of the production of specific virulence factors in biosensor strains, several potential sources for obtaining this new class of anti-virulence metabolites had been identified. In this regard, Tan and Zhang indicated that among the factors that may hinder the development of new anti-virulence therapies based on molecules QQ, is the presence of several false positives in the *in vitro* assays, which suggests an urgent need for standardization to identify true QQ activity and discard the effect of molecules on the expression of phenotypes that are co-dependent on other non-QS factors and/or depend on the metabolic activity of the cells [64].

Also, to date there are limited studies to identify the molecular targets of QQ molecules. The main target often suggested for some metabolites derived from natural products is the antagonistic effect on AhI-receptor proteins and molecular docking analysis has been the most-used tool. However, this technique has the limitation that it is only predictive and studies are needed to confirm the results. In addition, only a limited number of ligands for the known protein structures have been reported. Another aspect to be considered for the development of anti-virulence therapy refers to the lack of studies aimed at understanding the possible side effects of QQ molecules on the beneficial bacterial communities that interact with the host, and changes in the expression QS regulated phenotypes due the use of molecules QQ. More importantly, there is a clear need for studies in animal and chronic infection models in order to assess the performance of some promising molecules under close-to-real conditions [63].

Also for the future, there is a need for more mechanistic studies that would contribute to the rational design of specific QSIs, so far as discussed, a number of studies have shown QQ activity from bacterial, fungal and other non-plant extracts (Table **2**). In this regard, culturable microbes (bacteria, fungi) are particularly attractive as they represent a relatively unexplored source of QSIs that could help to overcome the 'supply issue' that usually limits the applicability prospects of natural products. In spite of the huge potential of plant secondary metabolites in the discovery of novel QSIs, the exploration of microbial sources is encouraged, as they represent a rich source of natural compounds without the supply limitations imposed by other natural sources. Nevertheless although it has been neglected until recently [192], it is important to evaluate the possibility of resistance generation towards QQ compounds, especially since at least for brominated furanones, that are one of the canonical QQ molecules, resistance can be easily obtained by the overexpression of efflux pumps and by a decrease in bacterial permeability for the compounds in *P. aeruginosa* laboratory and clinical strains [193-196]. In addition, it has demonstrated that environmental stress also selects the presence of active QS systems [197], which may be an important driving force for the selection of resistant strains [198]. Interestingly, besides furanones, resistance against 5-fluorouracil, an anticancer compound with QQ activity [1, 199] has also been found in *P. aeruginosa* clinical isolates [195]; hence, it is necessary to evaluate more QQ compounds in more bacterial species and to seriously consider the eventual appearance of QQ-resistant bacteria, able to tolerate several QQ compounds simultaneously [200].

Besides inhibition of processes like biofilm formation, bacterial virulence or proliferation; the fight against antibiotic-resistant bacteria may benefit from advances in stimulation of the host immune response. Current research on this field includes development of recombinant vaccines, new vaccine strategies, engineered antibodies for passive immunization, and the use of drugs that target host cells proteins relevant for the infectious process.

In spite of the great success of vaccination, it has result ineffective for some bacterial pathogens like those residing inside the host cells *e.g., M. tuberculosis*, those that do not induce permanent immunity after infection, *e.g., P. aeruginosa*, or those causing persistent infections, *e.g., S. aureus* [159]. Other bacteria for which efficient vaccines are needed are those whose prevalence are increasing or whose antibiotic resistant phenotype represents serious health problems like Group A and Group B *Streptococcus, Shigella*, pathogenic *E.coli, Salmonella, Chlamydia, Klebsiella pneumoniae* and *Clostridium difficile* [159]. In order to develop prophylactic and therapeutic vaccines against these bacteria, it is necessary a deeper understanding of the pathogen-host interactions, mechanism of pathogenicity and the type of immune response required for protection. For each particular pathogen is necessary to find ways to elicit the most effective balance of humoral and cellular immune responses. To reach this goal, more work is needed on development of new adjuvants, types of antigens, types of vectors, new vaccine formulations, co-expression or co-administration of the appropriate immunomodulatory citokines and chemokines; the order, routes and intervals of vaccine administration in heterologous prime-boost regimes. Progress on these aspects will certainly enable the development of specialized vaccine formulations for different patients populations (infants, children, adolescents, adults, elderly, pregnant women or immunocompromised patients) for prophylactic or therapeutic use. Furthermore, selection of vaccines formulations and administration regimes may be based on predictive biomarkers of vaccine efficacy for each subject.

Some of the new vaccines technologies currently under investigation are being developed predominantly for viral pathogens or cancer cells, thus, it is necessary also to exploit them for antibiotic resistant and other challenging bacteria.

Besides research on therapeutic vaccine formulations, treatments of infected patients will benefit from basic and clinical research on development of engineered antibodies for passive immunization, local stimulation of NETs activity and the use of immunomodulatory drugs.

CONFLICT OF INTEREST

The author confirms that he has no conflict of interest to declare for this publication.

ACKNOWLEDGEMENTS

We apologize for not discussing numerous studies published by our colleagues in recent years due to space constraints.

This work was supported by grants from SEP/CONACyT Mexico no.152794 and PAPIIT UNAM no. IA201116 to R-GC, HIM 2015-053 SSA 1183 and HIM 2016-026 SSA 1222 to HQ, Fideicomiso-COLPOS 167304 and Cátedras-CONACyT program to I C-J and by the Army Research Office (W911NF-14-1-0279) to TKW. TKW is the Biotechnology Endowed Chair at the Pennsylvania State University. C.D.L.F.-N. received a scholarship from the Fundación "la Caixa" and Fundación Canadá (Spain)-and is currently funded by Fundación Ramón Areces (Spain). C.D.L.F.-N is a co-inventor of a provisional patent application on the use of cationic anti-biofilm and innate defense regulator (IDR) peptides (U.S. Patent Application No. 61/870,655). A.J.M-R. acknowledges PLOCAN for a 2+2 fellowship and funding from the Spanish Ministry of Economy and Competitiveness, grant CTQ2014-55888-C03-01.

REFERENCES

[1]　Rangel-Vega A, Bernstein LR, Mandujano-Tinoco EA, García-Contreras SJ, García-Contreras R. Drug repurposing as an alternative for the treatment of recalcitrant bacterial infections. Front Microbiol 2015; 6: 282.

[2]　Costerton JW, Stewart PS, Greenberg EP. Bacterial biofilms: a common cause of persistent infections. Science 1999; 284(5418): 1318-22.

[3]　Hall-Stoodley L, Costerton JW, Stoodley P. Bacterial biofilms: from the natural environment to infectious diseases. Nat Rev Microbiol 2004; 2(2): 95-108.

[4]　de la Fuente-Nunez C, Reffuveille F, Fernandez L, Hancock RE. Bacterial biofilm development as a multicellular adaptation: antibiotic resistance and new therapeutic strategies. Curr Opin Microbiol 2013; 16(5): 580-9.

[5]　Bjarnsholt T, Ciofu O, Molin S, Givskov M, Hoiby N. Applying insights from biofilm biology to drug development - can a new approach be developed? Nat Rev Drug Discov 2013; 12(10): 791-808.

[6]　Pratt LA, Kolter R. Genetic analysis of *Escherichia coli* biofilm formation: roles of flagella, motility, chemotaxis and type I pili. Mol Microbiol 1998; 30(2): 285-93.

[7]　Otto M. Staphylococcal biofilms. Curr Top Microbiol Immunol 2008; 322: 207-28.

[8]　Beloin C, Roux A, Ghigo JM. *Escherichia coli* biofilms. Curr Top Microbiol Immunol 2008; 322: 249-89.

[9]　Caiazza NC, O'Toole GA. SadB is required for the transition from reversible to irreversible attachment during biofilm formation by *Pseudomonas aeruginosa* PA14. J Bacteriol 2004; 186(14): 4476-85.

[10]　Romero D, Aguilar C, Losick R, Kolter R. Amyloid fibers provide structural integrity to *Bacillus subtilis* biofilms. Proc Natl Acad Sci U S A 2009; 107(5): 2230-4.

[11]　Steinberger RE, Holden PA. Extracellular DNA in single- and multiple-species unsaturated biofilms. Appl Environ Microbiol 2005; 71(9): 5404-10.

[12]　Kaplan JB. Biofilm dispersal: mechanisms, clinical implications, and potential therapeutic uses. J Dent Res 2010; 89(3): 205-18.

[13]　Kostakioti M, Hadjifrangiskou M, Hultgren SJ. Bacterial biofilms: development, dispersal, and therapeutic strategies in the dawn of the postantibiotic era. Cold Spring Harb Perspect Med 2013; 3(4): a010306.

[14]　Cusumano CK, Pinkner JS, Han Z, *et al.* Treatment and prevention of urinary tract infection with orally active FimH inhibitors. Sci Transl Med 2011; 3(109): 109ra15.

[15]　Aberg V, Almqvist F. Pilicides-small molecules targeting bacterial virulence. Org Biomol Chem 2007; 5(12): 1827-34.

[16]　Cegelski L, Pinkner JS, Hammer ND, *et al.* Small-molecule inhibitors target *Escherichia coli* amyloid biogenesis and biofilm formation. Nat Chem Biol 2009; 5(12): 913-9.

[17]　Chorell E, Pinkner JS, Bengtsson C, *et al.* Mapping pilicide anti-virulence effect in *Escherichia coli*, a comprehensive structure-activity study. Bioorg Med Chem 2012; 20(9): 3128-42.

[18]　Adams H, Horrevoets WM, Adema SM, *et al.* Inhibition of biofilm formation by Camelid single-domain antibodies against the flagellum of *Pseudomonas aeruginosa*. J Biotechnol 2014; 186: 66-73.

[19]　Ren D, Zuo R, Gonzalez Barrios AF, *et al.* Differential gene expression for investigation of *Escherichia coli* biofilm inhibition by plant extract ursolic acid. Appl Environ Microbiol 2005; 71(7): 4022-34.

[20] Kim S, Song M, Roh BD, Park SH, Park JW. Inhibition of *Streptococcus mutans* biofilm formation on composite resins containing ursolic acid. Restor Dent Endod 2013; 38(2): 65-72.

[21] Qin N, Tan X, Jiao Y, *et al.* RNA-Seq-based transcriptome analysis of methicillin-resistant *Staphylococcus aureus* biofilm inhibition by ursolic acid and resveratrol. Sci Rep 2014; 4: 5467.

[22] Zhou L, Ding Y, Chen W, Zhang P, Chen Y, Lv X. The *in vitro* study of ursolic acid and oleanolic acid inhibiting cariogenic microorganisms as well as biofilm. Oral Dis 2013; 19(5): 494-500.

[23] Kurek A, Markowska K, Grudniak AM, Janiszowska W, Wolska KI. The effect of oleanolic and ursolic acids on the hemolytic properties and biofilm formation of *Listeria monocytogenes*. Pol J Microbiol 2013; 63(1): 21-5.

[24] Qin Z, Yang L, Qu D, Molin S, Tolker-Nielsen T. *Pseudomonas aeruginosa* extracellular products inhibit staphylococcal growth, and disrupt established biofilms produced by *Staphylococcus epidermidis*. Microbiology 2009; 155(Pt 7): 2148-56.

[25] Pihl M, Davies JR, Chavez de Paz LE, Svensater G. Differential effects of *Pseudomonas aeruginosa* on biofilm formation by different strains of *Staphylococcus epidermidis*. FEMS Immunol Med Microbiol 2010; 59(3): 439-46.

[26] Bendaoud M, Vinogradov E, Balashova NV, Kadouri DE, Kachlany SC, Kaplan JB. Broad-spectrum biofilm inhibition by *Kingella kingae* exopolysaccharide. J Bacteriol 2011; 193(15): 3879-86.

[27] Valle J, Da Re S, Henry N, *et al.* Broad-spectrum biofilm inhibition by a secreted bacterial polysaccharide. Proc Natl Acad Sci U S A 2006; 103(33): 12558-63.

[28] Bernal P, Llamas MA. Promising biotechnological applications of antibiofilm exopolysaccharides. Microb Biotechnol 2012; 5(6): 670-3.

[29] Travier L, Rendueles O, Ferrieres L, Herry JM, Ghigo JM. *Escherichia coli* resistance to nonbiocidal antibiofilm polysaccharides is rare and mediated by multiple mutations leading to surface physicochemical modifications. Antimicrob Agents Chemother 2013; 57(8): 3960-8.

[30] Hancock RE, Sahl HG. Antimicrobial and host-defense peptides as new anti-infective therapeutic strategies. Nat Biotechnol 2006; 24(12): 1551-7.

[31] de la Fuente-Nunez C, Mansour SC, Wang Z, *et al.* Anti-Biofilm and immunomodulatory activities of peptides that inhibit biofilms formed by pathogens isolated from cystic fibrosis patients. Antibiotics (Basel) 2014; 3(4): 509-26.

[32] Overhage J, Campisano A, Bains M, Torfs EC, Rehm BH, Hancock RE. Human host defense peptide LL-37 prevents bacterial biofilm formation. Infect Immun 2008; 76(9): 4176-82.

[33] de la Fuente-Nunez C, Korolik V, Bains M, *et al.* Inhibition of bacterial biofilm formation and swarming motility by a small synthetic cationic peptide. Antimicrob Agents Chemother 2012; 56(5): 2696-704.

[34] Amer LS, Bishop BM, van Hoek ML. Antimicrobial and antibiofilm activity of cathelicidins and short, synthetic peptides against *Francisella*. Biochem Biophys Res Commun 2010; 396(2): 246-51.

[35] Pompilio A, Scocchi M, Pomponio S, *et al.* Antibacterial and anti-biofilm effects of cathelicidin peptides against pathogens isolated from cystic fibrosis patients. Peptides 2011; 32(9): 1807-14.

[36]   de la Fuente-Nunez C, Reffuveille F, Haney EF, Straus SK, Hancock RE. Broad-spectrum anti-biofilm peptide that targets a cellular stress response. PLoS Pathog 2014; 10(5): e1004152.

[37]   Dosler S, Karaaslan E. Inhibition and destruction of *Pseudomonas aeruginosa* biofilms by antibiotics and antimicrobial peptides. Peptides 2014; 62: 32-7.

[38]   Reffuveille F, de la Fuente-Nunez C, Mansour S, Hancock RE. A broad-spectrum antibiofilm peptide enhances antibiotic action against bacterial biofilms. Antimicrob Agents Chemother 2014; 58(9): 5363-71.

[39]   Sieprawska-Lupa M, Mydel P, Krawczyk K, *et al.* Degradation of human antimicrobial peptide LL-37 by *Staphylococcus aureus*-derived proteinases. Antimicrob Agents Chemother 2004; 48(12): 4673-9.

[40]   Fjell CD, Hiss JA, Hancock RE, Schneider G. Designing antimicrobial peptides: form follows function. Nat Rev Drug Discov 2012; 11(1): 37-51.

[41]   de la Fuente-Nunez C, Reffuveille F, Mansour SC, *et al.* D-enantiomeric peptides that eradicate wild-type and multidrug-resistant biofilms and protect against lethal *Pseudomonas aeruginosa* infections. Chem Biol 2015; 22(2): 196-205.

[42]   Potrykus K, Cashel M. (p)ppGpp: still magical? Annu Rev Microbiol 2008; 62: 35-51.

[43]   Maisonneuve E, Castro-Camargo M, Gerdes K. (p)ppGpp controls bacterial persistence by stochastic induction of toxin-antitoxin activity. Cell 2013; 154(5): 1140-50.

[44]   Lewis K. Persister cells. Annu Rev Microbiol 2010; 64: 357-72.

[45]   Chen X, Schluesener HJ. Nanosilver: a nanoproduct in medical application. Toxicol Lett 2008; 176(1): 1-12.

[46]   Yamanaka M, Hara K, Kudo J. Bactericidal actions of a silver ion solution on *Escherichia coli*, studied by energy-filtering transmission electron microscopy and proteomic analysis. Appl Environ Microbiol 2005; 71(11): 7589-93.

[47]   Kalishwaralal K, BarathManiKanth S, Pandian SR, Deepak V, Gurunathan S. Silver nanoparticles impede the biofilm formation by *Pseudomonas aeruginosa* and *Staphylococcus epidermidis*. Colloids Surf B Biointerfaces 2010; 79(2): 340-4.

[48]   Palanisamy NK, Ferina N, Amirulhusni AN, *et al.* Antibiofilm properties of chemically synthesized silver nanoparticles found against *Pseudomonas aeruginosa*. J Nanobiotechnology 2014; 12: 2.

[49]   Secinti KD, Ozalp H, Attar A, Sargon MF. Nanoparticle silver ion coatings inhibit biofilm formation on titanium implants. J Clin Neurosci 2011; 18(3): 391-5.

[50]   Lee JH, Kim YG, Cho MH, Lee J. ZnO nanoparticles inhibit *Pseudomonas aeruginosa* biofilm formation and virulence factor production. Microbiol Res 2014; 169(12): 888-96.

[51]   García-Lara B, Saucedo-Mora MA, Roldan-Sanchez JA, *et al.* Inhibition of quorum-sensing-dependent virulence factors and biofilm formation of clinical and environmental *Pseudomonas aeruginosa* strains by ZnO nanoparticles. Lett Appl Microbiol 2015; 61(3): 299-305.

[52]   Schaible UE, Kaufmann SH. Iron and microbial infection. Nat Rev Microbiol 2004; 2(12): 946-53.

[53]   Bonchi C, Imperi F, Minandri F, Visca P, Frangipani E. Repurposing of gallium-based drugs for antibacterial therapy. Biofactors 2014; 40(3): 303-12.

[54]   Kaneko Y, Thoendel M, Olakanmi O, Britigan BE, Singh PK. The transition metal gallium disrupts *Pseudomonas aeruginosa* iron metabolism and has antimicrobial and antibiofilm activity. J Clin Invest 2007; 117(4): 877-88.

[55] DeLeon K, Balldin F, Watters C, *et al.* Gallium maltolate treatment eradicates *Pseudomonas aeruginosa* infection in thermally injured mice. Antimicrob Agents Chemother 2009; 53(4): 1331-7.

[56] Antunes LC, Imperi F, Minandri F, Visca P. *In vitro* and *in vivo* antimicrobial activities of gallium nitrate against multidrug-resistant *Acinetobacter baumannii*. Antimicrob Agents Chemother 2012; 56(11): 5961-70.

[57] Banin E, Lozinski A, Brady KM, *et al.* The potential of desferrioxamine-gallium as an anti-*Pseudomonas* therapeutic agent. Proc Natl Acad Sci U S A 2008; 105(43): 16761-6.

[58] García-Contreras R, Perez-Eretza B, Lira-Silva E, *et al.* Gallium induces the production of virulence factors in *Pseudomonas aeruginosa*. Pathog Dis 2014; 70(1): 95-8.

[59] García-Contreras R, Lira-Silva E, Jasso-Chavez R, *et al.* Isolation and characterization of gallium resistant *Pseudomonas aeruginosa* mutants. Int J Med Microbiol 2013; 303(8): 574-82.

[60] Bonchi C, Frangipani E, Imperi F, Visca P. Pyoverdine and proteases affect the response of *Pseudomonas aeruginosa* to gallium in human serum. Antimicrob Agents Chemother 2015; 59(9): 5641-6.

[61] Ross-Gillespie A, Weigert M, Brown SP, Kummerli R. Gallium-mediated siderophore quenching as an evolutionarily robust antibacterial treatment. Evol Med Public Health 2014; 2014(1): 18-29.

[62] Antunes LC, Ferreira RB, Buckner MM, Finlay BB. Quorum sensing in bacterial virulence. Microbiology 2010; 156(Pt 8): 2271-82.

[63] Castillo-Juárez I, Maeda T, Mandujano-Tinoco EA, *et al.* Role of quorum sensing in bacterial infections. World J Clin Cases 2015; 3(7): 575-98.

[64] Tang K, Zhang XH. Quorum quenching agents: resources for antivirulence therapy. Mar Drugs 2014; 12(6): 3245-82.

[65] Monciardini P, Iorio M, Maffioli S, Sosio M, Donadio S. Discovering new bioactive molecules from microbial sources. Microb Biotechnol 2014; 7(3): 209-20.

[66] Genilloud O. Current challenges in the discovery of novel antibacterials from microbial natural products. Recent Pat Antiinfect Drug Discov 2012; 7(3): 189-204.

[67] Pelaez F. The historical delivery of antibiotics from microbial natural products--can history repeat? Biochem Pharmacol 2006; 71(7): 981-90.

[68] Brown DG, Lister T, May-Dracka TL. New natural products as new leads for antibacterial drug discovery. Bioorg Med Chem Lett 2014; 24(2): 413-8.

[69] Wright GD. Something old, something new: revisiting natural products in antibiotic drug discovery. Can J Microbiol 2014; 60(3): 147-54.

[70] Harvey AL, Edrada-Ebel R, Quinn RJ. The re-emergence of natural products for drug discovery in the genomics era. Nat Rev Drug Discov 2015; 14(2): 111-29.

[71] Tay SB, Yew WS. Development of quorum-based anti-virulence therapeutics targeting Gram-negative bacterial pathogens. Int J Mol Sci 2013; 14(8): 16570-99.

[72] Spoel SH, Dong X. How do plants achieve immunity? Defence without specialized immune cells. Nat Rev Immunol 2012; 12(2): 89-100.

[73] Jones JD, Dangl JL. The plant immune system. Nature 2006; 444(7117): 323-9.

[74] Newman MA, Sundelin T, Nielsen JT, Erbs G. MAMP (microbe-associated molecular pattern) triggered immunity in plants. Front Plant Sci 2013; 4: 139.

[75] Hartmann A, Rothballer M, Hense BA, Schroder P. Bacterial quorum sensing compounds are important modulators of microbe-plant interactions. Front Plant Sci 2014; 5: 131.

[76]   Zoratti L, Karppinen K, Luengo Escobar A, Haggman H, Jaakola L. Light-controlled flavonoid biosynthesis in fruits. Front Plant Sci 2014; 5: 534.

[77]   Brango-Vanegas J, Costa GM, Ortmann CF, *et al.* Glycosylflavonoids from *Cecropia pachystachya* Trecul are quorum sensing inhibitors. Phytomedicine 2014; 21(5): 670-5.

[78]   Martin-Rodriguez AJ, Ticona JC, Jimenez IA, Flores N, Fernandez JJ, Bazzocchi IL. Flavonoids from *Piper delineatum* modulate quorum-sensing-regulated phenotypes in *Vibrio harveyi*. Phytochemistry 2015; 117: 98-106.

[79]   Vasavi HS, Arun AB, Rekha PD. Anti-quorum sensing activity of *Psidium guajava* L. flavonoids against *Chromobacterium violaceum* and *Pseudomonas aeruginosa* PAO1. Microbiol Immunol 2014; 58(5): 286-93.

[80]   Gopu V, Meena CK, Shetty PH. Quercetin influences quorum sensing in food borne bacteria: in-vitro and in-silico evidence. PLoS One 2015; 10(8): e0134684.

[81]   Vasavi HS, Arun AB, Rekha PD. Anti-quorum sensing activity of flavonoid-rich fraction from *Centella asiatica L*. against *Pseudomonas aeruginosa* PAO1. J Microbiol Immunol Infect 2016; 49(1): 8-15.

[82]   Kim HS, Lee SH, Byun Y, Park HD. 6-Gingerol reduces *Pseudomonas aeruginosa* biofilm formation and virulence *via* quorum sensing inhibition. Sci Rep 2015; 5: 8656.

[83]   Kumar NV, Murthy PS, Manjunatha JR, Bettadaiah BK. Synthesis and quorum sensing inhibitory activity of key phenolic compounds of ginger and their derivatives. Food Chem 2014; 159: 451-7.

[84]   Al-Sohaibani S, Murugan K. Anti-biofilm activity of *Salvadora persica* on cariogenic isolates of *Streptococcus mutans*: *in vitro* and molecular docking studies. Biofouling 2012; 28(1): 29-38.

[85]   Li G, Yan C, Xu Y, *et al.* Punicalagin inhibits *Salmonella* virulence factors and has anti-quorum-sensing potential. Appl Environ Microbiol 2014; 80(19): 6204-11.

[86]   Gutierrez-Barranquero JA, Reen FJ, McCarthy RR, O'Gara F. Deciphering the role of coumarin as a novel quorum sensing inhibitor suppressing virulence phenotypes in bacterial pathogens. Appl Microbiol Biotechnol 2015; 99(7): 3303-16.

[87]   Musthafa KS, Voravuthikunchai SP. Anti-virulence potential of eugenyl acetate against pathogenic bacteria of medical importance. Antonie Van Leeuwenhoek 2015; 107(3): 703-10.

[88]   Kim YG, Lee JH, Kim SI, Baek KH, Lee J. Cinnamon bark oil and its components inhibit biofilm formation and toxin production. Int J Food Microbiol 2015; 195: 30-9.

[89]   Chang CY, Krishnan T, Wang H, *et al.* Non-antibiotic quorum sensing inhibitors acting against N-acyl homoserine lactone synthase as druggable target. Sci Rep 2014; 4: 7245.

[90]   Joshi JR, Burdman S, Lipsky A, Yariv S, Yedidia I. Plant phenolic acids affect the virulence of *Pectobacterium aroidearum* and *P. carotovorum* subsp brasiliense *via* quorum-sensing regulation. Mol Plant Pathol 2015; (epub ahead of print).

[91]   Sybiya Vasantha Packiavathy IA, Agilandeswari P, Musthafa KS, Karutha Pandian S, Veera Ravi A. Antibiofilm and quorum sensing inhibitory potential of *Cuminum cyminum* and its secondary metabolite methyl eugenol against Gram negative bacterial pathogens. Food Res Int 2012; 45(1): 85-92.

[92]   Duarte A, Alves AC, Ferreira S, Silva F, Domingues FC. Resveratrol inclusion complexes: Antibacterial and anti-biofilm activity against *Campylobacter* spp. and *Arcobacter butzleri*. Food Res Int 2015; 77(Pt 2): 244-50.

[93]   Annapoorani A, Umamageswaran V, Parameswari R, Pandian SK, Ravi AV. Computational discovery of putative quorum sensing inhibitors against LasR and RhlR receptor proteins of *Pseudomonas aeruginosa*. J Comput Aided Mol Des 2012; 26(9): 1067-77.

[94]   Henry LK, Gutensohn M, Thomas ST, Noel JP, Dudareva N. Orthologs of the archaeal isopentenyl phosphate kinase regulate terpenoid production in plants. Proc Natl Acad Sci U S A 2015; 112(32): 10050-5.

[95]   Mumm R, Posthumus MA, Dicke M. Significance of terpenoids in induced indirect plant defence against herbivorous arthropods. Plant Cell Environ 2008; 31(4): 575-85.

[96]   Ahmad A, Viljoen AM, Chenia HY. The impact of plant volatiles on bacterial quorum sensing. Lett Appl Microbiol 2015; 60(1): 8-19.

[97]   Husain FM, Ahmad I, Khan MS, *et al.* Sub-MICs of *Mentha piperita* essential oil and menthol inhibits AHL mediated quorum sensing and biofilm of Gram-negative bacteria. Front Microbiol 2015; 6: 420.

[98]   Pejin B, Ciric A, Glamoclija J, Nikolic M, Sokovic M. *In vitro* anti-quorum sensing activity of phytol. Nat Prod Res 2015; 29(4): 374-7.

[99]   Burt SA, Ojo-Fakunle VT, Woertman J, Veldhuizen EJ. The natural antimicrobial carvacrol inhibits quorum sensing in *Chromobacterium violaceum* and reduces bacterial biofilm formation at sub-lethal concentrations. PLoS One 2014; 9(4): e93414.

[100]   Guo X, Zhang LY, Wu SC, *et al.* Andrographolide interferes quorum sensing to reduce cell damage caused by avian pathogenic *Escherichia coli*. Vet Microbiol 2014; 174(3-4): 496-503.

[101]   Ma L, Liu X, Liang H, *et al.* Effects of 14-alpha-lipoyl andrographolide on quorum sensing in *Pseudomonas aeruginosa*. Antimicrob Agents Chemother 2012; 56(12): 6088-94.

[102]   Tan SY, Liu Y, Chua SL, *et al.* Comparative systems biology analysis to study the mode of action of the isothiocyanate compound Iberin on *Pseudomonas aeruginosa*. Antimicrob Agents Chemother 2014; 58(11): 6648-59.

[103]   Borges A, Serra S, Cristina Abreu A, Saavedra MJ, Salgado A, Simoes M. Evaluation of the effects of selected phytochemicals on quorum sensing inhibition and *in vitro* cytotoxicity. Biofouling 2014; 30(2): 183-95.

[104]   Vadekeetil A, Kaur G, Chhibber S, Harjai K. Applications of thin-layer chromatography in extraction and characterisation of ajoene from garlic bulbs. Nat Prod Res 2015; 29(8): 768-71.

[105]   Kasper SH, Samarian D, Jadhav AP, Rickard AH, Musah RA, Cady NC. S-aryl-L-cysteine sulphoxides and related organosulphur compounds alter oral biofilm development and AI-2-based cell-cell communication. J Appl Microbiol 2014; 117(5): 1472-86.

[106]   Choi SC, Zhang C, Moon S, Oh YS. Inhibitory effects of 4-hydroxy-2,5-dimethyl-3(2H)-furanone (HDMF) on acyl-homoserine lactone-mediated virulence factor production and biofilm formation in *Pseudomonas aeruginosa* PAO1. J Microbiol 2014; 52(9): 734-42.

[107]   Defoirdt T, Miyamoto CM, Wood TK, *et al.* The natural furanone (5Z)-4-bromo-5-(bromomethylene)-3-butyl-2(5H)-furanone disrupts quorum sensing-regulated gene expression in *Vibrio harveyi* by decreasing the DNA-binding activity of the transcriptional regulator protein luxR. Environ Microbiol 2007; 9(10): 2486-95.

[108]   Ravichandiran V, Shanmugam K, Anupama K, Thomas S, Princy A. Structure-based virtual screening for plant-derived SdiA-selective ligands as potential antivirulent agents against uropathogenic *Escherichia coli*. Eur J Med Chem 2012; 48: 200-5.

[109] Ding X, Yin B, Qian L, *et al.* Screening for novel quorum-sensing inhibitors to interfere with the formation of *Pseudomonas aeruginosa* biofilm. J Med Microbiol 2011; 60(Pt 12): 1827-34.

[110] Padmavathi AR, Abinaya B, Pandian SK. Phenol, 2,4-bis(1,1-dimethylethyl) of marine bacterial origin inhibits quorum sensing mediated biofilm formation in the uropathogen *Serratia marcescens*. Biofouling 2014; 30(9): 1111-22.

[111] Lee JH, Lee J. Indole as an intercellular signal in microbial communities. FEMS Microbiol Rev 2010; 34(4): 426-44.

[112] Li X, Yang Q, Dierckens K, Milton DL, Defoirdt T. RpoS and indole signaling control the virulence of *Vibrio anguillarum* towards gnotobiotic sea bass (*Dicentrarchus labrax*) larvae. PLoS One 2014; 9(10): e111801.

[113] Lee JH, Wood TK, Lee J. Roles of indole as an interspecies and interkingdom signaling molecule. Trends Microbiol 2015; 23(11): 707-18.

[114] Lee J, Bansal T, Jayaraman A, Bentley WE, Wood TK. Enterohemorrhagic *Escherichia coli* biofilms are inhibited by 7-hydroxyindole and stimulated by isatin. Appl Environ Microbiol 2007; 73(13): 4100-9.

[115] Hidalgo-Romano B, Gollihar J, Brown SA, *et al.* Indole inhibition of N-acylated homoserine lactone-mediated quorum signalling is widespread in Gram-negative bacteria. Microbiology 2014; 160(Pt 11): 2464-73.

[116] Figueroa M, Jarmusch AK, Raja HA, *et al.* Polyhydroxyanthraquinones as quorum sensing inhibitors from the guttates of *Penicillium restrictum* and their analysis by desorption electrospray ionization mass spectrometry. J Nat Prod 2014; 77(6): 1351-8.

[117] Witso IL, Benneche T, Vestby LK, Nesse LL, Lonn-Stensrud J, Scheie AA. Thiophenone and furanone in control of *Escherichia coli* O103:H2 virulence. Pathog Dis 2014; 70(3): 297-306.

[118] Benneche T, Herstad G, Rosenberg M, Assev S, Scheie AA. Facile synthesis of 5-(alkylidene)thiophen-2(5H)-ones. A new class of antimicrobial agents. RSC Adv 2011; 1(2): 323-32.

[119] Defoirdt T, Benneche T, Brackman G, Coenye T, Sorgeloos P, Scheie AA. A quorum sensing-disrupting brominated thiophenone with a promising therapeutic potential to treat luminescent vibriosis. PLoS One 2012; 7(7): e41788.

[120] Srivastava A, Singh BN, Deepak D, Rawat AK, Singh BR. Colostrum hexasaccharide, a novel *Staphylococcus aureus* quorum-sensing inhibitor. Antimicrob Agents Chemother 2015; 59(4): 2169-78.

[121] Bobadilla Fazzini RA, Skindersoe ME, Bielecki P, Puchalka J, Givskov M, Martins sos Santos VA. Protoanemonin: a natural quorum sensing inhibitor that selectively activates iron starvation response. Environ Microbiol 2013; 15(1): 111-20.

[122] Easwaran N, Karthikeyan S, Sridharan B, Gothandam KM. Identification and analysis of the salt tolerant property of AHL lactonase (AiiA) of *Bacillus* species. J Basic Microbiol 2014; 54: 1-12.

[123] Sakr MM, Aboshanab KM, Aboulwafa MM, Hassouna NA. Characterization and complete sequence of lactonase enzyme from *Bacillus weihenstephanensis* isolate P65 with potential activity against acyl homoserine lactone signal molecules. Biomed Res Int 2013; 2013: 192589.

[124] Kim MH, Choi WC, Kang HO, *et al.* The molecular structure and catalytic mechanism of a quorum-quenching N-acyl-L-homoserine lactone hydrolase. Proc Natl Acad Sci U S A 2005; 102(49): 17606-11.

[125] Liu D, Momb J, Thomas PW, *et al.* Mechanism of the quorum-quenching lactonase (AiiA) from *Bacillus thuringiensis.* 1. Product-bound structures. Biochemistry 2008; 47(29): 7706-14.

[126] Simanski M, Babucke S, Eberl L, Harder J. Paraoxonase 2 acts as a quorum sensing-quenching factor in human keratinocytes. J Invest Dermatol 2012; 132(9): 2296-9.

[127] Draganov DI, Teiber JF, Speelman A, Osawa Y, Sunahara R, La Du BN. Human paraoxonases (PON1, PON2, and PON3) are lactonases with overlapping and distinct substrate specificities. J Lipid Res 2005; 46(6): 1239-47.

[128] Wahjudi M, Papaioannou E, Hendrawati O, *et al.* PA0305 of *Pseudomonas aeruginosa* is a quorum quenching acylhomoserine lactone acylase belonging to the Ntn hydrolase superfamily. Microbiology 2011; 157(Pt 7): 2042-55.

[129] Ochiai S, Yasumoto S, Morohoshi T, Ikeda T. AmiE, a novel N-acylhomoserine lactone acylase belonging to the amidase family, from the activated-sludge isolate *Acinetobacter* sp. strain Ooi24. Appl Environ Microbiol 2014; 80(22): 6919-25.

[130] Pennartz A, Genereux C, Parquet C, Mengin-Lecreulx D, Joris B. Substrate-induced inactivation of the *Escherichia coli* AmiD N-acetylmuramoyl-L-alanine amidase highlights a new strategy to inhibit this class of enzyme. Antimicrob Agents Chemother 2009; 53(7): 2991-7.

[131] Uroz S, Chhabra SR, Camara M, Williams P, Oger P, Dessaux Y. N-Acylhomoserine lactone quorum-sensing molecules are modified and degraded by *Rhodococcus erythropolis* W2 by both amidolytic and novel oxidoreductase activities. Microbiology 2005; 151(Pt 10): 3313-22.

[132] Chan KG, Atkinson S, Mathee K, *et al.* Characterization of N-acylhomoserine lactone-degrading bacteria associated with the *Zingiber officinale* (ginger) rhizosphere: co-existence of quorum quenching and quorum sensing in *Acinetobacter* and *Burkholderia.* BMC Microbiol 2011; 11: 51.

[133] Chowdhary PK, Keshavan N, Nguyen HQ, Peterson JA, Gonzalez JE, Haines DC. *Bacillus megaterium* CYP102A1 oxidation of acyl homoserine lactones and acyl homoserines. Biochemistry 2007; 46(50): 14429-37.

[134] Hume ME. Historic perspective: prebiotics, probiotics, and other alternatives to antibiotics. Poult Sci 2011; 90(11): 2663-9.

[135] Gaggia F, Mattarelli P, Biavati B. Probiotics and prebiotics in animal feeding for safe food production. Int J Food Microbiol 2010; 141(Suppl 1): S15-28.

[136] Brugere JF, Borrel G, Gaci N, Tottey W, O'Toole PW, Malpuech-Brugere C. Archaebiotics: proposed therapeutic use of archaea to prevent trimethylaminuria and cardiovascular disease. Gut Microbes 2014; 5(1): 5-10.

[137] Reid G, Sanders ME, Gaskins HR, *et al.* New scientific paradigms for probiotics and prebiotics. J Clin Gastroenterol 2003; 37(2): 105-18.

[138] Kim JE, Kim JY, Lee KW, Lee HJ. Cancer chemopreventive effects of lactic acid bacteria. J Microbiol Biotechnol 2007; 17(8): 1227-35.

[139] Callaway TR, Edrington TS, Anderson RC, *et al.* Probiotics, prebiotics and competitive exclusion for prophylaxis against bacterial disease. Anim Health Res Rev 2008; 9(2): 217-25.

[140] Montalto M, Curigliano V, Santoro L, *et al.* Management and treatment of lactose malabsorption. World J Gastroenterol 2006; 12(2): 187-91.

[141] Conway P, Wang X. Specifically targeted probiotics can reduce antibiotic usage in animal production. Asian-Australian J Animal Sci 2000; 13(Suppl): 358-61.

[142] Sakshi D, Krishnendra SN, Priyanka P, Priyanka S, Neelofar S, Jitendra N. Antagonistic activity of lactic acid bacteria from dairy products. Int J Pure App Biosci 2013; 1(1): 28-32.

[143] Cummins J, Ho M-W. Genetically modified probiotics should be banned. Microb Ecol Health D 2005; 17(2): 66-8.

[144] Besselink MG, van Santvoort HC, Buskens E, *et al.* Probiotic prophylaxis in predicted severe acute pancreatitis: a randomised, double-blind, placebo-controlled trial. Lancet 2008; 371(9613): 651-9.

[145] Roberfroid M. Prebiotics: the concept revisited. J Nutr 2007; 137(3 Suppl 2): 830s-7s.

[146] Wasilewski A, Zielinska M, Storr M, Fichna J. Beneficial effects of probiotics, prebiotics, synbiotics, and psychobiotics in inflammatory bowel disease. Inflamm Bowel Dis 2015; 21(7): 1674-82.

[147] DSM Nutritional Products Ltd [homepage on the Internet]. Canton of Aargau: Eubtiotics: Definition and different concepts [updated: 25th March 2014; cited: 29th February 2016]. DSM in Animal Nutrition & Health Information Center; [about 4 screens]. Available from: http://www.dsm.com/markets/anh/en_US/infocenter-news/2014/03/Eubiotics_Definition_and_different_concepts.html

[148] Pinna C, Biagi G. The utilisation of prebiotics and synbiotics in dogs. Ital J Animal Sci 2014; 13(1): 169-78.

[149] Marco ML, Tachon S. Environmental factors influencing the efficacy of probiotic bacteria. Curr Opin Biotechnol 2013; 24(2): 207-13.

[150] Chukwu E, Nwaokorie F, Coker A. Role of anaerobes as probiotic organisms. Int J Food Nutr Safety 2014; 5(2): 74-97.

[151] Brashears MM, Jaroni D, Trimble J. Isolation, selection, and characterization of lactic acid bacteria for a competitive exclusion product to reduce shedding of *Escherichia coli* O157:H7 in cattle. J Food Prot 2003; 66(3): 355-63.

[152] Sang Y, Blecha F. Antimicrobial peptides and bacteriocins: alternatives to traditional antibiotics. Anim Health Res Rev 2008; 9(2): 227-35.

[153] Perez RH, Zendo T, Sonomoto K. Novel bacteriocins from lactic acid bacteria (LAB): various structures and applications. Microb Cell Fact 2014; 13(Suppl 1): S3.

[154] Zacharof MP, Lovitt RW. Bacteriocins produced by lactic acid bacteria a review article. APCBEE Procedia 2012; 2: 50-6.

[155] Brogden KA. Antimicrobial peptides: pore formers or metabolic inhibitors in bacteria? Nat Rev Microbiol 2005; 3(3): 238-50.

[156] Deshmukh PV, Thorat PR. Bacteriocins: a new trend in antimicrobial food packaging. Int J Adv Res Eng Appl Sci 2013; 2(1): 1-12.

[157] Lin J. Novel approaches for *Campylobacter* control in poultry. Foodborne Pathog Dis 2009; 6(7): 755-65.

[158] Riley MA, Wertz JE. Bacteriocin diversity: ecological and evolutionary perspectives. Biochimie 2002; 84(5-6): 357-64.

[159] Delany I, Rappuoli R, De Gregorio E. Vaccines for the 21st century. EMBO Mol Med 2014; 6(6): 708-20.

[160] Nascimento IP, Leite LC. Recombinant vaccines and the development of new vaccine strategies. Braz J Med Biol Res 2012; 45(12): 1102-11.

[161] Palucka K, Banchereau J. Cancer immunotherapy *via* dendritic cells. Nat Rev Cancer 2012; 12(4): 265-77.

[162] Sanchez-Ramon S, de Diego RP, Dieli-Crimi R, Subiza JL. Extending the clinical horizons of mucosal bacterial vaccines: current evidence and future prospects. Curr Drug Targets 2014; 15(12): 1132-43.

[163] de Cassan SC, Draper SJ. Recent advances in antibody-inducing poxviral and adenoviral vectored vaccine delivery platforms for difficult disease targets. Expert Rev Vaccines 2013; 12(4): 365-78.

[164] Rollier CS, Reyes-Sandoval A, Cottingham MG, Ewer K, Hill AV. Viral vectors as vaccine platforms: deployment in sight. Curr Opin Immunol 2011; 23(3): 377-82.

[165] Gnjatic S, Sawhney NB, Bhardwaj N. Toll-like receptor agonists: are they good adjuvants? Cancer J 2010; 16(4): 382-91.

[166] Brinkmann V, Reichard U, Goosmann C, *et al.* Neutrophil extracellular traps kill bacteria. Science 2004; 303(5663): 1532-5.

[167] Halverson TW, Wilton M, Poon KK, Petri B, Lewenza S. DNA is an antimicrobial component of neutrophil extracellular traps. PLoS Pathog 2015; 11(1): e1004593.

[168] Owen J, Punt J, Strandford S. Infectious diseases and vaccines. In: Owen J, Punt J, Strandford S, Eds. Kuby Immunolgy. 7th ed. New York: W H Freeman and Company 2013; pp. 553-88.

[169] Ferraro B, Morrow MP, Hutnick NA, Shin TH, Lucke CE, Weiner DB. Clinical applications of DNA vaccines: current progress. Clin Infect Dis 2011; 53(3): 296-302.

[170] Seib KL, Zhao X, Rappuoli R. Developing vaccines in the era of genomics: a decade of reverse vaccinology. Clin Microbiol Infect 2012; 18(Suppl 5): 109-16.

[171] Schubert-Unkmeir A, Christodoulides M. Genome-based bacterial vaccines: current state and future outlook. BioDrugs 2013; 27(5): 419-30.

[172] McLellan JS, Chen M, Joyce MG, *et al.* Structure-based design of a fusion glycoprotein vaccine for respiratory syncytial virus. Science 2013; 342(6158): 592-8.

[173] Carleton HA. Pathogenic bacteria as vaccine vectors: teaching old bugs new tricks. Yale J Biol Med 2010; 83(4): 217-22.

[174] Bouvet JP, Fischetti VA. Diversity of antibody-mediated immunity at the mucosal barrier. Infect Immun 1999; 67(6): 2687-91.

[175] Kono M, Nakamura Y, Suda T, *et al.* Enhancement of protective immunity against intracellular bacteria using type-1 polarized dendritic cell (DC) vaccine. Vaccine 2012; 30(16): 2633-9.

[176] Sievers SA, Scharf L, West AP Jr., Bjorkman PJ. Antibody engineering for increased potency, breadth and half-life. Curr Opin HIV AIDS 2015; 10(3): 151-9.

[177] Schnepp BC, Johnson PR. Adeno-associated virus delivery of broadly neutralizing antibodies. Curr Opin HIV AIDS 2014; 9(3): 250-6.

[178] Menegazzi R, Decleva E, Dri P. Killing by neutrophil extracellular traps: fact or folklore? Blood 2012; 119(5): 1214-6.

[179] Floros T, Tarhini AA. Anticancer cytokines: biology and clinical effects of interferon-alpha2, interleukin (IL)-2, IL-15, IL-21, and IL-12. Semin Oncol 2015; 42(4): 539-48.

[180] Galluzzi L, Vacchelli E, Bravo-San Pedro JM, *et al.* Classification of current anticancer immunotherapies. Oncotarget 2014; 5(24): 12472-508.

[181] Freyne B, Marchant A, Curtis N. BCG-associated heterologous immunity, a historical perspective: experimental models and immunological mechanisms. Trans R Soc Trop Med Hyg 2015; 109(1): 46-51.

[182] Bekker LG, Haslett P, Maartens G, Steyn L, Kaplan G. Thalidomide-induced antigen-specific immune stimulation in patients with human immunodeficiency virus type 1 and tuberculosis. J Infect Dis 2000; 181(3): 954-65.

[183] Travar M, Petkovic M, Verhaz A. Type I, II, and III Interferons: Regulating Immunity to *Mycobacterium tuberculosis* Infection. Arch Immunol Ther Exp (Warsz) 2016; 64(1): 19-31.

[184] Flesch IE, Kaufmann SH. Stimulation of antibacterial macrophage activities by B-cell stimulatory factor 2 (interleukin-6). Infect Immun 1990; 58(1): 269-71.

[185] Erdag G, Morgan JR. Interleukin-1alpha and interleukin-6 enhance the antibacterial properties of cultured composite keratinocyte grafts. Ann Surg 2002; 235(1): 113-24.

[186] Yang D, Chen Q, Hoover DM, *et al.* Many chemokines including CCL20/MIP-3alpha display antimicrobial activity. J Leukoc Biol 2003; 74(3): 448-55.

[187] Dragoi AM, Talman AM, Agaisse H. Bruton's tyrosine kinase regulates *Shigella flexneri* dissemination in HT-29 intestinal cells. Infect Immun 2013; 81(2): 598-607.

[188] Napier RJ, Rafi W, Cheruvu M, *et al.* Imatinib-sensitive tyrosine kinases regulate mycobacterial pathogenesis and represent therapeutic targets against tuberculosis. Cell Host Microbe 2011; 10(5): 475-85.

[189] Stanley SA, Barczak AK, Silvis MR, *et al.* Identification of host-targeted small molecules that restrict intracellular *Mycobacterium tuberculosis* growth. PLoS Pathog 2014; 10(2): e1003946.

[190] Giamarellos-Bourboulis EJ, Poulaki H, Kostomitsopoulos N, *et al.* Effective immunomodulatory treatment of *Escherichia coli* experimental sepsis with thalidomide. Antimicrob Agents Chemother 2003; 47(8): 2445-9.

[191] Giamarellos-Bourboulis EJ, Bolanos N, Laoutaris G, *et al.* Immunomodulatory intervention in sepsis by multidrug-resistant *Pseudomonas aeruginosa* with thalidomide: an experimental study. BMC Infect Dis 2005; 5: 51.

[192] Defoirdt T, Boon N, Bossier P. Can bacteria evolve resistance to quorum sensing disruption? PLoS Pathog 2010; 6(7): e1000989.

[193] Maeda T, García-Contreras R, Pu M, *et al.* Quorum quenching quandary: resistance to antivirulence compounds. ISME J 2011; 6(3): 493-501.

[194] García-Contreras R, Maeda T, Wood TK. Resistance to quorum-quenching compounds. Appl Environ Microbiol 2013; 79(22): 6840-6.

[195] García-Contreras R, Martinez-Vazquez M, Velazquez Guadarrama N, *et al.* Resistance to the quorum-quenching compounds brominated furanone C-30 and 5-fluorouracil in *Pseudomonas aeruginosa* clinical isolates. Pathog Dis 2013; 68(1): 8-11.

[196] García-Contreras R, Perez-Eretza B, Jasso-Chavez R, *et al.* High variability in quorum quenching and growth inhibition by furanone C-30 in *Pseudomonas aeruginosa* clinical isolates from cystic fibrosis patients. Pathog Dis 2015; 73(6): ftv040.

[197] García-Contreras R, Nunez-Lopez L, Jasso-Chavez R, *et al.* Quorum sensing enhancement of the stress response promotes resistance to quorum quenching and prevents social cheating. ISME J 2014; 9(1): 115-25.

[198] Garcia-Contreras R, Maeda T, Wood TK. Can resistance against quorum-sensing interference be selected? ISME J 2016; 10(1): 4-10.

[199]   Ueda A, Attila C, Whiteley M, Wood TK. Uracil influences quorum sensing and biofilm formation in *Pseudomonas aeruginosa* and fluorouracil is an antagonist. Microb Biotechnol 2009; 2(1): 62-74.

[200]   Koul S, Prakash J, Mishra A, Kalia VC. Potential Emergence of Multi-quorum Sensing Inhibitor Resistant (MQSIR) Bacteria. Indian J Microbiol 2016; 56(1): 1-18.

[201]   Murugan K, Sekar K, Sangeetha S, Ranjitha S, Sohaibani SA. Antibiofilm and quorum sensing inhibitory activity of *Achyranthes aspera* on cariogenic *Streptococcus mutans*: an *in vitro* and *in silico* study. Pharm Biol 2013; 51(6): 728-36.

[202]   Vasavi HS, Arun AB, Rekha PD. Anti-quorum sensing potential of *Adenanthera pavonina*. Pharmacognosy Res 2015; 7(1): 105-9.

[203]   Abd-Alla MH, Bashandy SR. Production of quorum sensing inhibitors in growing onion bulbs infected with *Pseudomonas aeruginosa* E (HQ324110). ISRN Microbiol 2012; 2012: 161890.

[204]   Castillo-Juarez I, Garcia-Contreras R, Velazquez-Guadarrama N, Soto-Hernandez M, Martinez-Vazquez M. *Amphypterygium adstringens* anacardic acid mixture inhibits quorum sensing-controlled virulence factors of *Chromobacterium violaceum* and *Pseudomonas aeruginosa*. Arch Med Res 2013; 44(7): 488-94.

[205]   Murugan K, Sangeetha S, Kalyanasundaram VB, Saleh A-S. *In vitro* and *in silico* screening for *Andrographis paniculata* quorum sensing mimics: New therapeutic leads for cystic fibrosis *Pseudomonas aeruginosa* biofilms. Plant Omics 2013; 6(5): 340-6.

[206]   Lou Z, Hong Y, Liu Y, *et al.* Effect of ethanol fraction of burdock leaf on biofilm formation and bacteria growth. Eur Food Res Technol 2014; 239(2): 305-11.

[207]   Truchado P, Gimenez-Bastida JA, Larrosa M, *et al.* Inhibition of quorum sensing (QS) in *Yersinia enterocolitica* by an orange extract rich in glycosylated flavanones. J Agric Food Chem 2012; 60(36): 8885-94.

[208]   Amaya S, Pereira JA, Borkosky SA, Valdez JC, Bardon A, Arena ME. Inhibition of quorum sensing in *Pseudomonas aeruginosa* by sesquiterpene lactones. Phytomedicine 2012; 19(13): 1173-7.

[209]   Castillo S, Heredia N, Arechiga-Carvajal E, García S. Citrus extracts as inhibitors of quorum sensing, biofilm formation and motility of *Campylobacter jejuni*. Food Biotechnol 2014; 28(2): 106-22.

[210]   Hasan S, Danishuddin M, Adil M, Singh K, Verma PK, Khan AU. Efficacy of *E. officinalis* on the cariogenic properties of *Streptococcus mutans*: a novel and alternative approach to suppress quorum-sensing mechanism. PLoS One 2012; 7(7): e40319.

[211]   Cech NB, Junio HA, Ackermann LW, Kavanaugh JS, Horswill AR. Quorum quenching and antimicrobial activity of goldenseal (*Hydrastis canadensis*) against methicillin-resistant *Staphylococcus aureus* (MRSA). Planta Med 2012; 78(14): 1556-61.

[212]   Sepahi E, Tarighi S, Ahmadi FS, Bagheri A. Inhibition of quorum sensing in *Pseudomonas aeruginosa* by two herbal essential oils from *Apiaceae family*. J Microbiol 2015; 53(2): 176-80.

[213]   Salini R, Sindhulakshmi M, Poongothai T, Pandian SK. Inhibition of quorum sensing mediated biofilm development and virulence in uropathogens by *Hyptis suaveolens*. Antonie Van Leeuwenhoek 2015; 107(4): 1095-106.

[214]   Chenia HY. Anti-quorum sensing potential of crude *Kigelia africana* fruit extracts. Sensors (Basel) 2013; 13(3): 2802-17.

[215] Yap PS, Krishnan T, Yiap BC, Hu CP, Chan KG, Lim SH. Membrane disruption and anti-quorum sensing effects of synergistic interaction between *Lavandula angustifolia* (lavender oil) in combination with antibiotic against plasmid-conferred multi-drug-resistant *Escherichia coli*. J Appl Microbiol 2014; 116(5): 1119-28.

[216] Gemiarto AT, Ninyio NN, Lee SW, *et al.* Isoprenyl caffeate, a major compound in manuka propolis, is a quorum-sensing inhibitor in *Chromobacterium violaceum*. Antonie Van Leeuwenhoek 2015; 108(2): 491-504.

[217] Olivero-Verbel J, Barreto-Maya A, Bertel-Sevilla A, Stashenko EE. Composition, anti-quorum sensing and antimicrobial activity of essential oils from *Lippia alba*. Braz J Microbiol 2014; 45(3): 759-67.

[218] Alvarez MV, Ortega-Ramirez LA, Gutierrez-Pacheco MM, *et al.* Oregano essential oil-pectin edible films as anti-quorum sensing and food antimicrobial agents. Front Microbiol 2014; 5: 699.

[219] Jaramillo-Colorado B, Olivero-Verbel J, Stashenko EE, Wagner-Dobler I, Kunze B. Anti-quorum sensing activity of essential oils from Colombian plants. Nat Prod Res 2012; 26(12): 1075-86.

[220] Alvarez MV, Moreira MR, Ponce A. Antiquorum sensing and antimicrobial activity of natural agents with potential use in food. J Food Safety 2012; 32(3): 379-87.

[221] Tan LY, Yin WF, Chan KG. Silencing quorum sensing through extracts of *Melicope lunu-ankenda*. Sensors (Basel) 2012; 12(4): 4339-51.

[222] Pellegrini MC, Alvarez MV, Ponce AG, Cugnata NM, De Piano FG, Fuselli SR. Anti-quorum sensing and antimicrobial activity of aromatic species from South America. J Essent Oil Res 2014; 26(6): 458-65.

[223] Bai AJ, Vittal RR. Quorum sensing inhibitory and anti-biofilm activity of essential oils and their *in vivo* efficacy in food systems. Food Biotechnol 2014; 28(3): 269-92.

[224] Hossain MA, Park JY, Kim JY, Suh JW, Park SC. Synergistic effect and antiquorum sensing activity of *Nymphaea tetragona* (water lily) extract. Biomed Res Int 2014; 2014: 562173.

[225] Tan LY, Yin WF, Chan KG. *Piper nigrum*, *Piper betle* and *Gnetum gnemon*--natural food sources with anti-quorum sensing properties. Sensors (Basel) 2013; 13(3): 3975-85.

[226] Ghosh R, Tiwary BK, Kumar A, Chakraborty R. Guava leaf extract inhibits quorum-sensing and *Chromobacterium violaceum* induced lysis of human hepatoma cells: whole transcriptome analysis reveals differential gene expression. PLoS One 2014; 9(9): e107703.

[227] Musthafa KS, Sahu SK, Ravi AV, Kathiresan K. Anti-quorum sensing potential of the mangrove *Rhizophora annamalayana*. World J Microbiol Biotechnol 2013; 29(10): 1851-8.

[228] Zhang J, Rui X, Wang L, Guan Y, Sun X, Dong M. Polyphenolic extract from *Rosa rugosa* tea inhibits bacterial quorum sensing and biofilm formation. Food Control 2014; 42: 125-31.

[229] Sarkar R, Chaudhary SK, Sharma A, *et al.* Anti-biofilm activity of Marula - a study with the standardized bark extract. J Ethnopharmacol 2014; 154(1): 170-5.

[230] Song C, Ma H, Zhao Q, Song S, Jia Z. Inhibition of quorum sensing activity by ethanol extract of *Scutellaria baicalensis* Georgi. J Plant Pathol Microbiol 2012; S7:001

[231] Krishnan T, Yin WF, Chan KG. Inhibition of quorum sensing-controlled virulence factor production in *Pseudomonas aeruginosa* PAO1 by Ayurveda spice clove (*Syzygium aromaticum*) bud extract. Sensors (Basel) 2012; 12(4): 4016-30.

[232]   Sarabhai S, Harjai K, Sharma P, Capalash N. Ellagic acid derivatives from *Terminalia chebula* Retz. increase the susceptibility of *Pseudomonas aeruginosa* to stress by inhibiting polyphosphate kinase. J Appl Microbiol 2015; 118(4): 817-25.

[233]   Sarabhai S, Sharma P, Capalash N. Ellagic acid derivatives from *Terminalia chebula* Retz. downregulate the expression of quorum sensing genes to attenuate *Pseudomonas aeruginosa* PAO1 virulence. PLoS One 2013; 8(1): e53441.

[234]   Husain FM, Ahmad I, Khan MS, Al-Shabib NA. *Trigonella foenum-graceum* (seed) extract interferes with quorum sensing regulated traits and biofilm formation in the strains of *Pseudomonas aeruginosa* and *Aeromonas hydrophila*. Evid Based Complement Alternat Med 2015; 2015: 879540.

[235]   Gonzalez-Ortiz G, Quarles Van Ufford HC, Halkes SB, *et al.* New properties of wheat bran: anti-biofilm activity and interference with bacteria quorum-sensing systems. Environ Microbiol 2014; 16(5): 1346-53.

[236]   Kim HS, Park HD. Ginger extract inhibits biofilm formation by *Pseudomonas aeruginosa* PA14. PLoS One 2013; 8(9): e76106.

[237]   Ta CA, Freundorfer M, Mah TF, *et al.* Inhibition of bacterial quorum sensing and biofilm formation by extracts of neotropical rainforest plants. Planta Med 2014; 80(4): 343-50.

[238]   Rajesh PS, Ravishankar Rai V. Quorum quenching activity in cell-free lysate of endophytic bacteria isolated from *Pterocarpus santalinus* Linn., and its effect on quorum sensing regulated biofilm in *Pseudomonas aeruginosa* PAO1. Microbiol Res 2014; 169(7-8): 561-9.

[239]   Fuente Mde L, Miranda CD, Jopia P, *et al.* Growth inhibition of bacterial fish pathogens and quorum-sensing blocking by bacteria recovered from chilean salmonid farms. J Aquat Anim Health 2015; 27(2): 112-22.

[240]   Lopes RB, Costa LE, Vanetti MC, de Araujo EF, de Queiroz MV. Endophytic bacteria isolated from common bean (*Phaseolus vulgaris*) exhibiting high variability showed antimicrobial activity and quorum sensing inhibition. Curr Microbiol 2015; 71(4): 509-16.

[241]   Linthorne JS, Chang BJ, Flematti GR, Ghisalberti EL, Sutton DC. A direct pre-screen for marine bacteria producing compounds inhibiting quorum sensing reveals diverse planktonic bacteria that are bioactive. Mar Biotechnol (NY) 2015; 17(1): 33-42.

[242]   Alasil SM, Omar R, Ismail S, Yusof MY. Inhibition of quorum sensing-controlled virulence factors and biofilm formation in *Pseudomonas aeruginosa* by culture extract from novel bacterial species of *Paenibacillus* using a rat model of chronic lung infection. Int J Bacteriol 2015; 2015: 671562.

[243]   Durai S, Vigneshwari L, Balamurugan K. *Caenorhabditis elegans*-based *in vivo* screening of bioactives from marine sponge-associated bacteria against *Vibrio alginolyticus*. J Appl Microbiol 2013; 115(6): 1329-42.

[244]   Fu P, Liu P, Gong Q, Wang Y, Wang P, Zhu W. α-Pyrones from the marine-derived actinomycete *Nocardiopsis dassonvillei* subsp. *dassonvillei* XG-8-1. RSC Adv 2013; 3(43): 20726-31.

[245]   Singh VK, Kavita K, Prabhakaran R, Jha B. Cis-9-octadecenoic acid from the rhizospheric bacterium *Stenotrophomonas maltophilia* BJ01 shows quorum quenching and anti-biofilm activities. Biofouling 2013; 29(7): 855-67.

[246]   Sokovic M, Ciric A, Glamoclija J, Nikolic M, van Griensven LJ. *Agaricus blazei* hot water extract shows anti quorum sensing activity in the nosocomial human pathogen *Pseudomonas aeruginosa*. Molecules 2014; 19(4): 4189-99.

[247] Martin-Rodriguez AJ, Reyes F, Martin J, *et al.* Inhibition of bacterial quorum sensing by extracts from aquatic fungi: first report from marine endophytes. Mar Drugs 2014; 12(11): 5503-26.

[248] Glamoclija J, Stojkovic D, Nikolic M, *et al.* A comparative study on edible *Agaricus* mushrooms as functional foods. Food Funct 2015; 6(6): 1900-10.

[249] Jha B, Kavita K, Westphal J, Hartmann A, Schmitt-Kopplin P. Quorum sensing inhibition by *Asparagopsis taxiformis*, a marine macro alga: separation of the compound that interrupts bacterial communication. Mar Drugs 2013; 11(1): 253-65.

[250] Batista D, Carvalho AP, Costa R, Coutinho R, Dobretsov S. Extracts of macroalgae from the Brazilian coast inhibit bacterial quorum sensing. Botanica Mar 2014; 57(6): 441-7.

[251] Singh BN, Prateeksha, Pandey G, *et al.* Development and characterization of a novel Swarna-based herbo-metallic colloidal nano-formulation - inhibitor of *Streptococcus mutans* quorum sensing. RSC Adv 2015; 5(8): 5809-22.

[252] Tello E, Castellanos L, Arevalo-Ferro C, Duque C. Disruption in quorum-sensing systems and bacterial biofilm inhibition by cembranoid diterpenes isolated from the octocoral *Eunicea knighti*. J Nat Prod 2012; 75(9): 1637-42.

CHAPTER 2

Antibiotic Resistance: Global Trends, Policies, and Novel Solutions

Balagangadhar R. Totapally* and Andre Raszynski

Nicklaus Children's Hospital, Miami, FL 33155, USA and Herbert Wertheim College of Medicine, Florida International University, Miami, FL, USA

Abstract: Antibacterial agents such as sulfonamides, penicillin, and streptomycin became available in the 1930s and 1940s and were quickly adopted into clinical practice. It was noted early on that bacteria, when exposed to antimicrobial agents, rapidly developed strategies to resist them. Penicillin resistance in *Staphylococcus aureus* was detected as early as in 1945. From the 1950s onwards, a large number of antimicrobial drugs became clinically available and had a major impact on the treatment of infections. Most recently, bacterial antibiotic resistance has grown exponentially along with the increasing use of antimicrobial agents, while at the same time the development of new antimicrobial agents has decreased dramatically. This has led to major global crises of infections with drug-resistant microbes, increased morbidity, and mortality, and increased health care costs.

Antibiotic resistance results from mutations or acquisition of new genes in bacteria that reduce or eliminate the effectiveness of antibiotics. According to the CDC, every year more than 2 million people in the US develop an illness due to antibiotic resistant bacteria and 23,000 of them die. There are multiple reasons for the development and spread of antibiotic-resistant bacteria. Overuse and inappropriate use of antibiotics are prevalent in clinical practice. The spread of resistant bacteria in hospitalized patients raises grave concerns for increased local antibiotic resistance. Non-human use of antibiotics for animal growth promotion is a major cause of development of global antibiotic resistance.

A multifaceted approach is needed to detect, prevent, and control antibiotic resistance at local, national, and global levels. *The National Action Plan for Combating Antibiotic-resistant Bacteria* was developed by the CDC, and it provides a roadmap to guide the US in rising to this challenge. Implementation of antimicrobial stewardship programs, diligent surveillance for resistant bacteria, rigorous implementation of infection control practices, restriction of antibiotics for non-human and non-infectious purposes are needed to combat the growing threat of antibiotic resistance. Another important strategy to counter the menace of antimicrobial resistance is to develop new antibiotics with novel mechanisms of action.

*Corresponding author Balagangadhar R. Totapally: Nicklaus Children's Hospital, Miami, FL, USA; Tel: 1-3056622639; Fax: 1-3056630530; E-mail: bala.totapally@mch.com

Atta-ur-Rahman (Ed.)
All rights reserved-© 2016 Bentham Science Publishers

This chapter describes the global threat of antibiotic resistance, the mechanisms of development of antimicrobial resistance, the major causes of increased incidence of this problem, and the possible local, national, and global solutions to fight the scourge of antibiotic resistance.

Keywords: Antibiotics, antimicrobials, antibiotic resistance, infections, healthcare associated infection.

INTRODUCTION

Antibiotics or antimicrobials are chemicals/compounds that kill bacteria and other microbes. The discovery of penicillin in England by Sir Alexander Fleming in 1928 and of the first sulfonamide (Prontosil) in Germany by Gerhard Domagk in 1932 initiated the modern era of combating infections. Widespread utilization of antibiotics began in the 1940s and has saved countless lives since then. Bacteria have been in existence for billions of years before human evolution and they overwhelmingly outnumber the human population. Antimicrobial substances are also naturally produced by other microbes and plants; bacteria have adapted by developing resistance to antimicrobial substances throughout evolution. As early as in 1955, it was shown that resistance to antibiotics developed spontaneously by mutations [1]. Following the widespread use of antibiotics, many bacteria adapted by developing resistance- some to multiple antibiotics, thus making antibiotics less effective or even useless in combating the illnesses caused by these bacteria. Added to the problem of increased antibiotic resistance, the rate of new antibiotic development has slowed down. We are thus at a risk of returning to the pre-antibiotic era, with no effective treatments of bacterial infections.

According to Centers for Disease Control and Prevention's (CDC's) National Healthcare Safety Network, a growing number of healthcare-associated infections (HAI) are caused by bacteria which are resistant to antibiotics. These include methicillin-resistant *Staphylococcus aureus* (MRSA), vancomycin resistant *Enterococcus* (VRE), extended-spectrum cephalosporin-resistant *Klebsiella pneumoniae* (and *K. oxytoca*), *E. coli* and *Enterobacter* spp., and carbapenem-resistant *P. aeruginosa, K. pneumonia* (and *K. oxytoca*), *E. coli,* and *Enterobacter* spp.

It is estimated that between 40% and 50% of pathogens causing surgical site infections and 27% of pathogens causing infections after chemotherapy are resistant to standard prophylactic antibiotics available in the USA [2]. It was estimated that, in the USA, a 30% reduction in the efficacy of antibiotic prophylaxis for these procedures would result in 120,000 additional surgical site infections and post-chemotherapy associated infections per year and 6,300 infection-related deaths [2].

If left unaddressed, antibiotic resistance could make invasive surgeries very risky and patients could die from simple bacterial infections [3]. Widespread antibiotic resistance would lead to an increased socioeconomic burden from prolonged illness, increased cost of treatment, and higher mortality rate.

Warnings of increased resistance are not new [4, 5]. As early as 1945, when antibiotics were not yet widely available, Alexander Fleming, in his Nobel Prize acceptance speech, warned about microbes developing resistance [5]. In his speech, he said that "it is not difficult to make microbes resistant to penicillin in the laboratory by exposing them to concentrations not sufficient to kill them…there is the danger that the ignorant man may easily under-dose himself and, by exposing his microbes to nonlethal quantities of the drug, make them resistant" [5].

We are not winning the war against the scourge of antibiotic-resistant bacteria. There are several reasons why bacteria can outmaneuver humans in this fight:

- Bacteria have been in existence for 3.5 billion years, compared to a modern man who evolved about 250,000 years back, and bacteria have been adjusting to the changing world ever since.

- Bacteria are ubiquitous and outnumber humans exponentially. For example, during the course of a human life, the number of *E. coli* in the gut of each human being far exceeds the total number of people that now live and have ever lived [6].

- Bacteria can survive in extremes of temperatures, in frozen glaciers to high temperature of 650 °F at the bottom of the sea [6].

- Compared to humans, bacteria multiply in minutes. Thereby, they are more effective at adapting to a novel environment.

- With widespread, inappropriate, and sometimes indiscriminate use of antibiotics, both in humans and in animals, there is a huge "selection" pressure for bacteria to evolve and develop resistance.

- Bacteria can transmit resistance both vertically (to offsprings) and horizontally (to other bacteria).

- There is a discovery gap of new classes of antibiotics because antibiotic development takes a long time, is very expensive, and is not as profitable for the pharmaceutical companies as compared to other drugs such as cardiovascular medicines.

THE SPREAD OF ANTIBIOTIC RESISTANCE

Selective Pressure from Inappropriate Use of Antibiotics

Antibiotic resistance arises from mutations in bacterial genes and selection pressure from the inappropriate or improper use of antibiotics. Once bacteria develop resistance to any antibiotic, the resistant organisms survive and multiply, then spread within the community and globally.

Horizontal Transfer of Antibiotic Resistance Genes Among the Bacteria

Resistant bacteria also spread their resistance genes horizontally to other bacterial species through plasmids, and therefore neighboring bacterial species may also develop resistance and spread in the community. This spread is facilitated by interspecies gene transmission, poor sanitation and lack of hygiene in communities and hospitals, and the increased frequency of global travel and trade [7].

Local and Global Spread of Resistant Bacteria

The emergence and spread of antibiotic resistance are easily facilitated with the intensive use of antimicrobial agents and the international trade of both animals and food products used in the modern food production. Exposure or consumption of the contaminated food products, as well as contact with contaminated environment and transferable genes in commensals between food animals and humans, are the main routes of transmission of resistant pathogenic bacteria [8]. The exposure of humans to antimicrobial resistance from food animals can be controlled by either limiting the selective pressure from antimicrobial usage or by limiting the spread of the bacteria/genes [8]. With increased global trade and travel it is easy to spread resistant bacteria from one country to the other in a short period of time.

Global Map of Antibiotic Resistance

Antibiotic resistance has become a global problem due to the ubiquitous availability and easy access to antibiotics, a high burden of bacterial illnesses in low and middle-income countries, misuse and overuse of antibiotics, and non-human and nontherapeutic use of antibiotics.

The Enterobacteriaceae bacteria such as *E. coli, K. pneumoniae,* and other species, are part of the human gut flora and frequently cause hospital-acquired infections [9]. Carbapenem resistance in Enterobacteriaceae was first observed in Greece and in the U.S. and has now spread throughout the world; it has become an increasing clinical challenge with major public health implications [10-13]. Resistance to carbapenems amongst Enterobacteriaceae is usually mediated by transferable beta-lactamase enzymes through plasmids [14], which also confer resistance to most penicillins and cephalosporins [11].

In 2014, the World Health Organization (WHO) has published for the first time a global report of surveillance of antimicrobial resistance [15]. The central finding of the WHO report was that very high rates of resistance were observed in bacteria that cause common healthcare associated and community-acquired infections (*e.g.* urinary tract infection, pneumonia) in all WHO regions [15]. High rates of resistance to 3rd generation cephalosporins were reported for *E. coli* and *K. pneumoniae* in all regions of the WHO [15]. This has required a shift to the use of carbapenems as a first line for the treatment of these infections. Of great concern, is that *K. pneumoniae* resistant to carbapenems have also been identified in most of these countries, with as high as 54% resistance reported in some areas [15]. High rates of MRSA were found in many parts of the world; the implication is that in many countries the treatment of suspected or verified severe *S. aureus* infections, such as common skin and wound infections must rely on the use of second-line drugs. This also means that standard prophylaxis for surgical procedures with currently used first-line drugs will have limited effect in many settings. Second-line drugs for *S. aureus* are more expensive, have severe side-effects, and many require drug level monitoring which increase costs even further [15]. In addition, the global report on surveillance of antibiotic resistance by the WHO notes that there are limitations in effective oral treatment options for some common community-acquired infections in several countries [15].

Globally, 3.6% of new cases of tuberculosis (TB) and 20.2% of previously treated cases are estimated to be multi-drug resistant TB (MDR-TB), with much higher rates in Eastern Europe and central Asia [15]. A total of 84,000 cases of MDR-TB were reported to WHO in 2012. In spite of recent progress in the detection and treatment of MDR-TB, this represented only about 21% of the MDR-TB cases estimated to have developed in the world that year [15].

Antibiotic Resistance in the US

In a population- and laboratory-based active surveillance system in 7 U.S. states, the incidence of carbapenem-resistant Enterobacteriaceae (CRE) was 2.93 per 100,000 populations. There was a wide variation in the standardized incidence ratio of CRE between the seven states in the surveillance report, with highest incidence in Georgia (1.65) and lowest in Oregon (0.28) [16]. According to the National Nosocomial Infection Surveillance report, in 2003, the prevalence of methicillin resistance among coagulase-negative staphylococci was 89% (an increase of 1% compared to previous 5 years), and methicillin resistance in *Staphylococcus aureus* was 59.5% (an increase of 11% compared to previous 5 years) [17]. Approximately 29% of enterococci were resistant to vancomycin, 30% of Pseudomonas were resistant to 3rd generation cephalosporins, imipenem, or quinolones, and 31% of Enterobacter species were resistant to 3rd generation cephalosporins [17]. In 2013, the CDC published a report on the top 18 drug-resistant threats to the U.S. [16]. These threats were categorized based on level of concern: urgent, serious, and concerning (Table **1**).

Table 1. CDC report on drug-resistant threats to the United States [16].

Threats	Health Consequences
Urgent Threats	
Clostridium difficile (*C. difficile*)	*C. difficile* causes almost half a million infections among patients in the United States in a single year. An estimated 15,000 deaths are directly attributable to *C. difficile* infections [18].
Carbapenem-resistant Enterobacteriaceae (CRE)	CRE have become resistant to all or nearly all the antibiotics we have today and infections from CRE bacteria are on the rise among patients in medical facilities. Almost half of hospital patients who get bloodstream infections from CRE bacteria die from the infection.
Neisseria gonorrhoeae	The CDC estimates that more than 800,000 cases of gonococcal infections occur annually in the United States, 246,000 of which are drug resistant.
Serious Threats	
Multidrug-resistant Acinetobacter	Gram-negative bacteria which can cause pneumonia or bloodstream infections in critically ill patients. Many of these bacteria have become very resistant to antibiotics. Sixty three percent of healthcare-associated infections due to Acinetobacter are multidrug resistant. There are an estimated 7,300 infections and 500 deaths caused each year in the US by multidrug-resistant acinetobacter.
Drug-resistant campylobacter	*Campylobacter* is estimated to cause approximately 1.3 million infections, 13,000 hospitalizations, and 120 deaths each year in the United States. CDC reports resistance to ciprofloxacin in almost 25% of *Campylobacter* tested and resistance to azithromycin in about 2%.

Table 1: contd…

Fluconazole-resistant Candida	CDC estimates 3,400 fluconazole-resistant candida blood stream infections and 220 deaths annually in the US.
Extended-spectrum beta-lactamase (ESBL) producing Enterobacteriaceae	Nearly 26,000 (or 19%) healthcare-associated *Enterobacteriaceae* infections and 1,700 deaths are caused by ESBL-producing *Enterobacteriaceae* each year in the US.
Vancomycin-resistant Enterococcus (VRE)	An estimated 66,000 healthcare-associated *Enterococcus* infections occur in the United States each year with an overall 20,000 VRE occurred among hospitalized patients each year, with approximately 1,300 deaths attributed to these infections.
Multidrug-resistant *Pseudomonas aeruginosa*	An estimated 51,000 healthcare-associated *Pseudomonas aeruginosa* infections occur in the United States each year. More than 6,000 (or 13%) of these are multidrug-resistant, with roughly 400 deaths per year attributed to these infections.
Drug-resistant, non-typhoidal Salmonella	Non-typhoidal *Salmonella* causes approximately 1.2 million infections (100,000 drug-resistant), 23,000 hospitalizations, and 450 deaths each year in the United States. Non-typhoidal *Salmonella* is demonstrating resistance to ceftriaxone, ciprofloxacin, and other antibiotics.
Drug-resistant *Salmonella typhi*	*Salmonella typhi* causes approximately 21.7 million infections worldwide. In the United States, it causes approximately 5,700 infections and 620 hospitalizations each year. *Salmonella* typhi is becoming resistant to ceftriaxone, azithromycin, and ciprofloxacin (resistance is so common that it cannot be routinely used).
Drug-resistant Shigella	*Shigella* causes approximately 500,000 diarrheal illnesses (27,000 drug-resistant), 5,500 hospitalizations, and 40 deaths each year in the United States. *Shigella* is developing resistance to ciprofloxacin and azithromycin.
Methicillin-resistant *Staphylococcus aureus* (MRSA)	Staphylococci are the leading cause of healthcare-associated infections. CDC estimates that 80,461 invasive MRSA infections and 11,285 related deaths occurred in 2011. However, the incidence of serious MRSA infections has decreased over the last few years.
Drug-resistant *Streptococcus pneumoniae*	*S. pneumoniae* has developed resistance to drugs in the penicillin and erythromycin groups. It causes 4 million infections and 22,000 deaths annually. In 30% of severe *S. pneumoniae* cases, the bacteria are fully resistant to one or more clinically relevant antibiotics; thus, more than one million illnesses and 7,000 deaths per year are caused by resistant *S. pneumoniae*.
Drug-resistant tuberculosis	Tuberculosis (TB) is one of the most common infectious diseases and a frequent cause of death worldwide. Some TB is multidrug-resistant (MDR), showing resistance to at least INH and rifampicin (RMP), two essential first-line drugs and some TB is XDR TB, defined as MDR TB plus resistance to any fluoroquinolone and to any of the three second-line injectable drugs (*i.e.*, amikacin, kanamycin, capreomycin). Of a total of 10,528 cases of TB in the United States reported in 2011, antibiotic resistance was identified in 1,042, or 9.90%, of all TB cases.

Table 1: contd...

Concerning Threat	
Vancomycin-resistant *Staphylococcus aureus* **(VRSA)**	A total of 13 cases of vancomycin-resistant *Staphylococcus aureus* (VRSA) have been identified in the United States since 2002.
Erythromycin-resistant Group A Streptococcus (GAS)	GAS has developed resistance to clindamycin and macrolides. Currently, GAS is not resistant to treatment with penicillin. Of GAS bacterial samples tested at CDC from 2010 and 2011, 10% were erythromycin-resistant (and therefore resistant to other macrolides), while 3.4% were clindamycin-resistant.
Clindamycin-resistant Group B Streptococcus (GBS)	GBS has developed resistance to clindamycin and erythromycin. Forty-nine percent of GBS isolates (samples) tested were erythromycin-resistant, and 28% were clindamycin-resistant. Each year in the United States, clindamycin-resistant Group B Strep causes an estimated 7,600 illnesses and 440 deaths.

Antibiotic Resistance in Europe

The incidence of extended-spectrum β-lactamase (ESBL)-producing isolates in Europe was 11% in patients with intra-abdominal sepsis [19]. However, resistance to carbapenems was low, with all isolates exhibiting 99.3% ertapenem susceptibility [19]. National experts from 39 European countries reported, in an online survey performed in 2013, that the incidence of carbapenemase-producing Enterobacteriaceae is continuing to rise [11]. In the late 2000s, a new strain of β-lactamase, the New Delhi metallo-β-lactamase, emerged in the Indian subcontinent. The New Delhi metallo-β-lactamase was first isolated in 2008 from a Swedish patient who acquired the infection in India. Organisms carrying this new β-lactamase were also found in the United Kingdom, in ill patients who had either have travelled to or had links with the Indian subcontinent [20]. Since then, it has been detected in many countries including the USA, Japan, and Canada. With global travel, antibiotic resistance along with many communicable diseases can easily and rapidly spread to various parts of the world.

Interestingly, an examination of drinking water and seepage water around New Delhi showed that the gene coding for the New Delhi metallo-β-lactamase enzyme was found in 50 out of 50 drinking water samples and 51 out of 171 seepage water samples [21]. None of the samples from the Cardiff area had this gene. This has a major risk implication for people living in the New Delhi area for development of infections with these types of resistant organisms.

Antibiotic Resistance in Developing Countries

In developing countries, the risk of health-care-associated infections is two to twenty times higher compared to that in developed countries and the proportion of infected patients frequently exceeds 25% [22]. The prevalence of health-care-associated infections in developing countries was found to be 15.5 per 100 patients in a systematic meta-analysis study [23]. This rate is at least twice the rate published by the European Centre for Disease Prevention and Control [24]. In addition, the incidence of health-care-associated infections acquired in intensive care units in developing countries was 34.2 per 1,000 patient-days, triple the rates reported from the USA [23, 24].

An International Nosocomial Infection Control Consortium (INICC) surveillance study from January 2007 thru December 2012 in 503 intensive care units in Latin America, Asia, Africa, and Europe showed that the pooled rate of central line-associated bloodstream infections (CLABSIs) was 4.9 per 1,000 central line days, nearly 5-fold higher than the 0.9 per 1,000 central line days reported from comparable U.S. ICUs [25]. A High prevalence of HAI is associated with a higher incidence of infections with antibiotic resistant bacteria [26]. Frequencies of isolates of Pseudomonas resistant to amikacin (42.8% *vs* 10%) and imipenem (42.4% *vs* 26.1%) and isolates of *K. pneumoniae* resistant to ceftazidime (71.2% *vs* 28.8%) and imipenem (19.6% *vs* 12.8%) were also higher in the INICC's ICUs compared with the ICUs in the U.S., respectively [25].

HAI affect a very large number of patients worldwide each year with detrimental impact on patients, their families and healthcare systems. There are methods to assess the extent and the nature of the HAI problem which will help create a basis for monitoring of action. Most HAI are due to multiple causes related to systems issues such as processes of provision of care, economic constraints, and human behavior. Solutions and interventions to prevent HAI are available, and most are simple and inexpensive. Lastly, several hospitals and healthcare practices have succeeded in reducing the risk to patients [22]. Reduction of HAI is a major priority to not only to improve patient outcomes but also to curb antibiotic resistance.

The World Alliance for Patient Safety was launched in October 2004 to galvanize global commitment and action on a patient safety topic that represents a significant risk for all 192 WHO member states. The topic chosen for the First Challenge is the prevention of HAI. Under the banner 'Clean Care is Safer Care', the Challenge was launched in October 2005 and consists of actions in five major areas: blood safety, clinical procedure safety, injection safety, sanitation and safety of waste management, and promotion of safe hand hygiene practices during patient care [22, 27]. Key elements of hand hygiene practice improvement include staff education and motivation, adoption of an alcohol-based hand rub as the gold standard, use of performance indicators, and strong commitment by all stakeholders, such as frontline staff, managers and healthcare leaders [27].

Antibiotic Resistance in the Asia and Asia Pacific Region

Antibiotic resistance is increasing at an alarming rate in the Asia Pacific region. In India, approximately 60% of *Klebsiella pneumoniae* are resistant to carbapenems in 2013 compared to 30% in 2008 [28].

Data from Study for Monitoring Antimicrobial Resistance Trends (SMART) studies show that the level of antimicrobial resistance differs by geographic region, but is highest in Asia-Pacific countries [29-35]. SMART, initiated in 2002, is a global surveillance program designed to longitudinally monitor the epidemiological trends and *in vitro* antimicrobial susceptibilities to ertapenem and 11 other antimicrobial agents of a variety of aerobic and facultative Gram-negative bacilli isolated from patients with intra-abdominal infections (IAIs) [36]. The recent SMART report from Asia demonstrated a trend towards continuously increasing antimicrobial resistance among IAI pathogens in this region [36]. Reports from SMART have shown that the levels of antimicrobial resistance are highest in the Asia-Pacific region [32, 34, 36, 37]. Resistance rates were generally higher in Enterobacteriaceae isolated from Asian centers than those isolated from Oceania centers as per the 2004 SMART report [37]. The prevalence of ESBLs increased from 13% in 2002 to 28% in 2006 among the isolates that were prospectively collected from patients with intra-abdominal infections in the Asia/Pacific region [34]. In an another report from SMART, of all gram-negative bacilli collected from intra-abdominal infections in the Asia-Pacific region during 2007, 42.2% and 35.8% of *Escherichia coli* and *Klebsiella* species, respectively, were ESBL positive [32]. Moreover, ESBL rates in India for *E. coli*, *Klebsiella pneumoniae*, and *Klebsiella oxytoca* were 79.0%, 69.4%, and 100%, respectively [32]. ESBL-positive *E. coli* rates were also relatively high in China (55.0%) and Thailand (50.8%) [32]. The occurrence of extended-spectrum β-lactamases in patients from China has increased rapidly, especially in *E. coli* (from 20.8% in 2002 to 64.9% in 2009) and susceptibility rates of all tested third- and fourth-generation cephalosporins against Enterobacteriaceae declined by 30% during 2002 to 2009 [38].

Antibiotic Resistance in Africa

As with other regions of the world, antibiotic resistance is also increasing in the Africa region. During 2004-2009, three centralized clinical microbiology laboratories serving 59 private hospitals in three large South African cities collected 1,218 gram negative bacteria from complicated intra-abdominal infections and tested them for susceptibility to 12 antibiotics according to the 2011 Clinical Laboratory Standards Institute guidelines [39]. The highest ESBL rate was documented in *Klebsiella pneumoniae* (41.2%) isolates. This study also documented substantial resistance to standard antimicrobial therapy in gram-negative bacteria commonly isolated from complicated intra-abdominal infections in South Africa [39].

In summary, antibiotic resistance is widespread, and not a single region is immune to it. The prevalence of antibiotic resistance varies widely across the globe with higher prevalence in developing countries, especially in Asia-Pacific countries.

HEALTH AND ECONOMIC BURDEN DUE TO ANTIBIOTIC RESISTANCE

Systematic reviews of published studies reveal that infections with antibiotic resistant bacteria increase morbidity and mortality [15]. The health outcomes of patients with various antibiotic resistant bacteria based on systematic reviews are summarized in Table 2. [15]. The cost of care for infections caused by resistant strains are consistently greater than those for infections caused by susceptible strains [15].

Table 2. Health outcomes of patients with various antibiotic resistant bacteria based on systematic reviews [15].

Organism	Associated Health Outcomes
Third-generation cephalosporin-resistant (including extended spectrum beta-lactamase (ESBL)) *E. coli* infections	• A significant twofold increase in all-cause mortality, bacterium-attributable mortality and, in 30-day mortality • No significant increase in length of stay (LOS), ICU admission and post-infection LOS
Fluoroquinolone-resistant *E. coli* infections	• A significant twofold increase in both all-cause mortality and 30-day mortality for patients with fluoroquinolone-resistant *E. coli* infections • A significant twofold risk increase in infection attributable ICU admission, and a significant increase in incidence of septic shock
Third-generation cephalosporin-resistant *K. pneumoniae* infections	• A significant increase in all-cause mortality, bacterium-attributable mortality and 30-day mortality, and in the risk of ICU admission

Table 2: contd...

Carbapenem-resistant *K. pneumoniae* infections	• A significant increase in all-cause mortality and 30-day mortality
Methicillin-resistant *S. aureus* infections (MRSA)	• A significant increase in: - All-cause mortality, bacterium-attributable mortality and ICU mortality - Post-infection LOS and ICU LOS - Septic shock - Discharge to long-term care for MRSA compared to methicillin-susceptible *S. aureus* (MSSA), and more than twofold risk increase for discharge to long-term care for MRSA compared to MSSA

A single center study from a Chicago teaching hospital reported that 13.5% of the enrolled patients had antibiotic-resistant infections [40]. The medical costs attributable to antibiotic-resistant infection ranged from $18,588 to $29,069 per patient, and excess duration of hospital stay was 6.4-12.7 days, and attributable mortality was 6.5%. This resulted in a total cost of $13.35 million in 2008 dollars in that patient cohort alone [40].

The total economic cost of antibiotic resistance to the U.S. economy, although difficult to calculate, is estimated to be as high as $20 billion in excess direct health care costs, with additional costs to society of lost productivity as high as $35 billion a year (2008 dollars) [16, 40, 41]. The global cost of antibiotic resistance is enormous.

DEVELOPMENT AND SPREAD OF ANTIBIOTIC RESISTANCE

Overuse and misuse of antibiotics have led to selective growth of resistant bacteria and subsequent spread of resistant bacteria. In addition, resistant bacteria can transmit their resistance to neighboring bacteria. Nonhuman use of antibiotics, especially in dairy and poultry industries, has led to the development of resistant bacteria in animals which can be easily transmitted to humans *via* animal products or through water and soil contamination (Fig. **1**).

Improper Antibiotic Therapy

According to the Center for Disease Control and Prevention (CDC), an estimated 2 million people are infected with resistant bacteria each year, approximately 23,000 of which die as a direct result of these infections [16]. The use of antibiotics is the single most important cause of development of antibiotic resistance. Antibiotics are one of the most commonly prescribed medications. About 50% of hospitalized patients receive antibiotics [43]. However, up to 50%

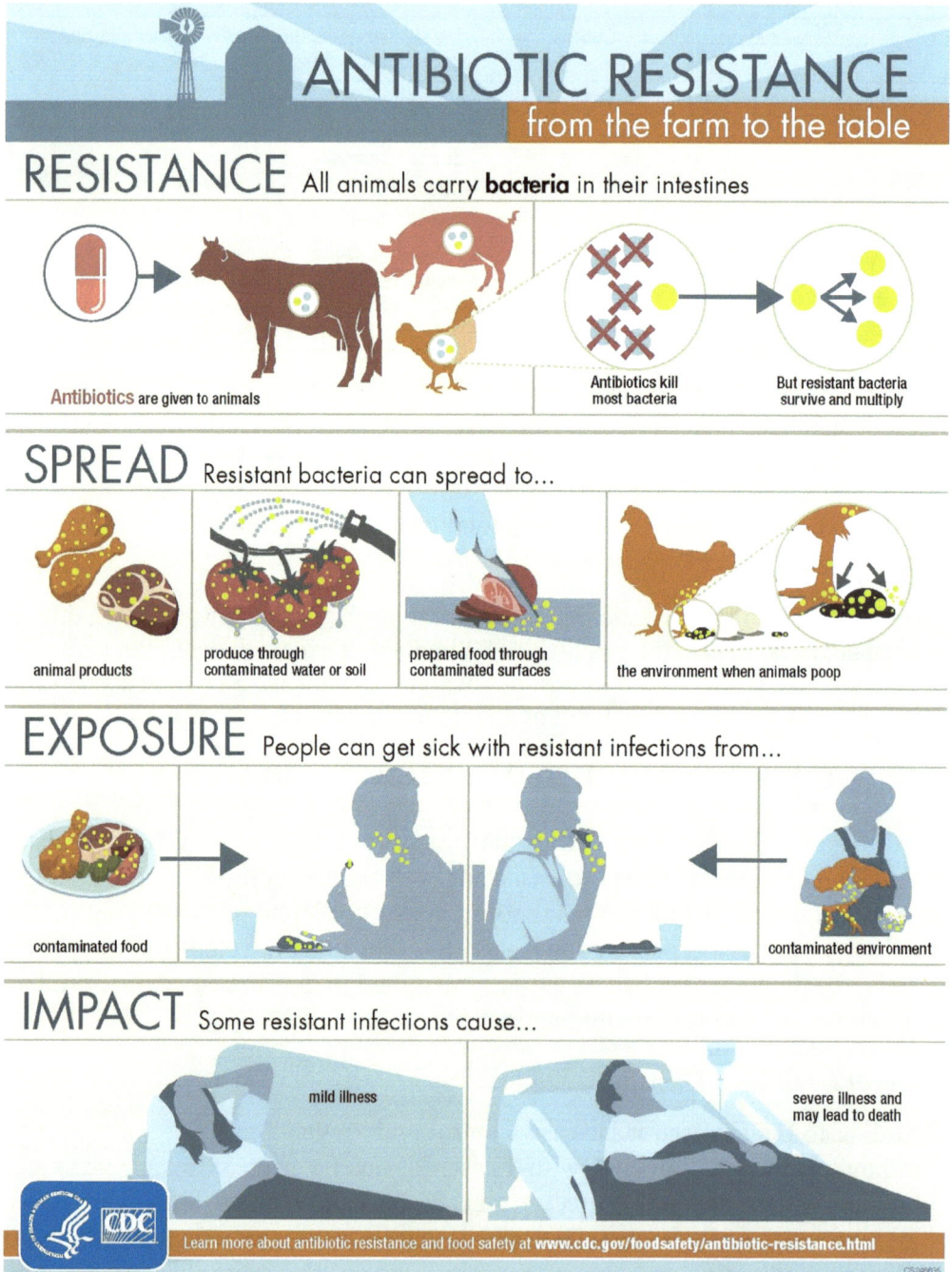

Figure 1: Antibiotic resistance from farm to the table. (Reproduced with permission from the Centers for Disease Control and Prevention [42]).

of the antibiotics are prescribed inappropriately or unnecessarily. In 2009, it was estimated that 10.7 billion dollars were spent on antibiotics in the US [44]. Approximately 60% of antibiotics expenditure occurs in the outpatient setting, where most patients have viral illnesses for which antibiotics are ineffective [44, 45]. Healthcare providers prescribed 262.5 million courses of antibiotics in 2011 (842 prescriptions per 1,000 persons). There was a significant geographic variation with a higher prescribing rate in the South census region (931 prescriptions per 1,000 persons) compared to that in the West (647 prescriptions per 1,000 persons) [46].

Per capita use of all antibiotics is high in South Africa, United Kingdom, and the United States [28]. Use of antibiotics was examined in the National Health and Nutrition Examination Survey (NHANES; 1999-2012). Use of an antibiotic in the past 30 days of the survey was one of the main outcome variables in the NHANES study. The percentage of the US population that used a prescription antibiotic had significantly declined from 6.1% in 1999-2002 to 4.1% in 2011-2012. Declines were identified among all age groups, both sexes, non-Hispanic white and non-Hispanic black persons, persons with and without insurance and among those who currently had asthma [47]. Unfortunately, similar trends are not seen elsewhere in the world. The recent rise in antibiotic consumption is seen in Brazil, Russia, India, China, and South Africa [28]. Between 2000 and 2010, consumption of antibiotic drugs increased by 36% (from ~ 54 billion standard units to ~ 73 billion standard units; antibiotic consumption is measured in standard units which are defined as the equivalent of one pill, capsule or ampoule.). Brazil, Russia, India, China, and South Africa accounted for 76% of this increase [48].

Another problem regarding antibiotic misuse is the public awareness of the role of antibiotics in the treatment of common viral illness and the side effects of the antibiotics. A recent survey by the Pew Health Group found that 36% of people surveyed in the United States mistakenly believed that antibiotics were effective in treating colds and 41% said they had heard only a little, or nothing at all, about antibiotic resistance [49]. This sort of misinformation may be more prevalent in the developing countries which only leads to misuse, overuse, and inappropriate use of antibiotics.

An analysis of a national administrative database (MarketScan Hospital Drug Database) and CDC's Emerging Infections Program data showed that antibiotic prescribing for inpatients is common, and there are ample opportunities to improve antibiotic use by reducing inappropriate antibiotic prescribing [43]. In 2010, 55.7% of patients discharged from 323 hospitals received antibiotics during their hospitalization and review of patients' records from 183 hospitals revealed that antibiotic prescribing potentially could be improved in 37.2% of the most common prescription scenarios reviewed [43]. In addition, the study showed that there was threefold difference in usage rates among 26 medical/surgical wards reporting to the National Healthcare Safety Network. Models estimated that a 30% reduction in use of broad-spectrum antibiotics could result in a 26% reduction in *C. difficile* infections [43].

Lack of in-depth knowledge of antibiotics and limited specialty resources in developing countries are other barriers for appropriate antibiotic prescribing. Physicians, in some countries, receive information about antibiotics primarily from pharmaceutical companies [50, 51]. In some countries, pharmaceutical companies are still allowed to provide incentives for prescribing medications [51]. Limiting contact between the pharmaceutical industry and junior doctors can have a positive effect on subsequent clinical behavior. Restriction of contact with pharmaceutical sales representatives with physicians is still not universally implemented [52]. With ever increasing social and internet media, pharmaceutical companies are able to directly advertise their products to the consumer and the physician [53]. The direct advertisement to consumers leads to more prescription of advertised medications [54]. In addition, the direct advertisements have misleading claims, omission of adverse effects, and overstatement of efficacy. Consumers and the physicians should be aware of these issues and there should be more stringent oversight on direct advertisement [55].

Nonhuman and Nontherapeutic Use of Antibiotics

The use of antibiotics in food animal production in the US and many other countries is now well known [56, 57]. The use of antibiotics for growth promotion in farm animals is accomplished as a feed additive in a low concentration for a prolonged period. This is a major risk factor for the development of antibiotic resistance and contributes to the emergence of antibiotic-resistant bacteria in food-producing animals [57]. There is a growing concern that non-therapeutic use of antibiotics leads to emergence of resistance and spread to people. There is a large body of evidence that show increased antibiotic resistance in bacteria in animals receiving non-therapeutic antibiotics supplements in their food products. This resistance spreads to other animals and humans- directly by contact and indirectly *via* the food chain, water, air, and soils (Fig. **1**). This has led to restriction or complet ban of nontherapeutic use of antibiotics in food animals in various European countries [58].

Although hospital use of antimicrobials has been assumed to be the biggest risk factor for the development of resistance and transmission of resistant infections among hospitalized patients, the greater load of antimicrobial use is actually found in food animal production [56]. Current evidence indicates that the use of antibiotics in food animals is associated with antibiotic resistance among bacteria isolated from humans and outbreaks of infections in humans with antibiotics resistant bacteria [59-64]. Some reports have shown that the growth-promoting antibiotic avoparcin, a member of the same glycopeptides family as that of vancomycin, led to the selection of vancomycin-resistant *Enterococcus faecium* [65-67].

Use of antibiotics in food animal production started as early as in the 1940s [68]. It was claimed, as early as in 1951, that chickens gained more weight in a shorter amount of time, resulting in greater feed efficiency, but also resulted in more resistant bacteria [69]. Over a period, larger size animals were produced in a shorter time with less amount of feed with the use of nontherapeutic antibiotic supplementation in food animal production. For example, in 1925, a chicken of 1.13 kg could be produced in 112 days. However, by 1950, this time was cut to 70 days and by 2014, a chicken weighing greater than 2.7 kg can be produced in 47 days with a less amount of feed [70].

Although the use of antibiotics in food animal production was started in developed countries, now it has spread to developing countries such as China, Brazil, and India. It was calculated that 38.5 million kg of antibiotics was used in 2012 in China's production of swine and poultry [68]. In contrast, the total use of antimicrobials by weight in 2011 for animal production was 13.6 million kg in the USA [71]. Only 3.5 million kg antibiotics were sold for the treatment of human sickness during the same year in the USA. It is estimated that 73% of antibiotics sold in the USA are intended for use in food animal production [72].

Food animals serve as a reservoir of resistant pathogens and those resistant pathogens can directly or indirectly result in antibiotic resistant infections in humans [57]. Use of antibiotics in food-producing animals allows antibiotic-resistant bacteria to thrive while susceptible bacteria are suppressed or die and the resistant bacteria can be transmitted from food-producing animals to humans through the food supply leading to infections with antibiotic-resistant bacteria in humans resulting in serious adverse human health consequences (Fig. **1**) [57].

Sweden has banned all growth-promoting antibiotics for use in food animals in 1986, the European Union banned avoparcin in 1997, and other antibiotics such as bacitracin, spiramycin, tylosin and virginiamycin in 1999 [73]. The ban of growth promoters has reduced nontherapeutic use of antibiotics in farm animals but has led to deterioration in animal health, including increased diarrhea, weight loss and mortality due to infections in early post-weaning pigs, and increase in usage of therapeutic antibiotics in food animals with potential direct impact on humans. It is being argued that the theoretical and political benefit of the widespread ban of growth promoters needs to be more carefully weighed against the increasingly apparent adverse consequences [73].

ANTIBIOTIC DISCOVERY GAP

Another challenge in our fight against the scourge of antibiotic resistance is the lack of discovery of a new class of antibiotics in recent decades. The last major class of antibiotic that was discovered was daptomycin in 1987. There are no new classes of antibiotics discovered in the past two decades. Increasing resistance to the existing antibiotics and decreased discovery of new antibiotics can potentially lead us back to the pre-antibiotic era with increased mortality and morbidity from infections. The time line for the antibiotic discovery is presented in Table **3**.

Table 3. Timeline of antibiotic class discovery (Adapted from ref. [74]).

Year	Antibiotics Discovered
1928	Penicillin
1932	Sulfonamides
1943	Streptomycin
1945	Bacitracin
1946	Nitrofurans
1947	Chloramphenicol Polymyxin
1948	Chlortetracycline Cephalosporin
1950	Pleuromutilin
1952	Erythromycin Isoniazide
1953	Vancomycin Streptogramin
1955	Cycloserine

Table 3: contd…

1956	Novobiocin
1957	Rifamycin
1959	Metronidazole
1961	Nalidixic acid Trimethoprim Lincomycin Fusidic acid
1969	Fosfomycin
1971	Mupirocin
1976	Carbapenem
1978	Oxazolidinone (linezolid was discovered in the 1990s)
1981	Monobactam
1987	Daptomycin (cyclic lipopeptide class)
1987 to now	Discovery void for a new class of antibiotics

COMBATING ANTIBIOTIC RESISTANCE

Combating antibiotic resistance is a local, national, and worldwide priority. Countries that have implemented comprehensive national strategies have been the most successful in controlling antibiotic resistance.

Antibiotic Conservation

Antibiotic overuse is the main cause for the global increase in antibiotic resistance. Reducing the need for antibiotics and reducing inappropriate use of antibiotics will prolong the effectiveness of existing antibiotics [75]. Improving antibiotic prescribing practices, facilitating the early and prompt laboratory detection of antibiotic susceptibility pattern of microbes that caused infection can lead to the reduction of unnecessary prescriptions of antibiotics and early use of appropriate antibiotics where they are indicated. In developing countries, one of the reasons for excessive use of antibiotics is the presence of a high burden of bacterial illnesses. Reducing the burden of infection can decrease the need for antibiotics [75]. Reducing the burden of infection may be achieved by: (a) improving public health and sanitation, especially in low-income countries where antibiotics are used to fill the gap created by unsafe water, poor sanitation, and deficient public health; (b) expanding the use of existing vaccines and investing in new vaccines; and (c) improving hospital infection control [75].

Improving Antibiotic Prescription in Communities

Worldwide, most antimicrobial use occurs outside of hospitals [76]. Interventions to preserve the effectiveness of antimicrobials have focused on hospitals or providers, thereby missing non-prescription antimicrobial use [77]. Non-prescription human antibiotic use is common outside of North America and northern Europe and accounted for 19-100% of antibiotic usage in those areas [78]. The rates of non-prescription antimicrobial use is higher in developing nations, but not exclusive to low or middle-income countries. The estimated rates of non-prescription antimicrobial use in parts of southern and eastern Europe, for instance, are between 20% and 30% of total consumption [78, 79]. Antibiotic resistant bacteria are common in communities with frequent non-prescription use.

Use of non-prescription medications may be due to many factors, including demand side issues such as lack of availability of doctors, lack of rapid diagnostic tests, ignorance about antibiotic use, inappropriate use, large disease burden, but the issues can be on the supply side, such as easy availability of antibiotics over the counter and availability of antibiotics on the internet without any local restrictions [78, 79].

Large amounts of antibiotics are wasted on patients who do not need them, and on non-human use, and at the same time, essential antibiotics are not available in some communities for serious bacterial infections [80]. Inappropriate use of antibiotics is common in practice. In the US, over 27 million courses antibiotics out of 101 million prescriptions are wasted just in the treatment of respiratory illnesses alone [81]. Rapid diagnostic tools allow doctors to identify an infection in minutes instead of hours or days, have the potential to transform the diagnosis and treatment process from an empirical one into a precise one [80]. Lack of rapid diagnostic tests lead to world-wise overuse of antibiotics and the right drug at the right time is not always used due to the lack of rapid diagnostic tools [80]. Rapid diagnostic tools will tell us if the infection is caused by a bacteria or a virus, the type of bacteria causing the infection if the bacteria is resistant to any one or more antibiotics, and antibiotic susceptibility of the bacteria [80]. They ultimately lead to reduced costs to the patients, hospitals and healthcare system [80]. In addition, the decreased use and appropriate and timely use of antibiotics will lead to reduced risk of emergence of antibiotic resistance and reduced selection pressure for resistant organisms.

Severe pneumonia is the largest cause of death in children in the world. Integrated Management of Childhood Illness (IMCI) strategy has been introduced around the world in more than 75 countries since 1992. IMCI is an integrated approach to child health that focuses on the well-being of the whole child. IMCI approaches the management of childhood illnesses in an action-oriented classification and uses a case management system to treat a broader burden of diseases rather than using a single disease approach. IMCI does not recommend antibiotic treatment for non-severe pneumonia defined as tachypnea without retractions [82].

Stricter regulations of dispensing the antibiotics which allow sale of over the counter first generation antibiotics, but impose stricter regulations for newer-generation antibiotics along with healthcare worker and public education are potential solutions to improve conservation of antibiotics [75].

Sale of prescription medications on the internet started in the 1990s and is ever increasing. There are several problems with the online sale of antibiotics. Prescription medications may be available without prescription even in countries with some regulations, the antibiotics may be of poor quality, and there will be delays in getting these medications for urgent treatments [78, 79]. This is a global problem. Tackling the issue of online pharmacies require coordinated regulatory activities across national and organizational boundaries with the participation of governmental and non-governmental agencies [79, 83].

Antimicrobial Stewardship Program

There is an increase, mostly inappropriate, in the use of antibiotics in humans. Antibiotic overuse is the main root cause of development of antibiotic resistance. Resistance to nearly all classes of antimicrobial is increasing. In addition, there has been a decline in the development of new antimicrobials in recent years. These trends have led health care facilities to adopt antimicrobial stewardship programs (ASPs) and infection control programs (ICPs) to optimize antimicrobial therapy, reduce treatment-related costs, improve clinical outcomes and safety, and reduce or stabilize antimicrobial resistance [65, 84]. The Infectious Diseases Society of America (IDSA) and the Society of Healthcare Epidemiology of America (SHEA) published the guidelines for ASPs in 2007 [77]. ASPs are executed by multidisciplinary teams comprising physicians, pharmacists, microbiologists, infectious disease specialists, and epidemiologists, with adequate experience in their respective fields. Although there is no single template suitable for instituting an ASP in all hospitals, antibiotic stewardship programs can be implemented effectively in a wide variety of hospitals using the published guidelines; the success of ASPs is dependent the leadership role and the coordinated multidisciplinary approach [85]. The CDC has published recommendations regarding the core elements of an ASP and the checklists for those core elements [85]. The recommended core elements of a successful ASP are listed in Table **4**.

Table 4. Core elements of antibiotic stewardship programs [85].

Core Element	Description
Leadership Commitment	Leadership support is critical to the success of antibiotic stewardship programs. Dedicating necessary human, financial and information technology resources.
Accountability	Appointing a single leader responsible for program outcomes. Experience with successful programs show that a physician leader is effective.
Drug Expertise	Appointing a single pharmacist leader responsible for working to improve antibiotic use. Works as a co-leader.
Action	Implementing at least one recommended action. Examples of some actions are: antibiotic "time outs", prior authorization, dose optimization programs, drug substitution, clinical pathways, *etc.*
Tracking	Monitoring antibiotic prescribing and resistance patterns. Data collection is a key to making meaningful changes. Monitoring may include processes as well as outcomes.
Reporting	Regular reporting information on antibiotic use and resistance to doctors, nurses and relevant staff.
Education	Educating clinical staff about resistance and optimal prescribing.

A randomized controlled study which implemented a multidisciplinary antimicrobial utilization team in an urban teaching hospital showed improved antibiotic utilization when prescribers received input from the antimicrobial utilization team [86]. Implementation of the ASP in a community hospital was also associated with significant reductions in C. difficile infection (CDI) rate, antimicrobial use, and pharmacy costs [87]. Although ASPs have shown to improve antibiotic prescription practices and reduced CDI rates, they are constituted entirely in hospital scenes and are not widely implemented beyond high-income nations. There is an urgency to apply the concepts of antibiotic stewardship at a local level in hospitals and communities across all countries.

Prevention and Reduction of Communicable Diseases

The burden of infectious diseases is significantly high, especially among low and middle-income countries. This leads to increased use of antibiotics. There are several reasons for the high disease burden from infections. Poor sanitation, poor infection control practices, and poor vaccination coverage are among the main reasons for high disease burden in the developing world.

Vaccination

The burden of pneumococcal disease has decreased with the introduction of the pneumococcal conjugate vaccine, which has resulted in decreased use of antibiotics [75, 88]. Pneumococcal vaccination also lowered rates of invasive pneumococcal disease caused by penicillin-resistant strains [88]. In the United States, multiple drug resistant pneumococcal strains decreased by 59% between 1999 and 2004 from 4.1 to 1.7 cases per 100,000 [88]. However, the global coverage of pneumococcal vaccination was estimated only at 31%. It was introduced in 117 countries by the end of 2014, but it is not yet a part of the routine immunization programs in large countries like India and China [89-92]. In addition, pneumococcal vaccination rates vary across the regions with coverage levels of 83% in the Americas, 50% in the African Region, but only at 2% in the Western Pacific Region [93]. An estimated 18.7 million infants worldwide are still missing out on basic vaccines [89].

Increasing vaccination coverage in each region will prevent many communicable diseases and the need for and use of antibiotics. It will consequently reduce the selection pressure for the emergence of antibiotic resistance. Inadequate vaccination coverage is a global problem, but has many local and regional factors play in various areas of the world. Local and regional barriers to vaccination should be reviewed and strategies should be developed to overcome those barriers.

Early Detection of Infections

Developing rapid diagnostic tests that are easily accessible and affordable will help not only in early treatment of bacterial infections but also prevent excess and unnecessary use of antibiotics for illnesses that do not require antibiotics. Advances in genetics, genomics, and computing technology will help improve our way of diagnosing infections and resistance [94].

Improving Sanitation

Prevention of infection reduces disease burden, antibiotic load, and development of antibiotic resistance and its spread. Unsafe water and poor sanitation help to spread resistant organisms. According to the latest estimates of the WHO/UNICEF Joint Monitoring Program for Water Supply and Sanitation, 32 per cent of the world's population (2.4 billion people) lacked improved sanitation facilities, and 663 million people still used unimproved drinking water sources in 2015 [95]. UNICEF works in more than 100 countries around the world to improve water supplies and sanitation facilities in schools and communities and to promote safe hygiene practices. UNICEF works with many partners, including families, communities, governments and like-minded organizations. At the community level, improvement of sanitation, access to clean water, poverty reduction, and vaccination will have a huge effect on infectious disease incidence as well as transfer of and colonization with resistant genes and multidrug-resistant organisms [7]. Significant progress was made during the last decade with respect to water and sanitation in developing countries. The number of children dying from diarrheal diseases, which are strongly associated with poor water, inadequate sanitation and hygiene, have steadily fallen over the two last decades from approximately 1.5million deaths in 1990 to 600,000 in 2012. UNICEF's Millennium Development Goal to cut unsafe water and poor sanitation by half by 2015 was achieved with respect to drinking water but fell short with respect to sanitation [95].

Several local innovative programs, such as community-led total sanitation, are working to improve water and sanitation by creating sustained behavior change in many rural areas [96]. The Sarvajal project is a high-tech solution to supply clean water using "water-ATMs" [97]. Using a cloud-based technology along with reverse osmosis ultrafiltration units provide on demand clean water. They use local entrepreneurs in collaboration with government agencies, philanthropies and private organizations [97].

Improvements in toilet design, pit emptying, and sludge treatment as well as new ways to reuse waste, can help to meet the enormous challenge of providing quality sanitation [98]. The Bill and Mellinda Gates Foundation's Water, Sanitation and Hygiene program focuses on developing innovative approaches and technologies that can lead to sustainable improvements in sanitation in the developing world, such as South Asia and Sub-Saharan Africa [98].

Improving Infection Control Practices

Healthcare-associated infections (HCAI) are a major patient safety concern. They affect hundreds of millions of people across the world every year. They lead to avoidable patient deaths and disability. They also waste scarce health care resources. No country can claim to have solved the problem completely, although it is a greater challenge in low and middle-income countries. The risk of health care-associated infections in developing countries is 2 to 20 times that of in developed countries [27]. Good hand hygiene is a very simple practice that can greatly reduce health care-associated infections and associated risks. The World Alliance for Patient Safety has selected health care-associated infection as the topic for its first Global Patient Safety Challenge [27]. The Global Patient Safety Challenge for 2005-2006 brought together the WHO Guidelines on Hand Hygiene in Health Care [99] along with ongoing actions on blood safety, injection and immunization safety, safer clinical practices, and safe water, sanitation and waste management [27].

Although HCAI cannot be entirely eliminated, several low-cost, simple and effective strategies have proven to be effective in reducing the burden of this world scourge. Unfortunately, while many hospitals have succeeded in reducing HCAI, many have failed. There is a gap between the availability of effective patient safety measures and their implementation. The Global Patient Safety Challenge with the theme "Clean Care is Safer Care" is working worldwide to assist countries to reduce the burden of HCAI infection [27]. Its objectives are to increase awareness of patient safety issues, get commitment from member countries and to test implementation of Hand Hygiene in Health Care WHO guidelines [27].

Improvement of hand hygiene practice requires national commitment, institutional priority and education of the public and the healthcare workers. Leadership commitment is important at institutional and as well as a national level to improve outcomes. Inadequate access to soap and water and sinks are obstacles to performing hand hygiene during healthcare delivery in developing countries. The use of alcohol-based hand rubs is a practical solution to overcome these obstacles. Alcohol rubs can be distributed individually to staff or placed at the point of care [22]. Alcohol rub is known to reduce HCAI and is highly cost-effective [100, 101]. WHO has recommended two alcohol-based (ethanol or isopropyl alcohol) hand rub solutions that can be prepared locally [99, 102]. An Interventional study consisting of hand hygiene education, reminders, and group sessions in a Kuwaiti teaching hospital showed a reduction in HCAI and improved compliance with hand hygiene practices [103].

Use of gloves, gowns, and aprons may also be considered for prevention of HCAI although they do not replace meticulous hand hygiene practices [65]. One needs to be careful that the gloves or gowns of healthcare workers can be colonized with pathogens, and their use may give a false sense of good hygiene. Environmental cleaning in hospitals is also important and is associated with a reduction in the transmission of healthcare-associated pathogens [65]. The CDC and Hospital Infection Control Practices Advisory Committee presented guidelines for environmental infection control and sterilization in healthcare facilities [104], and these can be adapted to meet local requirements and feasibility.

Restriction of Nontherapeutic Antibiotic Use

Domestic animals raised for food consumption excrete an enormous quantity of antibiotic resistant bacteria as a consequence of non-therapeutic antibiotic use. A ban on non-therapeutic antibiotic use will not only help to reduce antibiotic resistance, but also help in better preservation of future antimicrobials [58]. The FDA supports the concept that the use of medically important antibiotics for non-therapeutic use in food animal production does not protect and promote public health. A non-binding guidance was released in 2010 that recommended measures to reduce the use of these antibiotics for animal food production to reduce antibiotic selection pressure [105]. Non-therapeutic or sub-therapeutic use was banned in several European countries. The ban of growth promoters has, however, revealed that these agents had important prophylactic activity, and their withdrawal was associated with a deterioration in animal health, including increased diarrhea, weight loss and mortality due to *Escherichia coli* and *Lawsonia intracellularis* in early post-weaning pigs, and clostridial necrotic enteritis in broilers [73]. However, the Danish experience demonstrated that any negative disease effects resulting from the ban on non-therapeutic antibiotic use were short-lived and that altering animal husbandry practices could counter the expected increases in disease frequency [106].

The *FAAIR Report* (*Facts about Antibiotics in Animals and the Impact on Resistance*) of the Alliance for the Prudent Use of Antibiotics (APUA) in 2002 recommended that: (1) antibiotics should not be used in agriculture in the absence of disease; (2) antibiotics should be administered to animals only when prescribed by a veterinarian; (3) quantitative data on antimicrobial use in agriculture should be made available to inform public policy; (4) the ecology of antimicrobial resistance should be considered by regulatory agencies in assessing human health risk associated with antimicrobial use in agriculture; (5) surveillance programs for antimicrobial resistance should be improved and expanded; and (6) the ecology of antimicrobial resistance in agriculture should be a research priority [107]. These recommendations are still valid for current efforts to limit nontherapeutic antibiotic use in food production.

Antibiotic Innovation

Even if antibiotics are used appropriately and we take all the precautions against overuse and improper use of antibiotics in humans and animals, bacteria will still develop resistance, albeit at a slower pace. This will necessitate the development of new antibiotics.

The main reason for a mismatch between the demand for new antibiotics and research and development of new classes of antibiotics is that the commercial return for any given new antibiotic is uncertain until resistance has emerged against a previous generation of drugs [108]. In other medical fields, a new drug usually is an improvement on the previous ones and once it is introduced to the market, it will quickly become the standard first choice for patients. That is often not true for a new antibiotic. A new antibiotic is most probably no more effective than an existing and cheap generic product in the market, except for patients with infections that are resistant to previous generations of drugs. By the time that new antibiotic becomes the standard first line of care, it might be near or beyond the end of its patent life. This means that the company which developed it will struggle to generate sufficient revenues to recoup its development costs [108]. It takes a long time (over 10 years) from the start of a preclinical trial to the approval of a new antibiotic, and also it is expensive (requires over 100 million US dollars just to reach the approval stage) to bring a new antibiotic to the market, and has a low (3.3%) success rate of bringing to the market [108].

Companies which develop new drugs are incentivized to sell more medications for profitability. This will lead to overuse and misuse [108]. Stricter regulations and market interventions such as increasing drug price are the two solutions to decrease unnecessary overuse. While these solutions may be effective, they may lead to other problems. A purely regulatory approach to conserving antibiotics could resist access to life-saving antibiotics, which is already a major problem for many of the poorest people in the world. For example, strict regulation of morphine led to poor access to cheap, affordable pain medication for palliative care [109]. At the same time an approach based solely on increasing the price of antibiotics to stimulate investment and reduce over-use would also not be sufficient. A balanced approach is suggested by the review from the United Kingdom that was established for the analysis of the global problems of antimicrobial resistance [108]. The Review recommended improved funding for early stages of antibiotic discovery, providing public platforms for clinical trials, and lastly, supporting a viable market for high priority antibiotics [108].

In the current model, the profitability is based on the volume of sales. It is essential that the profitability of antibiotic sales should be de-linked from the volume of sales. A suggested new model proposes a global buyer who purchases new antibiotics from the developer; after that, according to the societal value, the global buyer then supplies them to various nation states based on their need and demand. In this model, the companies forfeit the right to market, but will have guaranteed profits [108]. However, implementation of such model will be complex and requires buy-in from many countries. Another approach suggested is a hybrid of the two models, offering price by volume model and the global payer approach, where a global buyer pays out some monies to the company, and the company still retains some control over the market [108].

Funding for early stages of antibiotic discovery is lagging behind. Already many countries are working on increasing the research funding for antibiotic innovation and discovery. There is a need for a global dedicated funding for antimicrobial research [108]. This funding mechanism can address the gaps in the antibiotic discovery and innovation.

Harmonizing and simplifying antibiotic approval process can globally incentivize companies to search for new antibiotics. Currently, most governments require registrations in each of its jurisdiction for any new drug to be marketed. It is costly, cumbersome, and requires knowledge and manpower to access global market. Harmonizing the best standards of global regulatory processes will simplify global access for the companies to market. The World Health Organization could coordinate the approval of new antibiotics [108].

CAUSE FOR OPTIMISM

The problem of antibiotic resistance can be solved with the collective efforts of public and private sectors, and local and national governments.and governmental and non-governmental agencies. The reviewers of antimicrobial resistance have already noted some cause for optimism [94]. Researchers and biotech entrepreneurs are teaming up to solve this problem with new drug development, vaccine development, and development of alternate therapies. The WHO is taking the lead to develop a framework agreement between 194 countries to tackle the problem of antibiotic resistance. Advances in genetics, genomics, and computer sciences will lead to the development of techniques for early detection of infection and resistance. Tackling antibiotic resistance aligns with growth objectives of low and middle-income countries. Improvement of sanitation and basic healthcare infrastructure is essential for tackling antibiotic resistance as well as the growth of these nations. Several countries are making this as a priority. For example, the US President has issued an Executive Order to tackle the menace of antibiotic resistance [110].

The Infectious Disease Society of America (ISDA) had launched a program called the 10x20 initiative to encourage the government to approve 10 new antibiotics by 2020 [111]. The initiative seeks a global commitment to create an antibiotic R&D enterprise powerful enough to produce 10 new systemic antibiotics by the year 2020. In 2013, the U.S. Food and Drug Administration granted fast-track status for ceftolozane/tazobactam (CXA-201) antibiotic treatment for complicated intra-abdominal infections, hospital-acquired bacterial pneumonia, ventilator-associated bacterial pneumonia, and complicated urinary tract infections.

CONFLICT OF INTEREST

The authors confirm that they have no conflict of interest to declare for this publication.

ACKNOWLEDGEMENTS

Declared none.

REFERENCES

[1]   Cavalli-Sforza LL, Lederberg J. Isolation of pre-adaptive mutants in bacteria by sib selection. Genetics 1956; 41(3): 367.

[2]   Teillant A, Gandra S, Barter D, Morgan DJ, Laxminarayan R. Potential burden of antibiotic resistance on surgery and cancer chemotherapy antibiotic prophylaxis in the USA: a literature review and modelling study. Lancet Infect Dis 2015.

[3]   The Center for Disease Dynamics Economics and Policy. Antibiotic Resistance. [cited 2015 October 30]; Available from: http://cddep.org/research-area/antibiotic-resistance.

[4]   Huttner A, Harbarth S, Carlet J, *et al.,* Antimicrobial resistance: a global view from the 2013 World Healthcare-Associated Infections Forum. Antimicrob Resist Infect Control 2013; 2(1): 31.

[5]   Fleming A. Penicillin. Nobel Lecture, December 11, 1945. 1945 [cited 2015 November 1]; Available from: http://www.nobelprize.org/nobel_prizes/medicine/laureates/1945/fleming-lecture.pdf.

[6]   Gould SJ. Planet of the bacteria. 1996 [cited 2015 November 1]; Available from: http://www.stephenjaygould.org/library/gould_bacteria.html.

[7]   Laxminarayan R, Duse A, Wattal C, *et al.* Antibiotic resistance-the need for global solutions. Lancet Infect Dis. 2013 Dec;13(12):1057-98.

[8]   Aarestrup FM, Wegener HC, Collignon P. Resistance in bacteria of the food chain: epidemiology and control strategies. Expert Rev Anti Infect Ther 2008 Oct; 6(5): 733-50.

[9]   Gaynes R, Edwards JR. Overview of nosocomial infections caused by gram-negative bacilli. Clin Infect Dis 2005 Sep 15; 41(6): 848-54.

[10]   Tzouvelekis LS, Markogiannakis A, Psichogiou M, Tassios PT, Daikos GL. Carbapenemases in *Klebsiella pneumoniae* and other *Enterobacteriaceae*: an evolving crisis of global dimensions. Clin Microbiol Rev 2012; 25(4): 682-707.

[11]   Glasner C, Albiger B, Buist G, *et al.* Carbapenemase-producing *Enterobacteriaceae* in Europe: a survey among national experts from 39 countries, February 2013. Euro Surveill 2013; 18(28).

[12]   Nordmann P, Cuzon G, Naas T. The real threat of *klebsiella pneumoniae* carbapenemase-producing bacteria. Lancet Infect Dis 2009; 9(4): 228-36.

[13]   Nordmann P, Naas T, Poirel L. Global spread of carbapenemase-producing *Enterobacteriaceae*. Emerg Infect Dis 2011; 17(10): 1791-8.

[14]   Bratu S, Tolaney P, Karumudi U, *et al.* Carbapenemase-producing *Klebsiella pneumoniae* in brooklyn, NY: molecular epidemiology and in vitro activity of polymyxin B and other agents. J Antimicrob Chemother 2005; 56(1): 128-32.

[15]   World Health Organization. Antimicrobial resistance Global Report on Surveillance 2014 [cited 2015 October 31]; Available from: http://apps.who.int/iris/bitstream/10665/112642/1/9789241-564748_eng.pdf.

[16]   Guh AY, Bulens SN, Mu Y, *et al.* Epidemiology of carbapenem-resistant *Enterobacteriaceae* in 7 US communities, 2012-2013. JAMA 2015 ;314(14): 1479-87.

[17]   National Nosocomial Infections Surveillance (NNIS) System Report, data summary from January 1992 through June 2004, issued October 2004. Am J Infect Control. 2004; 32(8): 470-85.

[18]   Centers for Disease Control and Prevention. Nearly half a million Americans suffered from *Clostridium difficile* infections in a single year. 2015 [cited 2015 October 31]; Available from: http://www.cdc.gov/media/releases/2015/p0225-clostridium-difficile.html.

[19]   Hawser SP, Bouchillon SK, Lascols C, *et al.* Susceptibility of european *Escherichia coli* clinical isolates from intra-abdominal infections, extended-spectrum beta-lactamase occurrence, resistance distribution, and molecular characterization of ertapenem-resistant isolates (SMART 2008-2009). Clin Microbiol Infect 2012; 18(3): 253-9.

[20]   Kumarasamy KK, Toleman MA, Walsh TR, *et al.* Emergence of a new antibiotic resistance mechanism in India, Pakistan, and the UK: a molecular, biological, and epidemiological study. Lancet Infect Dis 2010; 10(9): 597-602.

[21]   Walsh TR, Weeks J, Livermore DM, Toleman MA. Dissemination of NDM-1 positive bacteria in the New Delhi environment and its implications for human health: an environmental point prevalence study. Lancet Infect Dis 2011; 11(5): 355-62.

[22]   Pittet D, Allegranzi B, Storr J, *et al.* Infection control as a major World Health Organization priority for developing countries. J Hosp Infect 2008; 68(4): 285-92.

[23]   Allegranzi B, Bagheri Nejad S, Combescure C, *et al.* Burden of endemic health-care-associated infection in developing countries: systematic review and meta-analysis. Lancet 2011; 377(9761): 228-41.

[24]   Rosenthal VD. Health-care-associated infections in developing countries. Lancet 2011; 377(9761):186-8.

[25]   Rosenthal VD, Maki DG, Mehta Y, *et al.* International Nosocomial Infection Control Consortium (INICC) report, data summary of 43 countries for 2007-2012. Device-associated module. Am J Infect Control 2014; 42(9): 942-56.

[26]   Rosenthal VD, Maki DG, Jamulitrat S, *et al.* International Nosocomial Infection Control Consortium (INICC) report, data summary for 2003-2008, issued June 2009. Am J Infect Control 2010; 38(2): 95-104 e2.

[27]   World Health Organization. The global patient safety challenge 2005–2006 "Clean Care is Safer Care". Geneva: World Health Organization; 2005 [cited 2015 November 5]; Available from: http://www.who.int/patientsafety/events/05/GPSC_Launch_ENGLISH_FINAL.pdf.

[28]   The Center for Disease Dynamics Economics and Policy. Resistance Map. [cited 2015 November 5]; Available from: http://resistancemap.cddep.org/resmap/resistance.

[29]   Lob SH, Badal RE, Bouchillon SK, Hawser SP, Hackel MA, Hoban DJ. Epidemiology and susceptibility of gram-negative appendicitis pathogens: SMART 2008-2010. Surg Infect (Larchmt) 2013; 14(2): 203-8.

[30]   Rossi F, Baquero F, Hsueh PR, *et al.* In vitro susceptibilities of aerobic and facultatively anaerobic Gram-negative bacilli isolated from patients with intra-abdominal infections worldwide: 2004 results from SMART (Study for Monitoring Antimicrobial Resistance Trends). J Antimicrob Chemother 2006; 58(1): 205-10.

[31]   Chen YH, Hsueh PR, Badal RE, *et al*. Antimicrobial susceptibility profiles of aerobic and facultative gram-negative bacilli isolated from patients with intra-abdominal infections in the Asia-Pacific region according to currently established susceptibility interpretive criteria. J Infect 2011; 62(4): 280-91.

[32]   Hawser SP, Bouchillon SK, Hoban DJ, Badal RE, Hsueh PR, Paterson DL. Emergence of high levels of extended-spectrum-beta-lactamase-producing gram-negative bacilli in the Asia-Pacific region: data from the Study for Monitoring Antimicrobial Resistance Trends (SMART) program, 2007. Antimicrob Agents Chemother 2009; 53(8): 3280-4.

[33]   Hsueh PR, Badal RE, Hawser SP, *et al*. Epidemiology and antimicrobial susceptibility profiles of aerobic and facultative gram-negative bacilli isolated from patients with intra-abdominal infections in the Asia-Pacific region: 2008 results from SMART (Study for Monitoring Antimicrobial Resistance Trends). Int J Antimicrob Agents 2010; 36(5): 408-14.

[34]   Ko WC, Hsueh PR. Increasing extended-spectrum beta-lactamase production and quinolone resistance among gram-negative bacilli causing intra-abdominal infections in the Asia/Pacific region: data from the Smart Study 2002-2006. J Infect 2009; 59(2): 95-103.

[35]   Huang CC, Chen YS, Toh HS, *et al*. Impact of revised CLSI breakpoints for susceptibility to third-generation cephalosporins and carbapenems among *Enterobacteriaceae* isolates in the Asia-Pacific region: results from the Study for Monitoring Antimicrobial Resistance Trends (SMART), 2002-2010. Int J Antimicrob Agents 2012 Jun; 40 Suppl: S4-10.

[36]   Hsueh PR. Study for Monitoring Antimicrobial Resistance Trends (SMART) in the Asia-Pacific region, 2002-2010. Int J Antimicrob Agents 2012; 40 Suppl: S1-3.

[37]   Hsueh PR, Snyder TA, Dinubile MJ, Satischandran V, McCarroll K, Chow JW. *In vitro* susceptibilities of aerobic and facultative gram-negative bacilli isolated from patients with intra-abdominal infections in the Asia-Pacific region: 2004 results from SMART (Study for Monitoring Antimicrobial Resistance Trends). Int J Antimicrob Agents 2006; 28(3): 238-43.

[38]   Yang Q, Wang H, Chen M, *et al*. Surveillance of antimicrobial susceptibility of aerobic and facultative Gram-negative bacilli isolated from patients with intra-abdominal infections in China: the 2002-2009 Study for Monitoring Antimicrobial Resistance Trends (SMART). Int J Antimicrob Agents 2010; 36(6): 507-12.

[39]   Brink AJ, Botha RF, Poswa X, *et al*. Antimicrobial susceptibility of gram-negative pathogens isolated from patients with complicated intra-abdominal infections in South African hospitals (SMART Study 2004-2009): impact of the new carbapenem breakpoints. Surg Infect (Larchmt). 2012; 13(1): 43-9.

[40]   Roberts RR, Hota B, Ahmad I, *et al*. Hospital and societal costs of antimicrobial-resistant infections in a Chicago teaching hospital: implications for antibiotic stewardship. Clin Infect Dis 2009; 49(8): 1175-84.

[41]   Alliance for the Prudent Use of Antibiotics. The cost of antibiotic resistance to U.S. families and the health care system. 2010 [cited 2015 October 31]; Available from: http://www.tufts.edu/med/apua/consumers/personal_home_5_1451036133.pdf.

[42]   Centers for Disease Control and Prevention. Antibiotic resistance from farm to the table- Antibiotic resistance infographic 508c. [cited 2015 12/28/2015]; Available from: http://www.cdc.gov/foodsafety/pdfs/ar-infographic-508c.pdf.

[43]   Fridkin S, Baggs J, Fagan R, *et al*. Vital signs: improving antibiotic use among hospitalized patients. MMWR Morb Mortal Wkly Rep. 2014; 63(9): 194-200.

[44]   Suda KJ, Hicks LA, Roberts RM, Hunkler RJ, Danziger LH. A national evaluation of antibiotic expenditures by healthcare setting in the United States, 2009. J Antimicrob Chemother 2013; 68(3): 715-8.

[45]   The Pew Charitable Trusts. Antibiotic use in human health care. 2015 [cited 2015 October 30]; Available from: http://www.pewtrusts.org/~/media/assets/2015/02/antibioticoveruseinfographic_2-pgs.pdf?la=en.

[46]   Hicks LA, Bartoces MG, Roberts RM, *et al*. US outpatient antibiotic prescribing variation according to geography, patient population, and provider specialty in 2011. Clin Infect Dis. 2015 May 1;60(9):1308-16.

[47]   Frenk SM, Kit BK, Lukacs SL, Hicks LA, Gu Q. Trends in the use of prescription antibiotics: NHANES 1999-2012. J Antimicrob Chemother 2015.

[48]   Van Boeckel TP, Gandra S, Ashok A, *et al*. Global antibiotic consumption 2000 to 2010: an analysis of national pharmaceutical sales data. Lancet Infect Dis. 2014 Aug; 14 (8):742-50.

[49] The Pew Health Group. Americans' knowledge of and attitudes toward antibiotic resistance. 2012 [cited 2015 October 30]; Available from: http://www.pewtrusts.org/~/media/legacy/uploadedfiles/phg/content_level_pages/in_the_news/abxpollsummarypdf.pdf.

[50] Thriemer K, Katuala Y, Batoko B, *et al.* Antibiotic prescribing in DR Congo: a knowledge, attitude and practice survey among medical doctors and students. PLoS One 2013; 8(2): e55495.

[51] Kamal S, Holmberg C, Russell J, *et al.* Perceptions and attitudes of egyptian health professionals and policy-makers towards pharmaceutical sales representatives and other promotional activities. PLoS One 2015; 10(10): e0140457.

[52] Pokorny AM, Gittins CB. Dangerous liaisons: doctors-in-training and the pharmaceutical industry. Intern Med J 2015; 45(10): 1085-8.

[53] Tyrawski J, DeAndrea DC. Pharmaceutical companies and their drugs on social media: a content analysis of drug information on popular social media sites. J Med Internet Res 2015; 17(6): e130.

[54] Mintzes B, Barer ML, Kravitz RL, *et al.* How does direct-to-consumer advertising (DTCA) affect prescribing? A survey in primary care environments with and without legal DTCA. CMAJ 2003 Sep; 169(5): 405-12.

[55] Kannan S, Gowri S, Tyagi V, *et al.* Direct-to-physician and direct-to-consumer advertising: Time to have stringent regulations. Int J Risk Saf Med 2015; 27(2): 77-83.

[56] Silbergeld EK, Davis M, Leibler JH, Peterson AE. One reservoir: redefining the community origins of antimicrobial-resistant infections. Med Clin North Am 2008; 92(6): 1391-407, xi.

[57] Centers for disease control and prevention NARMSfEBN. Antibiotic use in food-producing animals. Tracking and reducing the public health impact. [cited 2015 October 31]; Available from: http://www.cdc.gov/narms/animals.html.

[58] Marshall BM, Levy SB. Food animals and antimicrobials: impacts on human health. Clin Microbiol Rev 2011; 24(4): 718-33.

[59] Angulo FJ, Nargund VN, Chiller TC. Evidence of an association between use of anti-microbial agents in food animals and anti-microbial resistance among bacteria isolated from humans and the human health consequences of such resistance. J Vet Med B Infect Dis Vet Public Health 2004; 51(8-9): 374-9.

[60] Glynn MK, Bopp C, Dewitt W, Dabney P, Mokhtar M, Angulo FJ. Emergence of multidrug-resistant Salmonella enterica serotype typhimurium DT104 infections in the United States. N Engl J Med 1998; 338(19): 1333-8.

[61] Nelson JM, Smith KE, Vugia DJ, *et al.* Prolonged diarrhea due to ciprofloxacin-resistant campylobacter infection. J Infect Dis 2004; 190(6): 1150-7.

[62] Sjolund-Karlsson M, Howie RL, Blickenstaff K, *et al.* Occurrence of beta-lactamase genes among non-Typhi Salmonella enterica isolated from humans, food animals, and retail meats in the United States and Canada. Microb Drug Resist 2013; 19(3) :191-7.

[63] Varma JK, Greene KD, Ovitt J, Barrett TJ, Medalla F, Angulo FJ. Hospitalization and antimicrobial resistance in salmonella outbreaks, 1984-2002. Emerg Infect Dis 2005; 11(6):943-6.

[64] Varma JK, Molbak K, Barrett TJ, *et al.* Antimicrobial-resistant nontyphoidal *Salmonella* is associated with excess bloodstream infections and hospitalizations. J Infect Dis 2005; 191(4): 554-61.

[65] Lee CR, Cho IH, Jeong BC, Lee SH. Strategies to minimize antibiotic resistance. Int J Environ Res Public Health 2013; 10(9): 4274-305.

[66] Capita R, Alonso-Calleja C. Antibiotic-resistant bacteria: a challenge for the food industry. Crit Rev Food Sci Nutr 2013; 53(1): 11-48.

[67] Bager F, Madsen M, Christensen J, Aarestrup FM. Avoparcin used as a growth promoter is associated with the occurrence of vancomycin-resistant *Enterococcus faecium* on Danish poultry and pig farms. Prev Vet Med 1997; 31(1-2): 95-112.

[68] Krishnasamy V, Otte J, Silbergeld E. Antimicrobial use in chinese swine and broiler poultry production. Antimicrob Resist Infect Control 2015; 4: 17.

[69] Starr MP, Reynolds DM. Streptomycin resistance of coliform bacteria from turkeys fed streptomycin. Am J Public Health Nations Health 1951; 41(11 Pt 1): 1375-80.

[70] National Chicken Council. U.S. broiler performance. 2015 [cited 2015 October 31]; Available from: http://www.nationalchickencouncil.org/about-the-industry/statistics/u-s-broiler-performance/.

[71] Food and Drug Administration. 2011 summary report on antimicrobials sold or distributed for use in food-producing animals. 2014 [cited 2015 October 31]; Available from:

http://www.fda.gov/downloads/ForIndustry/UserFees/AnimalDrugUserFeeActADUFA/UCM338170.pdf.

[72] Trusts TPC. Record-high antibiotic sales for meat and poultry production. 2013 [cited 2015 October 31]; Available from: http://www.pewtrusts.org/en/research-and-analysis/analysis/2013/02/06/recordhigh-antibiotic-sales-for-meat-and-poultry-production.

[73] Casewell M, Friis C, Marco E, McMullin P, Phillips I. The European ban on growth-promoting antibiotics and emerging consequences for human and animal health. J Antimicrob Chemother 2003; 52(2): 159-61.

[74] Silver LL. Challenges of antibacterial discovery. Clin Microbiol Rev 2011; 24(1): 71-109.

[75] Laxminarayan R. Antibiotic effectiveness: balancing conservation against innovation. Science 2014; 345(6202): 1299-301.

[76] Wise R, Hart T, Cars O, *et al.* Antimicrobial resistance. Is a major threat to public health. BMJ 1998; 317(7159): 609-10.

[77] Dellit TH, Owens RC, McGowan JE, Jr., *et al.* Infectious diseases society of america and the society for healthcare epidemiology of america guidelines for developing an institutional program to enhance antimicrobial stewardship. Clin Infect Dis 2007; 44(2): 159-77.

[78] Morgan DJ, Okeke IN, Laxminarayan R, Perencevich EN, Weisenberg S. Non-prescription antimicrobial use worldwide: a systematic review. Lancet Infect Dis 2011; 11(9): 692-701.

[79] The Review on Antimicrobial Resistance. Safe, secure and controlled: managing the supply chain of antimicrobials. 2015 [cited 2015 November 26]; Available from: http://amr-review.org/sites/default/files/Safe%2C%20secure%20and%20controlled%20-%20Managing%20the%20supply%20chain%20of%20antimicrobials.pdf.

[80] The Review on Antimicrobial Resistance. Rapid diagnostics: stopping unnecessary use of antibiotics. 2015 [cited 2015 November 26]; Available from: http://amr-review.org/sites/default/files/Rapid%20Diagnostics%20-%20%20Stopping%20Unnecessary%20use%20of%20Antibiotics.pdf.

[81] Shapiro DJ, Hicks LA, Pavia AT, Hersh AL. Antibiotic prescribing for adults in ambulatory care in the USA, 2007-09. J Antimicrob Chemother 2014 Jan; 69(1): 234-40.

[82] I.M.C.I. Integrated Management of Childhood Illness: Chart Booklet. Geneva: World Health Organization; 2014. Available from: http://apps.who.int/iris/bitstream/10665/104772/16/9789241506823_Chartbook_eng.pdf?ua=1.

[83] INTERPOL. INTERPOL-coordinated operation strikes at organized crime with seizure of 20 million illicit medicines. 2015 [cited 2015 November 26]; Available from: http://www.interpol.int/News-and-media/News/2015/N2015-082.

[84] Owens RC, Jr. Antimicrobial stewardship: concepts and strategies in the 21st century. Diagn Microbiol Infect Dis 2008; 61(1): 110-28.

[85] Centers for Disease Control and Prevention. Core elements of hospital antibiotic stewardship programs. 2014 [cited 2015 November 1]; Available from: http://www.cdc.gov/getsmart/healthcare/pdfs/core-elements.pdf.

[86] Camins BC, King MD, Wells JB, *et al.* Impact of an antimicrobial utilization program on antimicrobial use at a large teaching hospital: a randomized controlled trial. Infect Control Hosp Epidemiol 2009; 30(10): 931-8.

[87] Malani AN, Richards PG, Kapila S, Otto MH, Czerwinski J, Singal B. Clinical and economic outcomes from a community hospital's antimicrobial stewardship program. Am J Infect Control 2013; 41(2): 145-8.

[88] Kyaw MH, Lynfield R, Schaffner W, *et al.* Effect of introduction of the pneumococcal conjugate vaccine on drug-resistant *Streptococcus pneumoniae*. N Engl J Med 2006; 354(14): 1455-63.

[89] World Health Organization. Immunization coverage. Fact Sheet No 378. Updated September 2015. 2015 [cited 2015 November 4]; Available from: http://www.who.int/mediacentre/factsheets/fs378/en/.

[90] Indian Medical Association. Recommended immunization schedule followed in india. [cited 2015 November 4]; Available from: http://www.ima-india.org/page.php?page_id=42.

[91] Child immunization schedule in Jiangsu province of China [cited 2015 November 4]; Available from: http://www.dulwich-

suzhou.cn/uploaded/DCSZ_Documents/Child_immunization_schedule_in_Jiangsu_province_of_China.pdf.

[92] World Health Organization. WHO vaccine-preventable diseases: monitoring system. 2015 global summary. 2015 [cited 2015 November 4]; Available from: http://apps.who.int/immunization_monitoring/globalsummary/schedules.

[93] World Health Organization. Global Immunization Data 2015 [cited 2015 November 4]; Available from: http://www.who.int/immunization/monitoring_surveillance/Global_Immunization_Data.pdf?ua=1.

[94] The Review on Antimicrobial Resistance. Antimicrobial Resistance: Tackling a crisis for the health and wealth of nations. 2014 [cited 2015 November 26]; Available from: http://amr-review.org/sites/default/files/AMR%20Review%20Paper%20-%20Tackling%20a%20crisis%20for%20the%20health%20and%20wealth%20of%20nations_1.pdf.

[95] UNICEF. Water, sanitation and hygiene. 2015 [cited 2015 12/21/2015]; Available from: http://www.unicef.org/wash/.

[96] Community-led total sanitation. 2015 [cited 2015 12/21/2015]; Available from: https://en.wikipedia.org/wiki/Community-led_total_sanitation.

[97] Sarvajal. Water For All. Technology and market based social sector models that deliver drinking water to the last mile. Available from: http://www.sarvajal.com/#about.

[98] Bill and Mellinda Gates Foundation. Water, sanitation & hygiene. strategy review. 2015 [cited 2015 12/21/2015]; Available from: http://www.gatesfoundation.org/What-We-Do/Global-Development/Water-Sanitation-and-Hygiene.

[99] Pittet D, Allegranzi B, Boyce J. The World Health Organization guidelines on hand hygiene in health care and their consensus recommendations. Infect Control Hosp Epidemiol 2009; 30(7): 611-22.

[100] Pittet D, Hugonnet S, Harbarth S, *et al.* Effectiveness of a hospital-wide programme to improve compliance with hand hygiene. Infection Control Programme. Lancet 2000; 356(9238): 1307-12.

[101] Pittet D, Sax H, Hugonnet S, Harbarth S. Cost implications of successful hand hygiene promotion. Infect Control Hosp Epidemiol 2004; 25(3): 264-6.

[102] World Health Organization. WHO Guidelines on Hand Hygiene in Health Care. 2009 [cited 2015 November 27]; Available from: http://apps.who.int/iris/bitstream/10665/44102/1/9789241597906_eng.pdf.

[103] Salama MF, Jamal WY, Mousa HA, Al-Abdulghani KA, Rotimi VO. The effect of hand hygiene compliance on hospital-acquired infections in an ICU setting in a Kuwaiti teaching hospital. J Infect Public Health 2013; 6(1): 27-34.

[104] Centers for Disease Control and Prevention. Guideline for disinfection and sterilization in healthcare facilities, 2008 2008 [cited 2015 November 27]; Available from: http://www.cdc.gov/hicpac/pdf/guidelines/Disinfection_Nov_2008.pdf.

[105] Food and Drug Administration. The judicious use of medically important antimicrobial drugs in food-producing animals. Guidance 209. 2012 [cited 2015 12/21/2015]; Available from: http://www.fda.gov/downloads/AnimalVeterinary/GuidanceComplianceEnforcement/GuidanceforIndustry/UCM216936.pdf.

[106] Aarestrup FM, Jensen VF, Emborg HD, Jacobsen E, Wegener HC. Changes in the use of antimicrobials and the effects on productivity of swine farms in Denmark. Am J Vet Res 2010; 71(7): 726-33.

[107] Policy recommendations. Clin Infect Dis 2002; 34 Suppl 3: S76-7.

[108] The Review on Antimicrobial Resistance. Securing new drugs for future generations: the pipeline of antibiotics. 2015 [cited 2015 November 26]; Available from: http://amr-review.org/sites/default/files/SECURING%20NEW%20DRUGS%20FOR%20FUTURE%20GENERATIONS%20FINAL%20WEB_0.pdf.

[109] Shetty P. The parlous state of palliative care in the developing world. Lancet 2010; 376(9751): 1453-4.

[110] Executive Order 13676 of September 18, 2014; Combating Antibiotic-Resistant Bacteria Federal Register. 2014; 184 (79):56931-5

[111] IDSA. The 10 x '20 Initiative: pursuing a global commitment to develop 10 new antibacterial drugs by 2020. Clin Infect Dis 2010; 50(8): 1081-3.

CHAPTER 3

Drug Safety Approaches in Anti-Infective Drug Discovery and Development

Lucila I. Castro-Pastrana[1,*], Paola Serrano-Martínez[2] and Lenin Domínguez-Ramírez[1]

[1]*Department of Chemical and Biological Sciences, School of Sciences, Universidad de las Américas Puebla, Cholula, México and* [2]*Department of Cell Biology, University Medical Center Groningen, University of Groningen, Groningen, The Netherlands.*

Abstract: Anti-infective agents are some of the most widely used therapeutic drugs worldwide. Overall, the most common serious adverse events attributable to anti-infective agents include liver injury, nephrotoxicity, hypersensitivity reactions, cardiac arrhythmias, drug-drug interactions and therapeutic failure. In clinical practice, serious problems of toxicity limit the usefulness of antimicrobial drugs.

In order to improve the design of clinical trials and better conceptualize research plans for the development of anti-infective drugs, it is important to take into consideration cutting-edge drug safety approaches that can be implemented during discovery and early phase studies, as well as promising methods and models for clinical research advancement. In the present text, we describe a holistic perspective inspired by chemoinformatics, systems biology, and predictive clinical pharmacology, to discuss the utility of *in silico* methods, preclinical models, genomics, translational biomarkers and postmarketing surveillance strategies for safety evaluation and risk detection during anti-infective drug development.

Keywords: Adverse effect, adverse reaction, AMES test, animal model, anti-infective drug, biomarkers, cardiotoxicity, chemoinformatics, clinical trial, Cramer rules, drug development, drug discovery, drug-induced toxicity, environmental risk assessment, hepatotoxicity, humanized mice, nephrotoxicity, pharmacogenomics, pharmacovigilance, preclinical study, quantitative structure-activity relationship (QSAR), systems toxicology, translational medicine, verhaar scheme, zebrafish.

INTRODUCTION

Antimicrobial agents are some of the most widely used therapeutic drugs worldwide. Overall, the most common serious adverse events attributable to anti-

---

Corresponding author Lucila I. Castro-Pastrana: Department of Chemical and Biological Sciences, School of Sciences, Universidad de las Américas Puebla, CP. 72810 Cholula, México; Tel: +52-222-229-2605; E-mail: lucila.castro@udlap.mx

Atta-ur-Rahman (Ed.)
All rights reserved-© 2016 Bentham Science Publishers

infective agents include liver injury, nephrotoxicity, hypersensitivity reactions, cardiac arrhythmias, drug-drug interactions and therapeutic failure.

In order to improve the design of clinical trials and better conceptualize research plans for the development of anti-infective drugs, it is important to take into consideration cutting-edge drug safety approaches that can be implemented during discovery and early phase studies, as well as promising methods and models for clinical research advancement.

In drug discovery, as well as in drug optimization, the identification of structure-activity relationships for early detection of adverse effects and for the estimation of the mechanism of action of antimicrobial-induced toxicities, may help in successful clinical development of drug candidates. Quantitative structure-activity relationship (QSAR) models can be constructed for precise adverse effect clusters including efficacy against resistant pathogens. Moreover, chemoinformatics can also serve as a predictive tool for environmental risk of new anti-infective drugs by modeling toxicity to sentinel organisms and representing a more economical alternative to experimental toxicity testing.

In clinical practice, serious problems of toxicity limit the usefulness of antimicrobial drugs. During preclinical development, research involving the use of tissue and animal models of increased complexity and physiological relevance can prevent some of these toxicity issues. Clinical predictability of the human response depends on the ability of preclinical models to mimic the properties of absorption, distribution, metabolism, elimination and toxicity (ADMET); whether successful or not, these predictions reveal profound inter-species and inter-individual similarities and differences.

The use of genomic technologies such as chemogenomics, pharmacogenomics, and toxicogenomics combined with gene expression profiling for risk assessment can also increase the understanding of the molecular mechanisms that lead to antimicrobial-induced toxicity in order to optimize lead selection processes and to guide rational drug development.

Likewise, novel and emerging biomarkers with better sensitivity and specificity should be further identified and qualified to enable translation from preclinical species to human populations, to aid in the evaluation of drug safety and to predict toxicity. In addition, predictive biomarkers for acute as well as for long-term toxicity are needed. Toxicities detected in a timely manner in the preclinical models favor a more rigorous decision-making process concerning termination of development.

When a new antimicrobial candidate reaches clinical trials in humans, there are additional strategies like genotype-based subject stratification, safety signal identification, and risk-benefit profiling that complete the evaluation of its safety and efficacy. Also, drug delivery research becomes more important at this stage since efficient and rationally developed delivery systems may play a crucial role in clinical outcomes.

Finally, it is important that post-market commitments to drug safety surveillance activities be based on proactive methodologies that take advantage of clinical observations to improve the design of clinical trials and evaluate drug safety earlier in the drug development pipeline. Pharmacovigilance-guided drug design will adequately address the expectancies of translational medicine for novel anti-infective drugs only by means of effectively bringing real-world drug safety information back to drug discovery stages.

In the present text, we use a holistic perspective inspired by chemoinformatics, systems biology, and predictive clinical pharmacology, to discuss the utility of *in silico* methods, preclinical models, genomics, translational biomarkers and postmarketing surveillance strategies for safety evaluation and risk detection during anti-infective drug development.

DETERMINATION OF POTENTIAL DRUG TOXICITY AND SIDE EFFECTS WITH *IN SILICO* AND DATABASE ANALYSIS METHODS

Drug discovery is a costly, multidisciplinary enterprise whose goal is to design a chemical compound capable of modifying an enzymatic activity or a signal cascade in order to bring about a change in the metabolism of a given organism. In its most basic form, it involves the selection of a target, the design and synthesis of a molecule that will directly affect a defined target. A number of computational high-throughput methods have been in development and use since the 60's such as quantitative structure-activity relationship (QSAR) [1]. Target selection is then followed by preclinical development and clinical trials before seeking health agency approval and initiating its commercialization. The culmination of this process takes years and billions of dollars [2, 3].

The first steps in this process, target selection and drug design are where most emphasis is placed, as they constitute an intersection between basic and applied design. This intersection is attractive to both academia and industry since the former is usually more developed in academia while the latter is the province of industry. Currently, drug design involves a lot of bench work; automated, that is carried out by robots, or otherwise, requiring a lot of manpower. It also involves the use of computer power: chemical databases containing millions of compounds can be tested via docking against a given target biomolecule (protein or nucleic acid) and further refined via computational combinatorial chemistry before ever being synthesized [4, 5]. While the merits of this so-called *in silico* strategy are still under debate, it is an active area of research and development.

As the drug design pipeline progresses towards the approval of a drug, the requirement to assess its possible toxicology becomes pressing. Toxicity, defined as the capacity of a substance to produce injury has been proposed to be an important characteristic of any substance since early 1970 and has become an irreplaceable component of risk assessment. *In silico* toxicity predictions are not intended to substitute experimental data but to guide efforts to acquire the relevant information that will quantify the probable toxicity of a given drug or family of compounds.

The following section will focus on the *in silico* methods available to predict toxic effects caused by chemicals. It does not intend to cover all the current and potential methods for such predictions, but to offer an overview of the methods *i.e.* "decision tree" models as well as more general QSAR methodologies that have been created to replace decision making solely on the experience of individual chemists.

In general, decision tree methods are deceptively simple, consisting of a series of yes or no questions. The questions presented are based on current knowledge of metabolism and toxicity. Whereas, QSAR uses physicochemical descriptors that are pruned to create models aimed to correlate compound activity with individual structure or with families of compounds. However, to answer these questions as well as to apply QSAR models both chemical and biochemical knowledge is required. So, in a broad manner, these methods supplement human experience in the fields of chemistry, biochemistry, *etc.* as well as the intuition that develops with this experience, while adding a semiquantitative component.

Cramer Rules (Oral Toxicity)

A universal problem in drug development is that the demand for data concerning drug design and drug toxicity has grown faster than scientist's ability to supply it.

Analysis of a new compound is more complex and time intensive as a consequence of this lack of data. Cramer rules were originally introduced around 1978, as a systematic decision tree to unambiguously classify the toxicity of organic and organometallic compounds based on their structure as well as biochemical and physiological chemistry [6]. These rules were formulated using the codification of the then available chemical and biochemical knowledge and are used to guide the analysis that will prioritize research into the toxicity or usefulness of any given set of drugs or substances. The results of this analysis are the classification of a chemical in question into three classes according to its likelihood of toxicity:

(i)   **Class I** are substances with structures and data suggesting low oral toxicity. If combined with low exposure, these substances are a low priority for investigation.

(ii) **Class III** are substances that permit no strong initial presumption of safety or which suggest significant toxicity. By default, these become a high priority for further research.

(iii) **Class II** are intermediate between I and III.

The definitions used for the process are drawn from natural sciences but used in a broader context. Thus, Cramer rules are best used in conjunction with the Merck Index, Weurman Report and even Hawk's Physiological Chemistry. These three reference books cover, respectively, chemical, biochemical and physiological knowledge.

An example of one of these definitions, taken from the original reference, is as follows:

"A *Normal constituent of the body* means any systemic constituent present at a normal physiological level whether free or combined, except hormones."

This exemplifies a determining question from the decision tree that identifies normal constituents, which if answered yes, would then lead to a Class I rating for this substance (except in the case of hormones).

In order for this decision-making procedure to be performed effectively there are a few other rules:

(i) In borderline cases, II is chosen over I or III over II.

(ii) Functional groups are considered as entire groups not as individual fragments, *i.e.* "a thioamide is not a thione or amine."

While the decision tree is cumbersome to use at first, its implementation in computational tools such as Toxtree (Cramer class in [7]) make it more precise, systematic and faster to use. These tools also make it more accessible for use by undergraduate students. Furthermore, once any user has performed an evaluation, it can be easily reviewed and corrected by a more experienced user, when required.

Verhaar Scheme

(a well-established decision tree used to assess the risks of aquatic pollutants)

The Verhaar scheme is a classification method used to rank organic pollutants into four distinct classes and it is employed to estimate the environmental risks of these chemicals [8]. In contrast to Cramer rules, which are mostly applied to human health concerns, the Vehaar scheme focuses on the effects of chemicals on the environment and so, in a way, is more ecologically oriented.

For example, a parameter of this scheme known as Maximum Tolerable Concentration (MTC) is defined as an aquatic concentration at which only certain percentage of a species in a given ecosystem would be affected by a specific pollutant.

This scheme divides chemicals into four classes [8, 9]:

(i) Inert chemicals, Class 1, these are not reactive and do not interact with a specific receptor class in an organism. Their mode of action is acute aquatic toxicity, also known as *narcosis*. These chemicals are considered as those of minimal or baseline toxicity.

(ii) Less inert chemicals, Class 2, these are also not reactive but of higher toxicity than the baseline ones. Their mode of action is designated as *polar narcosis*; they are commonly characterized by possessing hydrogen bond donor activity.

(iii) Reactive chemicals, Class 3, these types encompass different modes of action: their reactivity is unspecific but affects common chemical motifs found in biomolecules such as cystines, peptide bonds, glycosidic bonds and others. They can be reactive *per se* or activated through biological metabolism.

(iv) Specifically acting chemicals, Class 4, these are those that are toxic because of their interactions with certain specific receptors like acetyl cholinesterase inhibitors or DDT.

In a similar way to the decision tree in the Cramer rules, a subset of rules must be applied to assign a class. If any chemical fails to be classified it cannot be analyzed by this scheme and no toxicity prediction can be made; for all others, LC_{50}, log P, and other properties can be calculated.

The Verhaar scheme is dependent on the availability of experimental data particularly with regard to the baseline toxicity. And, in order to have a common toxicity scale across its classes, it uses a Toxic Ratio derived from experimentally determined LC_{50} and its ratio to the calculated LC_{50} (based on log K_{ow} values). Thus, classification assignment is made on a numerical basis as well as a chemical/structural one.

For example, compounds classified as Class 1 do not contain iodine nor ionic groups. If a compound contains a halogen other than I, the compound must be acyclic and the halogen cannot be part of an unsaturated bond (for a full list of the rules, check references [8, 10]). A simple example of a compound from Class 2 would be a weakly acidic phenol, *i.e.* phenols with one nitro substituent, and/or one to three chlorine substituents. Class 3 compounds follow more complex rules and include functional groups such as ketenes, aldehydes, isothiocyanates, *etc*. In a way, Class 4 compounds are the easiest to classify since they have a known specific mechanism of action, as is the case for DDT, pyrethroids and others.

In the original paper describing the Verhaar scheme, a quantitative score called Toxic Ratio was also defined as the ratio of a QSAR-derived LC_{50} divided by an experimentally determined LC_{50} for *Poecilia reticulata* (guppy). As such, it was limited by the sensitivity of the animal model and can only be cautiously applied to other fish.

Modified Verhaar Scheme

In 2008, due to the interest in the computational applications of the Verhaar scheme, its rules were revised [11].

Changes were made in the following two main areas:

1) A Class 5 was added in order to assign a class to chemicals that do not conform to the Verhaar rules. That is, Class 5 represents chemicals outside the scope of the model but that are not considered harmless.

2) A subdivision of Classes 3 and 4 was added in order to enrich them with current knowledge of experimentally determined mechanisms of action.

As for any knowledge-based method, it will be further enriched as experimental data becomes available.

Skin Irritation or Corrosion Prediction

In contrast to the previous examples of toxicity prediction that are used to anticipate toxicity on a more general level, this particular method is specific for substances applied to the skin that cause characteristic levels of irritation effect (inflammation) or corrosion (irreversible skin damage). Despite this apparent limitation, this methodology is included in the present review since it is based on physicochemical properties such as molecular weight, melting point, vapor pressure, log P_{ow} and surface tension. Complementary to these parameters, a series of physicochemical limits have been defined that allow for the successful prediction of skin irritation or corrosion in compounds with a purity over >95%. These limits are based on a training dataset of compounds with known effects on skin obtained from studies in animal models. A simple example of these limits is the following: from examination of the European Union chemical regulations containing physicochemical and toxicological data on 1833 chemicals with purity of ≥95%, a limit of < 620 g/mol molecular weight was established for skin corrosion. Analysis conducted using this method revealed that skin irritants with higher molecular weight are only active because they readily hydrolyze or decompose into ions [12].

Another important characteristic of this prediction tool is that it has been scaled so that it can be expressed as the EU risk phrases for chemicals classified for skin irritation/corrosion namely, R34, R35 and R38 ('causes burns', 'causes severe burns' or 'irritating to skin', respectively). See Table **1** for a breakdown of a general set of limits as well as for two specific cases [13, 14].

Table 1. Skin irritation and corrosion rules (exclusion rules)

Risk	Rules for all Chemical Groups	Rules for all Chemical Groups Containing C, O, H, N and S.	Rules for all Chemical Groups Containing C, H, O and Halogens.
Not R34, R35, R38	Melting point below 200 °C		Molecular weight > 370 g/mol
Not R34, R35, R38	Log P_{ow} or log K_{ow} below -3.1		
Not R34, R35	Lipid solubility < 0.01 g/kg	Molecular weight > 620 g/mol	Molecular weight > 280 g/mol
Not R34, R35		Melting point > 50 °C	
Not R38		Melting point > 120 °C	

SMARTCyp – Cytochrome P450-Mediated Drug Metabolism and Metabolites Prediction

For drug design the activity of the drug and its specificity are of utmost importance; however, its pharmacokinetic properties are also relevant. It has been established that the kinetic profile of a compound is largely dependent on phase I metabolism in which cytochromes P450 (CYPs) play the main role. CYPs are a large family of heme-thiolate enzymes with at least 60 different isoforms in humans. While they are responsible for a number of reactions (such as cell detoxification), they are also the cause of the majority of drug-drug interactions leading to toxicity issues. Thus, predicting the sites of reaction in the chemical structure of drugs with CYPs is a hot topic. SMARTCyp has been developed as a tool based on quantum mechanics-derived data, transition state prediction as well as an energetic database relating interaction energies to 2D structures [15].

Several anti-infective drugs are substrates, inhibitors or inducers of CYP3A4, an isoform widely involved in xenobiotic metabolism (Fig. **1**). The SMARTCyp approach has been successfully employed to predict substrates of CYP3A4, correctly identifying 81% in the top three solutions. The few shortcomings of this method are due to the fact that it uses 2D information; it is, however, very fast and does not require a lot of computational power. Further improvements are in process, such as making it general enough for other CYPs.

Covalent Protein Binding as Related to Toxicity

Toxicity as related to covalent protein binding is a field that still is under development as it requires even more detailed experimental information than methods. As reviewed by Enoch and colleagues [16] two main methods have been used to derive structural alerts for chemical groups that could covalently bind to proteins: category formation and an expert system. For the expert systems, a set of rules derived from toxicological evidence are used; in particular, evidence for a specific endpoint must exist. An endpoint is described as a well-defined outcome such as skin sensitization, skin irritation or AMES mutagenicity. In contrast, categories are more closely related to initiating events as it uses chemical knowledge and relates it to toxicological data where available. These two methods are complementary and synergic: a double flag indicated by the expert and the category system suggests a high likelihood of toxicity. A single flag raised by the expert system without a clear category will be met with less confidence.

Mutagenicity Prediction Methods

The AMES test is a universally accepted standard for mutagenicity. It is an *in vitro* assay originally developed to test reverse mutations due to exposure to a given chemical [17]. Thus, the assay indirectly measured DNA damaged by different mechanisms (thymine dimerization, bond breakage and chemical modification, to mention a few) and attempted to quantify it through the number of colonies able to grow in a minimal medium. Since the number of spontaneous revertants is a known constant, the test was easy to perform as well as easy to interpret.

As it has been described for the previous examples of toxicity predictive strategies, mutagenicity and carcinogenicity predictions often rely on epidemiological information as well as on health statistics. However, to address the topic of mutagenicity prediction we will emphasize the use of QSAR derived methodologies to establish four very reliable models:

(i) Mutagenic potency in *Salmonella thyphimurium*,

(ii) Discrimination between mutagens and nonmutagens in *S. thyphimurium*,

(iii) Carcinogenicity potency in rodent models and,

(iv) Discrimination between rodent carcinogens and noncarcinogens.

i and ii seek to produce a computational equivalent to the experimental AMES test while iii and iv are applications specific for eukaryotic organisms. The use of

Salmonella thyphimurium as a sensor for the effect of aromatic amines as mutagens will be discussed in the following section.

In 1992, Debnath *et al.* [18] assayed the effect of about 200 aromatic and heteroaromatic amines on *S. thyphimurium*. They found that the mutagenic activity of these compounds was linearly dependent on their hydrophobicity as well as on the energies of their highest occupied molecular orbital (HOMO) and lowest unoccupied molecular orbital (LUMO). While this first study found a positive correlation for mutagenicity with 3 physicochemical properties, it was insufficient to discriminate nonmutagenic compounds from active mutagenic compounds. In 2007, a new study by Benigni and colleagues [19] used 229 amine compounds, to refine the model to a point where it can be used to discriminate between active and inactive mutagenic compounds as well as to grade their mutagenicity.

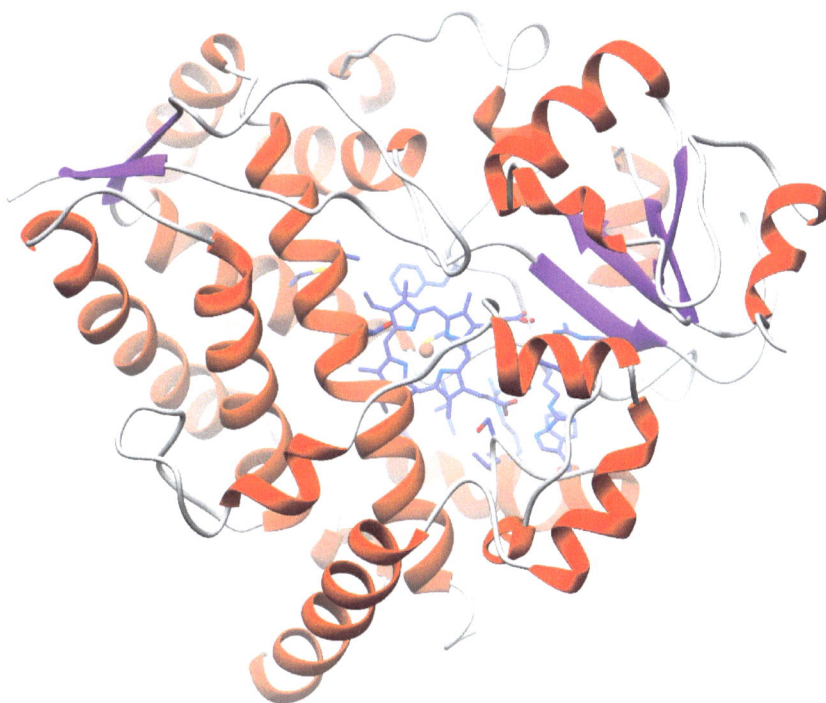

Figure 1: Cytochrome P450 3A4 bound to an inhibitor, tert-butyl {6-oxo-6-[(pyridin-3-ylmethyl)amino]hexyl}carbamate. CYP 3A4 is a key xenobiotic-metabolizing enzyme that oxidizes and clears the majority of drugs; its inhibition could be beneficial by enhancing the therapeutic efficiency of co-administered pharmaceuticals.

To offer a quantitative comparison between the QSAR model to predict mutagenicity levels and mutagenic activity, we present both equations.

Mutagenicity in *S. typhimurium* TA98 was modeled by:

$$log\ TA98 = 1.08\ log\ P + 1.28\ HOMO - 0.73\ LUMO + 1.46\ I_L + 7.20 \qquad \textbf{(1)}$$

where I_L is a variable that indicates if a compound has three or more fused rings ($I_L = 1$).

The discriminating function for mutagenicity on *S. typhimurium* TA98 was modeled by:

$$w = -0.34\ HOMO + 0.86\ LUMO - 0.28 MR_5 + 0.48 MR_6 + 0.67\ Idist^* \qquad \textbf{(2)}$$

Where MR_5 and MR_6 are Molar Refractivity contributions of substituents in positions 5 and 6 to the amino group. *Idist* is an adjustment parameter to account for amino groups with bulky substituents without mutagenic activity. For nonmutagens $w = 1.68$, for mutagens $w = -0.49$; thus, the threshold between mutagenic and nonmutagenic is $w = 0.59$.

It is immediately apparent that these two models differ by the use of logP, which is a good predictor for mutagenicity but does not help to discern between a mutagenic and a nonmutagenic compound. In contrast, both models include HOMO and LUMO energetic differences. In the form depicted above, both models are applicable after their scales are normalized. However, they can be parameterized to allow the use of non-normalized data; so, the ability to add new experimental information makes these models easier to re-parameterize.

From a broader perspective, not only that of drug design, these methods are extremely useful to predict the effects of compounds on humans and other animals. As can be appreciated from the examples given of the equations and data required to evaluate compound toxicity, these methods are powerful but difficult to implement by a novice user. This is why we turn next to a single application that allows any user, even an inexperienced one, to apply all of these methods in a quick, reproducible fashion.

---

*Note: The statistical details have been left out for clarity. Readers are advised to review them in their original publications.

Toxtree as a Platform to Perform *In Silico* Toxicology Predictions

Toxtree [7] is a user-friendly open-source application that categorizes chemicals and predicts various types of toxic effects by applying decision tree approaches, QSAR and other *in silico* methodologies. All of the methodologies mentioned above and many more are available within Toxtree. These applications have been commissioned by the European Union Reference Laboratory for Alternatives to Animal Testing (EURL ECVAM, https://eurl-ecvam.jrc.ec.europa.eu/laboratories-research/predictive _toxicology/qsar_tools/toxtree) and distributed as a Java application. So, it is cross-platform and can be run on Windows, Linux or Mac as a graphical interphase for all of these methods and databases. As with any other computational platform, Toxtree does not replace chemical, biochemical or biophysical knowledge on the part of the user, but allows for several methods based on different rules to be used in parallel on a single set of compounds (Table **2**). For example, a list of chemical compounds including pesticides, herbicides as well as plant extracts can be fed directly into Toxtree and then all of its methods be applied to estimate their toxicities. By taking this approach, toxicity predictions are not limited to any single protocol but are enriched and complemented by each different method.

Since the platform is open source, it can be readily extended by the original creator, the final user, as well as those responsible for its maintenance. Each independent user can take advantage of the existing toolset within Toxtree but refine it for a specific application or context; for example, for use in the cosmetic industry or as an initial threshold for selecting leads in drug design.

Table 2. Methods available within Toxtree.

The Cramer classification scheme
An Extended Cramer scheme
The Kroes TTC decision tree
The Verhaar scheme for aquatic modes of action
Modified Verhaar scheme
Rulebases for skin and eye irritation and corrosion
The Benigni-Bossa rulebase for mutagenicity and carcinogenicity
The ToxMic rulebase for the in vivo micronucleus assay
Structural alerts for covalent protein binding.
Structural alerts for identification of Michael Acceptors
The START rulebase for persistance / biodegradation potential
Structural alerts for the identification of organic functional groups (ISSFUNC rulebase)

in silico tools for toxicology prediction are diverse in terms of their rational and the specific scope of their predictions (*e.g.* skin irritation and corrosion versus carcinogenicity or mutagenesis). Nevertheless, their main goals are the same:

(i)   To reduce the cost involved in toxicology research as well as in regulatory decision making.

(ii) To facilitate the analysis, evaluation and re-evaluation of known compounds and predictions for new or previously unknown chemicals.

In silico tools are not meant to replace the so-called wet research, but to help in cost reduction and to reduce the use of animals in research.

The approach followed by the European Union Reference Laboratory for Alternatives to Animal Testing accomplish these goals by making these tools accessible to any computer savvy user on any of the three major computing platforms. Toxtree then makes it easy to analyze not only a few dozen compounds but often hundreds of thousands to millions and to then record that information for further reference.

Computer-Aided Discovery in Antimicrobial Research

Adverse drug reactions (ADRs) as well as drug-related toxicities are a major concern during drug development. As with all drugs, antimicrobial discovery is also burdened with the need to discern between interesting but ultimately toxic leads and those that pose minimal risk. It is important to bear in mind that any method employed to design a drug with antimicrobial activities must accomplish two main goals: to kill the target pathogen and to not be deleterious to the host of the pathogen *via* ADMET properties (absorption, distribution, metabolism, elimination, and toxicity).

The multitasking model for quantitative-structure biological effect relationships (mtk-QSBER) is similar to other QSAR methodologies in that it requires previously obtained data to create a model that simultaneously predicts antimicrobial activity and ADMET properties of drugs and/or chemicals. Recently this method has been used to develop models to aid in anti-infective drug design for *Pseudomonas spp.* and *E. coli*. Validation of this model was demonstrated by predicting the anti-*E. coli* activity and safety of avarofloxacin. The mtk-QSBER model was developed from a dataset of more than 37,800 cases (chemicals and animal/bacterial responses to them). It achieved an accuracy of over 95%. These results converged with the already available experimental evidence confirming the anti-*E. coli* activities and safety of this drug [20]. In another test of this method, a model was created for *Pseudomonas spp*. This time an antibacterial drug called delafloxacin was employed. The mtk-QSBER model was created using more than 54,000 cases and displayed accuracy higher than 90%, also demonstrating remarkable consistency with experimental data.

The application of this chemoinformatic approach to the virtual screening of new anti-infective agents could accelerate drug discovery in alliance with experimental methodologies [21]. It must be emphasized that mtk-QSBER model must be generated for each target pathogen, and thus, data must be already available, or the user must be able to obtain it. So far this is its only major limitation.

NOVEL ANIMAL MODELS FOR PRECLINICAL SAFETY EVALUATION OF ANTI-INFECTIVE DRUGS

In recent years, there has been a low output of successful pharmaceutical products; 9 out of 10 candidate drugs entering clinical development fail to reach the market. Approximately one-quarter to one-third of these failures are related to safety issues. Drug discovery is based on the principle "if you are going to fail, fail early" since every phase in the process of drug development implies high costs to the pharmaceutical industry [22]. Therefore, earlier detection of safety issues means a decrease in costs associated with drug development and an increase in successful clinical development of candidate drugs can be expected. In order to detect safety-related issues early on during drug development, preclinical evaluation using animal models is a crucial phase of the process.

It is a well-established practice to test anti-infective agents using animal models of infectious diseases, and it is an essential preclinical requisite of a future anti-infective therapy [23]. By law, new therapies have to be evaluated in animals before they can be tested in humans [24]. The long-standing use of animals in the laboratory and the sheer volume of data collected from animal studies have made laboratory animals the 'gold standard' for evaluating the safety of new drugs such as anti-infectives [24]. Animal models of infectious diseases are important tools that bridge the gap between *in vitro* studies and the clinical evaluation of anti-infectives [24, 25]. While *in vitro* testing determines the susceptibility of microorganisms to pharmacological agents, *in vivo* testing challenge the *in vitro* activities against a variety of host factors, like metabolic processes and anti-infective defense mechanisms [23]. These host factors can influence the toxicity and the generation of drug-induced adverse reactions. Since variability in treatment efficacy, effectiveness and toxicity is determined by complex relationships between host, infective agent and drug factors, the limitations of animal models should be considered [23, 26]. Given the differences in pharmacokinetic profiles, drug metabolism and anatomy between animals and humans, data obtained from toxicity studies in animals have led to incorrect predictions of anti-infective toxicity in humans. However, if these limitations are considered, toxicity testing done in experimental models can give clear predictions and indications of the clinical safety of anti-infectives [23]. Therefore, the challenge is to develop new animal models that can more closely mimic the course of human infectious diseases and improve clinical predictability of the safety of anti-infectives.

A large variety of animal models are used to determine the pharmacokinetics of anti-infective therapy and help in the prospective assessment of drug-induced adverse reactions and drug-drug interactions [27, 28]. In pharmacokinetics, considerations for selecting an animal model are based on broad similarities to humans in the physiological and biochemical parameters crucial for drug absorption, distribution, metabolism or excretion (ADME) processes [28]. Safety pharmacology has become an important aspect of the non-clinical safety assessment for new pharmacological agents [22]. Therefore, new animal screening models have recently been used in the early stages of the drug discovery process to generate predictive *in vivo* data for the safety assessment of anti-infectives.

Zebrafish

The zebrafish (*Danio rerio*) is a small tropical fish species that has become popular in research and drug discovery [22]. The popularity of this vertebrate model for use in the study of human disease is attributed to numerous advantages, including:

(i)   Their anatomical, molecular and genetic similarity to humans; the organization of the genome and the genetic pathways controlling signal transduction and development are highly conserved between zebrafish and human;

(ii)   The availability of a large genetic toolbox;

(iii)   Its high fecundity;

(iv)   Its rapid embryonic development *ex utero*, allowing for experimental manipulation and direct observation of tissue formation and organogenesis *in vivo*;

(v)   The ease and low-cost for maintaining a large stock of these animals;

(vi)   The optical transparency of embryos and larvae, that enables massive phenotype-based screens;

(vii) Very few ethical issues associated with the use of larvae up to the feeding stage;

(viii) Many pathological processes similar to various human diseases, and;

(ix)   No gender difference in larvae at early larval stages of development.

These properties have made the zebrafish an excellent model for the study of human diseases [29, 30].

In addition, the zebrafish larvae can potentially be used during the drug discovery process in toxicity studies for the analysis of drug safety. There is evidence confirming that mammalian and zebrafish toxicity profiles are very similar, and some protocols have been developed for the assessment of compound toxicity [31]. The small size of the fish and easy availability of large numbers of its larvae are some of the advantages of the use of the zebrafish for drug screening efficacy and which make it suitable for high throughput *in vivo* screening of drugs. The larvae can live in 50μL of fluid, in which only micrograms of a compound are needed for a screening analysis. Therefore, *in vivo* analysis of the effects of pharmacological agents can be conducted at earlier stages in drug development, with high throughput characteristics and a reduction in the material required for testing [29-31].

The zebrafish has been suggested as a model for hazard detection instead for risk assessment. In this way, the study on the zebrafish could be applied as a first screen in potential hazard detection, followed by risk assessment determined by more sophisticated tests in mammalian systems. This hazard detection assay should be considered as a rapid and simple screening method, and as a test to be used to prioritize compounds. A suitable model for use as a predictive assay needs to include the following characteristics [22]:

(i) Relevant to human toxicity;

(ii) Reliable;

(iii) Convenient;

(iv) It takes into account ethical considerations (*i.e.* reduction of the number of animals or the use of species with lower neurophysiological sensitivity);

(v) By early discovery of events of toxicity, it saves money, time and animals expended in the development of the compound.

The zebrafish model covers most of these characteristics; therefore, it can potentially be used in the early assessment of ADRs.

The Use of the Zebrafish Model for the Assessment of Anti-Infective Toxicity

There are a number of studies using the zebrafish model for the evaluation of hepatic, renal and cardiovascular toxicity, and drug-drug interactions, which are serious adverse events attributable to anti-infective therapy.

The general anatomy, organization, cellular composition and function of the zebrafish liver are almost the same as in mammals. The zebrafish completes its primary liver morphogenesis 48 hours post-fertilization and the liver is completely formed and functional by 72 hours post-fertilization. Moreover, the early embryonic stages of hepatogenesis are similar to those in mice. Disease phenotypes in zebrafish are comparable to those in mammals, as well as the presence of metabolizing enzymes [31]. CYP450 enzymes are important catalyzers of the drug metabolizing reactions and many drug-drug interactions that are clinically relevant are associated with inhibition or induction of these enzymes. Regarding the importance of the early detection of drug-drug interactions, the U.S. Food and Drug Administration (FDA) requires CYP assessment for drug approval [32]. It is known that certain antibiotics are CYP inducers or inhibitors. As an example, clotrimazole and rifampicin are human CYP3A inducers while erythromycin is a mammalian CYP3A inhibitor. There are several zebrafish cytochrome genes that have high homology to human genes or can cause catalyzing reactions similar to mammals. Therefore, these similarities allow the assessment of drug metabolism and toxicity using zebrafish CYP450. This assessment is performed using a zebrafish microplate assay which is highly sensitive, reproducible and offers high throughput. Results using this specific assay reported CYP effects of specific CYP inducers or inhibitors as being the same in mammals and zebrafish, as was proven for erythromycin. These data demonstrate that the zebrafish model has comparable cytochrome metabolism profiles as mammals; therefore, it is a powerful tool that can be used as the preliminary screen for anti-infective safety, in order to predict and avoid drug-drug interactions [32].

The hearts of mammals and zebrafish have similar functional characteristics, including blood flow directions, a high-pressure system driven by a specialized endocardium musculature, a heart rhythm regulated by an electrical system and a heartbeat associated with pacemaker activity [33]. Because of the transparency of the larval state, observation of the heart rhythm as well as the vasculature and circulation is possible in zebrafish and does not require physical intervention [34]. The zebrafish's pharmacological responses to well-characterized cardiotoxins have been assessed; the results obtained were satisfactory as the responses were similar to human reactions. Moreover, the use of the zebrafish for the evaluation of cardiovascular toxicity is supported by a study in which human cardiotoxic and non-cardiotoxic drugs were administered to the zebrafish by soaking or microinjection. The human non-cardiotoxic drugs used were tetracycline hydrochloride and gentamicin sulfate and resulted in a non-cardiotoxic response in the zebrafish as in the case of humans. Therefore, the zebrafish is a highly predictive animal model for assessing the cardiovascular toxicity of anti-infective drugs *in vivo* [33].

Kidney research using the zebrafish model is also relevant for the assessment of the toxicity caused by certain drugs, due to the fundamental elements of nephron structure and function conserved between vertebrates. The zebrafish embryo possesses a simple renal system that consists of a pronephros composed of two nephrons. In the case of the adult zebrafish, the organ is a more complex mesonephros with several nephrons [34]. The parameters required to evaluate the effects of drugs on the zebrafish renal function are based on morphological changes, the inflammatory response and the measurement of renal clearance [35]. Based on these parameters, the functional phenotype caused in the mammalian kidney by gentamicin is also observed in the zebrafish embryo pronephros. Gentamicin is an aminoglycoside antibiotic that is nephrotoxic in mammals. Injection of gentamicin into zebrafish embryos causes acute renal failure with typical features observed in higher organisms. Moreover, the renal failure in zebrafish is accompanied by an inflammatory response, which is an important component of acute kidney injury (AKI) [34-36]. Therefore, the simple renal system of the zebrafish with features similar to those in mammals and the possibility to use it for the assessment of renal failure, make the zebrafish a suitable *in vivo* model for early evaluation of the renal toxicity of anti-infectives.

As described above, the biology and pharmacological responses need to be sufficiently conserved between humans and zebrafish for this model to play a role in early drug safety assessment [35]. The great number of similarities in general anatomy, organization, cellular composition, function, metabolizing processes and disease phenotypes between the zebrafish and the mammals, place the zebrafish as a potential model for the assessment of early adverse drug events of anti-infectives related with renal, hepatic and cardiac toxicity.

3.2. Genetically Engineered Mouse Models

Humanized mice have recently emerged as powerful tools for the study of human disease. These are amenable animal models transplanted with human cells or tissues, and/or equipped with human transgenes, which have great utility in the investigation of human infection agents [37]. Mainly, two different approaches are used to generate humanized mouse models: (i) the introduction of human genes into the mouse genome to generate genetically humanized mouse models and (ii) the transplantation of human cells into competent recipients resulting in tissue humanized mouse models [38]. The success of the engraftment depends on avoiding rejection, which is ensured by the correct localization and support of the transplanted tissue by host factors. Humanized mice with high levels of human chimerism in various host organs and tissues have been successfully developed, providing a novel approach to be used in preclinical studies of human pathogens [37].

The Use of Humanized Mice to Predict Drug Metabolism and Toxicity

Another novel and promising application of these models is related to drug metabolism and toxicity. The prediction of human responses from *in vivo* studies is often limited by the interspecies differences in drug metabolism, which create qualitative and quantitative variance between drug metabolites produced in humans and animals. These differences lead to the inability to identify human-specific drug metabolites in preclinical stages. The identification of human-specific metabolites generated after drug intake allows for the determination of their toxicity. Therefore, species differences in drug metabolism have limited the relevance to humans of drug metabolism and toxicity data gathered from animal toxicology studies [38, 39].

It is possible to minimize the impact of the interspecies differences in drug metabolism by using one of the following two approaches to humanize mice. The first strategy consists of replacing single or multiple mouse genes with their human counterparts, such as mouse models expressing human receptors (replacing the mouse receptors), drug metabolizing enzymes and transporters. The liver plays an important role in drug metabolism and detoxification, so for the second strategy mice have been engineered with human hepatocytes engrafted in their livers [38]. This strategy entails two genetic modifications: (i) defects in the immune system of the mice, allowing them to accept transplanted human liver cells and (ii) a gene knockout or an expressed transgene for damaging the endogenous murine liver cells, which facilitates the engraftment of transplanted human liver cells. These genetic modifications enable the repopulation of the murine liver by the transplanted human liver cells, which can synthesize human proteins. Therefore, it has been possible to develop humanized mice models with high levels of human liver reconstitution, in which hepatic clearance and pharmacokinetic properties of drugs are similar to humans [39].

Assessment of Drug-Drug Interactions Using Humanized Mice

The enzymes involved in drug-drug interactions are those of the metabolic pathways in the liver. Many clinically important drug-drug interactions have not been predicted by the use of current *in vitro* or *in vivo* animal models. The results demonstrated with humanized mice models position them as powerful tools for the assessment of drug-drug interactions.

A new model system for human liver replacement was produced, by the expression of a herpes simplex virus type 1 thymidine kinase transgene within the liver of a highly immunodeficient mouse strain (NOG), producing the NOG mouse expressing a thymidine kinase transgene (TK-NOG). The humanized liver of the TK-NOG mice expresses mRNAs encoding human CYP450 enzymes, transporters and transcription factors affecting drug metabolism at levels similar to those in the donor human hepatocytes [40]. This humanized mouse model was used to predict whether a potential drug–drug interaction involving clemizole (candidate treatment for hepatitis C virus infection) would occur. Clemizole was coadministered with ritonavir to the TK-NOG mice to test the hypothesis that ritonavir could alter clemizole pharmacokinetics. As a drug-drug interaction was generated in the humanized mice, a similar type of interaction could be expected in humans and so the drug-drug interaction was predicted with this model. Based on this data, humanized mice can be used to predict and assess potential drug–drug interactions [38, 40].

3.2.3. Use of Humanized Mice in Pharmacogenetic Studies

Another important use of humanized mice during drug development is in the field of pharmacogenetics. Nowadays, pharmacogenetic information for drug selection or dose adjustment is being used increasingly to improve drug efficacy and to reduce drug toxicity. However, large and costly human clinical studies are required for testing pharmacogenetic hypotheses [38]. Humanized mice could offer a solution to this problem. For example, TK-NOG mice were used to examine the effect that genetic variations within CYP genes have on drug metabolism. CYP2C19 participates in the metabolism of many drugs and it is highly polymorphic in the human population, affecting drug metabolism. Donor human hepatocytes with CYP2C19 alleles that are associated with reduced, intermediate or ultrarapid rates of CYP2C19-mediated drug metabolism were transplanted into mice that were subsequently exposed to a certain drug. Statistically significant differences were observed in the rate of drug metabolism of the humanized mice reconstituted with different genotypes [41]. This model system could enable human pharmacogenetic analyses to be routinely performed. Moreover, advances in cellular reprogramming methodology which enables induced liver cells to be developed from individuals with specific genotypes, will amplify the scope of human pharmacogenetic studies that can be performed in humanized mice [38].

The Use of Humanized Mice for the Safety Assessment of Anti-Infectives

There are a number of human-specific infectious agents that can be studied using humanized mice. These include hepatitis viruses, HIV, cytomegalovirus (CMV), Epstein–Barr virus (EBV), dengue virus, *Neiserria gonorrhoea* and *Neisseria meningitidis*, measles virus, *P. falciparum* and *Ebola virus* [42-47]. The humanized mice developed for the study of these pathogens are suitable for research of the pathogenesis and prognosis of human disease. These models are powerful tools for drug development, and for determining the efficacy of anti-infective drugs however novel tests need to be developed in order to use them to study drug safety.

Chimeric mice with humanized livers are promising tools to assist in the prediction and assessment of ADRs, during the process of drug development. At present, no regulations or guidelines are required for the use of humanized mouse models in preclinical studies [41]. Thus, these specialized *in vivo* models can be used in research aimed at establishing them as the most suitable models for the assessment of anti-infective safety and efficacy.

BIOMARKER DRIVEN STRATEGIES FOR RISK PROFILING AND SAFETY PREDICTION

The Need for Safe and Effective Anti-Infective Agents

Antibiotic resistance is a growing threat to the modern world and the discovery of the next generation of safe and effective antibiotics remains a big challenge. Recent drug approvals like the antifungal isavuconazonium sulfate, the antibiotic oritavancin and the anti-leishmanial miltefosine bring hope to the race to develop a new anti-infective arsenal. However, these novel therapeutic approaches seem to share the same toxicity spectrum as their forerunners.

As drug-drug interactions can often contribute to drug safety problems, it is also interesting to note that some of these interactions are being incorporated into therapeutic strategies. As with the new drug cobicistat which is a potent inhibitor of cytochrome CYP3A and acts as a pharmacokinetic-enhancing agent when used in combination with antiviral drugs like atazanavir and darunavir. Moreover, novel compounds isolated from soil producing micro-organisms, as in the case of the antibiotic teixobactin, show promise to avoid development of resistance [48].

This timid but still optimistic scenario gets cloudier when taking into consideration the serious anti-infective-induced adverse drug reactions in post-marketing settings. To date, adverse findings in preclinical *in vivo* models provide around 70% concordance with human toxicities. Unfortunately, hepatic effects and hypersensitivity/cutaneous reactions show the poorest correlation and are seldom detected in the preclinical models. For that reason, early, predictive, and noninvasive biomarkers are needed that may be used *in vitro*, *in vivo* and then translated into the clinic [49].

Moreover, the discovery of novel biomarkers is a promising endeavor that can advance precision medicine and boost pharmaceutical innovation by helping to decrease non-clinical safety-related attrition. A biomarker-driven strategy facilitates the selection of potential drug candidates with an improved safety profile and accelerates all phases of the drug development process.

Those biomarkers could, if validated, serve as very useful tools for monitoring drug safety in the premarketing period, principally during phase III of the investigational new drug process, and in the early post-marketing period.

Ideally, the use of biomarkers for ADR detection combined with pharmacovigilance activities for their assessment should be embedded within a framework of integrated and comprehensive surveillance strategies whose effectiveness has been proven for the evaluation of post-approval safety.

These postmarketing strategies may include:

(i)   The use of large drug-specific or disease-specific registries.

(ii) The creation of networks linking multiple medical centers through pharmacovigilance databases.

(iii) Data mining of large electronic databases.

(iv) Periodic Safety Update Reports.

(v)   Epidemiological studies.

Active surveillance, drug or ADR targeted pharmacovigilance, trained surveillance clinicians, case-control methodology, standardized reporting and rigorous data analysis procedures have also been identified as strategic elements for more efficiently translating pharmacovigilance knowledge to clinical practice [50].

Translational Safety Biomarkers

Biomarker discovery and their use during preclinical and clinical trials as well as in clinical practice is becoming more important given that a distinction between 'adverse effects' and 'adverse reactions' has been recently claimed from a clinical endpoint perspective. Aronson JK defined an adverse drug effect as: "a potentially harmful effect resulting from an intervention related to the use of a medicinal product, which constitutes a hazard and may or may not be associated with a clinically appreciable adverse reaction and/or an abnormal laboratory test or clinical investigation, as a marker of an adverse reaction" and an adverse drug reaction as "an appreciably harmful or unpleasant reaction, resulting from an intervention related to the use of a medicinal product". In brief, an adverse effect constitutes a potential harm, and an adverse reaction implies appreciable damage. Thus, biomarkers can be related to adverse effects and surrogate endpoints to adverse reactions [51].

This distinction becomes very important when reporting adverse events in clinical trials as well as when interpreting pharmacovigilance signals and making clinical and regulatory decisions in 'real-world' healthcare practice. In clinical research, this definition could also play a significant role in adaptive trials by allowing early identification of risks and consequently the introduction of modifications to the initial study design [52].

Hepatotoxicity (32%) and cardiovascular toxicity, principally drug-induced malignant arrhythmias (33%) have been the major safety reasons for drug market withdrawals over the last three decades [53]. Therefore, many scientific and regulatory efforts are combining to better profile the liver and cardiac safety of drugs during the experimental phases of drug development. So, as can be expected, biomarkers are of utmost importance to help rule out low levels of risk for severe adverse drug events in these early phases, thereby decreasing development times, attrition rates and related costs.

Hepatotoxicity

In 1999, the U.S. FDA began a series of annual conferences to discuss issues related to drug-induced liver injury (DILI) [54]. Then in 2009, FDA´s Center for Drug Evaluation and Research (CDER) published the 'Guidance for Industry Drug-Induced Liver Injury: Premarketing Clinical Evaluation' [55] and created a software program termed '**e**valuation of **D**rug-**I**nduced **S**erious **H**epatotoxicity' or eDISH [56]. These efforts have prevented market withdrawals due to serious hepatotoxicity since 1997.

Serum alanine aminotransferase (ALT) activity is the biochemical benchmark of liver damage, but not all ALT increases necessarily progress to severe liver injury. For that reason, other biomarkers like glutamate dehydrogenase (GLDH), membrane-bound catechol-O-methyltransferase (MB-COMT) and retinol-binding protein 4 (RBP4), have been proposed as alternatives for earlier and/or more sensitive and specific detection of DILI [49, 57]. Furthermore, Hu and colleagues developed a hepatotoxicity panel containing 15 different liver-specific blood proteins that were identified as a toxicity signature by using proteomic platforms in a mouse model [57].

Of particular concern is idiosyncratic DILI, which is usually detected in a late stage of drug development. Identification of rare or idiosyncratic drug-induced hepatotoxicity during clinical trials could benefit from the gradual discovery of pharmacogenetic markers. For instance, different human leukocyte antigen (HLA) alleles have been found to be associated with hepatotoxicity induced by anti-infective drugs like abacavir (HLA-B*57:01), amoxicillin-clavulanate (HLA-A*02:01), flucloxacillin (HLA-B*57:01) and nevirapine (HLA-Cw8-B14, HLA-

Cw8, HLA-B*35:05, HLADRB*01:01, HLA-C*04:01) [58]. Idiosyncratic hepatotoxicants can also be identified from preclinical toxicological studies by measuring their effects on oxidative stress/reactive metabolite gene expression (OS/RM) in liver RNA samples. Recognized hepatotoxic anti-infectives like isoniazid, ketoconazole, sulfamethoxazole, and ritonavir, as well as chloramphenicol, an antimicrobial agent that was not previously labeled as hepatotoxicant, were recently defined as OS/RM-producing compounds [59]. Interestingly enough, most of these drugs are not acutely toxic in rats, which provide compelling evidence in favor of using this gene expression signature to avoid idiosyncratic liver toxicity of drug candidates.

Additionally, global gene-expression profiles are useful in the discovery of novel genes and pathways involved in antimicrobial toxicity. An example of the application of these toxicogenomic approaches in ADR research is the liver gene-expression profiling for trovafloxacin exposure on rats and mice which was able to determine that IFN-γ and IL-8 play critical roles in trovafloxacin-induced idiosyncratic liver injury (this drug has since been withdrawn from the European and U.S. markets) [60]. Thus, transcriptomic studies on drug-induced toxicity can provide valuable mechanistic insights into several ADRs but these studies need to be further validated in order to anticipate an idiosyncratic adverse response across species and in specific human subpopulations.

To meet the challenges of drug safety, multi-centre clinical trials, international consortia, regulatory agencies and other initiatives are working together to validate biomarkers, generate guidelines and concentrate evidence that will facilitate drug-induced hepatotoxicity identification and prediction from the very early phases of drug discovery and development. The Mechanism Based Integrated Systems for the Prediction of Drug-Induced Liver Injury (MIP-DILI) project supported by the European Union's Innovative Medicines Initiative, the U.S. Drug-Induced Liver Injury Network (DILIN), the international Drug-Induced Liver Injury Consortium (iDILIC), the Predictive Safety Testing Consortium (PSTC) and the SAFE-T Consortium (Safer and Faster Evidence-based Translation) are just a few of the many organizations that contribute to the efforts being made worldwide [61]. Lastly, when it comes to hepatic safety, antimicrobial drugs are always an issue, not only because of their structural features and unveiled toxicity mechanisms but because of deficiencies in their patterns of use and prescription in clinical settings and ambulatory care; hence, the need for research on DILI to remain an ongoing priority.

Cardiotoxicity

According to the Expert Working Group on Biomarkers of Drug-Induced Cardiac Toxicity established by the Center for Drug Evaluation and Research (CDER) of the U.S. FDA, the ideal toxicity biomarker should be specific, sensitive, predictive, robust, non-invasive, accessible and able to bridge across species [62]. Using this criteria, in 2004 they concluded that troponins T (cTnT) and I (cTnI) meet all these requirements by reflecting early myocardial damage as well as the extent of irreversible myocardial cell injury caused by anti-infective drugs and that serum cardiac troponins can be used as biomarkers of drug-induced cardiac injury in preclinical as well as in clinical studies. In order to serve as feasible models for screening compounds in drug development, biomarkers should also be suitable for detecting organ toxicity in sufficiently well-characterized animal species. Thus to date, cardiac troponin remains the most effective translational safety biomarker, but other biomarkers are highlighted as complementary and, therefore, useful in cardiac toxicity preclinical assessments *i.e.* interleukin 6, myeloperoxidase and soluble CD 40 ligand [49, 63].

Concerning cardiac toxicity, the ever-increasing number of cases of drug-induced torsade de pointes (TdP) associated with non-cardiac drugs was recently declared an iatrogenic epidemic [64]. QT prolongation, a surrogate marker for the risk of developing TdP, is an established side effect of certain anti-arrhythmic drugs and is also a rare side effect of a wide range of non-cardiac drugs. For many years, quinidine was the only anti-infective drug listed as responsible for QT prolongation and TdP. Later on, the antimalarial halofantrine was shown to have torsadogenic effects followed by many others *i.e.* fluoroquinolones, antimalarials, azole antifungals and antivirals [65, 66]. To date, more than 60 different anti-infective drugs have been reported as causative agents of drug-induced TdP in the U.S. FDA Adverse Event Reporting System. This adverse effect has been recognized as a complex regulatory and clinical problem leading to market withdrawals (grepafloxacin) or warnings (telithromycin) [67].

Worldwide, regulatory agencies acknowledge that QT prolongation is a convenient end-point to assess, but that it is only a surrogate marker of cardiotoxicity; no consensus exists on the degree of QT prolongation that becomes clinically significant [68]. The risk of developing TdP is proportional to the degree of QT prolongation, but there are reported cases of TdP in patients with apparently normal QT interval [69] while 20% of TdP cases often result in sudden death due to the development of ventricular fibrillation [67].

Based on this, cheminformatics modeling combined with systems biology tools have demonstrated to be useful strategies to link chemical structure to ADRs (*i.e.* drug-induced TdP) clustered in the context of their system organ classes. This approach provides valuable predictive information for compounds during the early phases of drug discovery because it can help to find appropriate biomarkers for severe ADRs, better understand possible ADRs for novel compounds sharing similar substructures and to estimate the most influencing substructural features for the predicted ADRs [70].

For candidate chemical template selection and to refine chemical structure design of novel anti-infective drugs, pharmacophore and ion channel structure modeling are promising tools to create better predictors of drug-induced TdP [71]. Early prediction of complex adverse events such as QT prolongation or hepatotoxicity can also be improved through *in silico* quantitative structure activity/property relationship (QSAR/QSPR) models. Likewise, it is also possible to screen for potential adverse effects of experimental drugs by using pharmacovigilance resources to generate multi-ADR predictor tools based on the integration of 3D pharmacophoric similarity data [72].

Investigation of drug toxicity using metabolite analysis (pharmacometabolomics) has also shown encouraging results for cardiac toxicity screening. After experimenting with guinea pigs that were administered three different doses of the fluoroquinolone sparfloxacin, Park and colleagues provided evidence that safety signals could be captured more frequently during premarketing clinical trials by using metabolic phenotypes to detect a predisposition to or risk of drug toxicity [73]. Metabolomic approaches helped them to select the endogenous metabolites that substantially contributed to the prediction of sparfloxacin-induced QT prolongation, to determine the dose dependency of the toxic response and to categorize the degree of toxicity based on the plasma levels of the metabolites.

Cytidine-59-diphosphate (CDP), deoxycorticosterone, L-aspartic acid and stearic acid were identified as determinants of the individualized QT prolongation caused by sparfloxacin [73]. Although this metabolic module is also related to various complex diseases, the equation obtained by Park *et al.*, allows for early prediction of QT prolongation in the preclinical settings and their approach can be applied to other antibiotics and can be further validated in humans.

The association between genetic biomarkers and drug toxicity is also being widely investigated, particularly in relation to the specific pharmacokinetic and pharmacodynamic factors that influence susceptibility for drug-induced QT interval prolongation. To date, the genes coding for CYP enzymes (CYP2B6, CYP2C9, CYP2C19, CYP2D6, CYP3A4), for P-glycoprotein (ABCB1), for the hERG potassium channel (KCNH2) and for other ion channels (genes CACNA1C, KCND3, KCNE1, KCNE2, KCNJ2, KCNJ5, KCNN3, KCNQ1, SCN4A, SCN4B, SCN5A) and proteins (ACN9, AKAP6, AKAP7, APLP2, ATP2A2, BRUNOL4, CALR, CASQ2, CERKL, JPH2, JPH3, NRG3, NOS1AP, NUBPL, PALLD, PPP2R3A, SLC22A23, SLCO3A1, ZFHX3) have been investigated for variants that confer risk for developing acquired QT prolongation when taking drugs and some degree of association with drug-induced QT prolongation or drug-induced TdP was found [74]. Specifically related to anti-infective drugs, clinical studies with moxifloxacin and levofloxacin contributed to find that Caucasians may be more sensitive to drug-induced QT prolongation than Asians. Niemeijer and colleagues emphasized the importance of studying genetic variation associated with QT prolongation in early-phase studies in order to be able to detect variants with large adverse effects and stratify risk, to gain a better understanding of ADR mechanisms and eventually result in genetic targeted marketing [74].

For a summary of all the factors that make certain patients susceptible to the effects of QT-prolonging drugs, we recommend Owens RC work on QT prolongation with antimicrobial agents for a comprehensive review of the electrophysiological basis of this adverse effect, its predisposing factors and the most relevant information on risk/benefit evaluations to safely prescribe anti-infectives [75].

Nephrotoxicity

Another safety concern with some groups of anti-infectives is drug-induced nephrotoxicity, particularly AKI. Since significant renal damage can exist with minimal or no change in serum creatinine levels this classic marker is considered a poor indicator of early renal dysfunction [76]. Elevated blood urea nitrogen (BUN) levels and total protein in urine have similar limitations. New biomarkers are in the spotlight of research looking to find ones whose performance are comparable across species and that are sensitive to species-specific drug responses and organ physiology. Burt and colleagues demonstrated these virtues for the emerging urinary biomarkers NGAL (neutrophil gelatinase-associated lipocalin) and KIM-1 (kidney injury molecule 1), which are also capable of differentiating the area of injury within the kidney as in the case of polymyxin B-treated dogs, monkeys and rats.

Furthermore, early genomic indicators of nephrotoxicity have recently been discovered, and their expression patterns are being validated in female cynomolgus monkeys treated with gentamicin and everninomicin (an experimental antibiotic). Waf-1, matrix metalloproteinase-9, vimentin, clusterin, osteopontin and hepatitis A virus cellular receptor-1 demonstrated a high degree of correlation between changes in gene expression and the probability of the development of histopathologic lesions. These results provide preliminary evidence for predicting the onset of drug-induced renal tubular damage in primate models [77].

Also, KIM-1 and NGAL have been monitored in healthy children to establish reference intervals and contribute to the rational design and interpretation of clinical trials using these emerging AKI biomarkers [78, 79]. Significant differences in gender, age, ethnic and daytime levels were found which provides important information for optimizing the diagnostic or prognostic qualification and use of these novel renal tubular markers in children. In premature neonates treated with gentamicin, KIM-1 demonstrated significant performance as an indicator of aminoglycoside-associated nephrotoxicity [80]. These investigations in pediatric populations provide very useful information that can later be used in adult clinical trials designed to contribute to the development of safer drugs for children.

In summary, the identification of more and better predictive biomarkers of organ damage is key for the generation of integrative and predictive toxicological information that can reduce attrition rates in drug development [81].

Environmental Toxicity

Drug safety has become an overarching framework for managing risk not only relevant to human health but also for the integrity of the ecosystem. For many years, regulatory agencies like the U.S. FDA, Health Canada and the European Medicines Agency (EMA) have increasingly required environmental risk assessments as part of the application process for marketing authorization of new medicinal products. However, 'ecopharmacovigilance' is a developing discipline defined as "the science and activities concerning detection, assessment, understanding and prevention of adverse effects or other problems related to the presence of pharmaceuticals in the environment, which affect both human and the other animal species" [82].

Based on this, the challenge of identifying relevant biomarkers for patient safety is expanding to include the need to discover significant biomarkers for environmental risk assessment and regulation.

In order to identify the potential risks that a medicinal product may pose to the environment, measurements of oxidative stress, DNA adducts and protein adducts, mutagenicity, genotoxicity, endocrine disruption, cytotoxicity and growth inhibition are conducted in model organisms (*i.e.* green and blue-green algae, fish species, aquatic invertebrates, earthworms, sediment-dwelling organisms, non-target plants, soil and sewage microorganisms). To date, the Organization for Economic Co-operation and Development (OECD) Guidelines for the Testing of Chemicals are followed worldwide to assess the potential effects of chemicals on human health and the environment.

Markedly, residues of antibiotics have been found in terrestrial and aquatic environments so that considering their global rates of consumption and their impact on the environment is now becoming a real concern.

The effects of the exposure of zebrafish to several antibiotics have been studied. Oxytetracycline and amoxicillin caused minimal sublethal effects in this organism as demonstrated by their level of modulation of the oxidative biomarkers catalase, glutathione-S-transferase, and lactate dehydrogenase [83]. In the case of norfloxacin, this antibiotic significantly increased the activity of glutathione peroxidase, glutathione-S-transferase and catalase, thus showing a negative impact on the specific biochemical processes related to oxidative stress [84]. Ciprofloxacin was also tested on zebrafish to assess its impact on growth, on the development of histopathological changes in selected organs (*i.e.* gills, kidney, liver) and on the activity of some oxidative stress parameters, where only these latter markers were affected [85].

The impact of antimicrobials on the terrestrial environment can be measured using the earthworm *Eisenia fetida*. This organism was exposed to tetracycline and chlortetracycline to demonstrate that the activities of superoxide dismutase and catalase are induced and that DNA damage (genotoxicity) occurs in a dose-dependent manner [86].

Biomarkers for environmental health risk assessment need to be systematically developed to be able to link exposure to disease end-points. Their added value consists of the information they can provide for the understanding of mechanisms of toxicity, which can then improve the design and outcome of preclinical and clinical studies.

The Systems Toxicology Approach

As an extension of systems biology, systems toxicology seeks to study the effects of toxicants (*i.e.* drugs) on molecular and cellular networks by integrating chemoinformatics, *in vitro* assays, pharmaco/toxicodynamics, pharmaco/toxicokinetics, pharmaco/toxicogenomics, physiology, clinical trial information, pharmacovigilance, public health and consumption data into quantitative models able to describe the relationship between drug exposure and response.

Since model parameters are selected based on available experimental data, accurate prediction can only occur when the information collected is complete and retrieved continuously for feedback and model optimization. In fact, mathematical modeling has increasingly been used in drug discovery and development and has the potential to impact every stage of the process from target screening and validation, to toxicity analysis and preclinical testing [87].

An integrated understanding of systems toxicology is recognized as a key component for the success of safety prediction. Drug development and clinical practice will thoroughly benefit from an approach that moves towards translational safety and can truly predict and prevent adverse outcomes in humans. That is the reason why early, accurate, quantitative and predictive biomarkers of tissue injury are desperately needed in preclinical and clinical studies. Moreover, these biomarkers need to be acceptable from the scientific and regulatory point of view. At present, the Predictive Safety Testing Consortium (PSTC) of the U.S. FDA's Critical Path Institute, and the Innovative Medicines Initiative (IMI) of the European Commission are using translational strategies to undertake major efforts to develop improved safety testing approaches and methods that will accelerate drug development.

One of the most challenging safety issues of anti-infective drugs is lack of efficacy. Microbial resistance accounts for a certain extent of therapeutic failure, but it is not the only factor involved. Drug quality, drug dosing, preparation and administration, prescription patterns, empirical antimicrobial use, non-compliance with antibiotic use guidelines and policies, and lack of knowledge of the indications and contraindications of anti-infectives, are mostly responsible for treatment inefficacy.

Inappropriate antibiotic dosing is of particular concern due to the possibility of therapeutic failure from underdosing or due to the development of ADRs associated with overdosing [88]. Thus, factors that may have a significant impact on antibiotic dosing in clinical practice include demographic, pharmacokinetic and physiological differences which should be explored in detail so they can be included in systems, toxicology-derived models and can be applied in a continuous process of monitoring and reassessment of a drug's safety throughout all its development phases.

One example of this can be found in the treatment of obesity. Since the incidence of obesity has increased rapidly worldwide, prescribing appropriate doses of drugs requiring weight-based dosing is challenging in the case of overweight patients due to a lack of data [88]. Specifically, obesity has been shown to be associated with treatment failure due to antibiotic underdosing.

Ghobadi and colleagues recently proposed a mechanistic predictive pharmacokinetic model that includes the physiological and biochemical changes associated with obesity and morbid obesity, and which allows the prediction of changes in drug clearance on the basis of *in vitro* data [89]. They used the Simcyp Population-based Simulator™ for predicting the population distribution of the pharmacokinetic outcome by integrating large demographic, genetic, physiological and pathological data collected on obese adults, together with *in vitro* data on human drug metabolism. Parameters considered were hepatic clearance, first-pass gut-wall metabolism, severity of obesity, age, gender, body mass index, body surface area, cardiac output, liver volume, hepatic blood flow, CYP450 enzyme activity, protein binding, haematocrit, kidney volume, renal function and gastrointestinal tract blood flow. This model requires further validation for specific anti-infective drugs so that it can be applied for appropriate trial design of population pharmacokinetic studies or for clinical management of drugs in obese patients.

In addition, Mahmood used total body weight and simple allometry to create a model that predicts drug clearance in the obese individuals using data obtained from normal weight subjects. Daptomycin, cefazoline, tobramycin and vancomycin were included in this retrospective analysis that can now be used to select the initial dose for a clinical trial of the obese subjects [90]. However, Le and colleagues found that in children, and at least for vancomycin, pharmacokinetic differences between obese and normal weight pediatric patients are small and not likely to be clinically relevant in dose variation [91]. Either way, there are still very few pharmacokinetic studies on obese children that can help to predict drug disposition of antimicrobial agents in this group [92].

In conclusion, continuous data generation, validation, and analysis as well as model re-formulation are essential to meet the needs of this new era in drug development.

Linking Pharmacovigilance with Pharmacogenomics to Find Drug Safety Solutions

Because of the well-known limitations of preclinical and clinical studies, post-marketing drug safety monitoring is crucial for the identification of risks, toxicity mechanisms and trigger factors that can be meticulously studied and then validated 'back into' the early stages of drug development.

Furthermore, improving pharmacovigilance methods is not only a concern for new drugs but also for the existing drugs that are being used in an off-label manner or which were not originally studied before approval under the clinical conditions in which they are being used today (*i.e.* comorbidities and polypharmacy) [50].

Considering that one of the most challenging factors in understanding variability in drug safety is individual susceptibility, linking pharmacogenomics with pharmacovigilance information which may be very helpful to identify potential drug safety solutions and their application in drug discovery.

One example of an initiative that uses this approach is the Canadian Pharmacogenomics Network for Drug Safety or CPNDS Consortium (formerly called GATC or 'Genotype-specific Approaches to Therapy in Childhood'), which has been investigating the associations between severe ADRs and genetic markers and then translating them to the clinic in order to prevent their occurrence. In a 4-year period study, the CPNDS database containing 326 pediatric reports of cutaneous adverse drug reactions (CADRs) was analyzed and it was found that 65.6% of these CADRs were classified as severe including: anaphylaxis, erythema multiforme, drug rash with eosinophilia and systemic symptoms syndrome (DRESS), serum sickness-like reaction (SSLR), Stevens-Johnson syndrome (SJS), rash cases covering 50% or more of the body surface area, as well as other CADRs with possible life-threatening indicators [93]. Antibacterials (n = 95, 41.8%) were the most common cause of these severe CADRs. Based on this, the identification of genetic markers conferring risk of developing the different types of CADRs is of great interest and even more so in pediatrics.

The main limitations for the collection of the data required to undertake such a pharmacovigilance/pharmacogenomics study are the underreporting rates within voluntary surveillance systems, the inappropriate ADR phenotyping (which *i.e.* is very common for CADRs), and the number of well-characterized cases and controls needed to obtain sufficient statistical power to detect genetic effects [50].

Nevertheless, the incorporation of pharmacogenomics into routine clinical practice is becoming a reality. In 2014 the Clinical Pharmacogenetics Implementation Consortium (CPIC) published their recommendations to properly prepare clinical guidelines for drug therapy optimization based on the patients' genotype [94]. So far therapeutic ineffectiveness and other severe ADRs are the main phenotypes already associated with specific genotypes in the CPIC guidelines, which are available for download from the Pharmacogenomics Knowledgebase (PharmGkb) website: www.pharmgkb.org [95]. Table **3** modestly summarizes the vast amount of information contained in the CPIC guidelines for anti-infective agents to date.

Table 3. Genetic variants that have been validated for their association with specific anti-infective drug-induced adverse reactions and which screening is currently recommended in the CPIC guidelines for drug selection and dosing according to patient's genotype [94-96].

Anti-Infective Drug	Adverse Reaction	Genotype(s)	Recommendation for Therapy
Abacavir	Life-threatening hypersensitivity reactions (affect 6% of patients)	HLA-B*57:01 positive (presence varies across ethnic groups)	Strong: If present, drug is not recommended, consider an alternative drug. Screening should be performed before initiation of therapy.
Atazanavir	Hyperbilirubinemia with jaundice (40-48% of patients with grade 3/grade 4 plasma indirect bilirubin elevation) with high risk of non-adherence and premature discontinuation	Poor metabolizer genotypes: UGT1A1 *28/*28; *28/*37; *37/*37; rs887829 T/T (*80/*80), *6/*6	Strong: Consider an alternative agent particularly where jaundice would be of concern to the patient.
Boceprevir PEG-IFN alfa – 2a	Unfavorable sustained virologic response to PEG-interferon-alpha-	IFNL3 (IL28B) rs12979860 CT or TT	Strong: Unfavorable effect on response

PEG-IFN alfa – 2b	containing regimens		rates.
Ribavirin			
Telaprevir			

In the field of idiosyncratic ADRs, other important findings have been made related to genetic variants in the human leukocyte antigen (HLA) region. Strong associations have been found for life-threatening hypersensitivity reactions induced by abacavir (HLA-B*57:01) and for carbamazepine (HLA-B*15:02 and HLA-A*31:01). The findings for abacavir were validated and lead to the creation of now available dosing guidelines (Table 3) [97], which is also the case for the association found between carbamazepine and the HLA-B*15:02 genotype [98]. Moreover, it has been suggested that HLA-A*31:01 is a predictive biomarker of carbamazepine-induced hypersensitivity across various ancestries [99] which underscores the relevance of doing further HLA genotyping studies in correlation with other drugs.

Although there is paucity *of available* information on genetic antimicrobial-safety markers already validated for their translation to the clinic, it is important to recognize that most ADRs result from a mixture of clinical, environmental, and genetic factors, and that before embarking on pharmacogenomic investigation, researchers are prompted to evaluate which ADRs are most likely to possess a genetic component that is feasible for study. To that end, a prioritization tool was recently proposed by Shaw and colleagues, to facilitate the selection of ideal study targets, as well as optimizing study design for successful discovery and replication of clinically relevant genetic biomarkers [100].

As suggested for other methods and strategies throughout this chapter, these tools and data can be used for the further investigation of drugs already on the market or during the research and development process of new medicines.

CONCLUDING REMARKS

In our globalized world, one would expect a rapid and efficient flow of information when a safety signal arises for drugs that are under development as well as for those already on the market. Unfortunately, most adverse events occurring in clinical practice remain underreported due to ineffective pharmacovigilance systems. Moreover, adverse events occurring in clinical trials are seldom published especially when a trial ends before completion. Stockmann and colleagues mined the ClinicalTrials.gov database for all registered antimicrobial research studies conducted since the year 2000 and found that only

7% of a total of more than 16,000 studies had reported results [101]. Regardless of the negative or inconclusive outcomes of a clinical trial, journal editors are presently offering many initiatives to foster the dissemination of clinical study results. Regulatory agencies should also encourage the publication of the results of clinical trials and adverse events occurring during research, in order to support antimicrobial development and evidence-based prescribing.

In any case, it is clear that safety issues related to anti-infective drugs must be identified promptly, all the way from research to clinical practice by taking advantage of the powerful tools that are now available to assess safety in the early stages of drug development.

It is well known that time, cost and regulatory requisites have increased for testing new drug candidates in humans. This situation has created much interest in the development of more suitable models that can provide predictive information about human drug metabolism and toxicity. *In silico* methods, humanized mouse models, translational biomarkers, and genomic technologies offer the possibility of confronting the current and future challenges of drug development, *i.e.* the implementation of personalized medicine strategies and the assessment of drug efficacy and safety of new anti-infectives developed for the treatment of emerging resistant human pathogens. These drug safety approaches will have a great impact on global health issues and the pharmacological industry, by increasing the output of successful pharmaceutical products intended to treat emerging and re-emerging infectious diseases.

CONFLICT OF INTEREST

The authors confirm that there are no known conflicts of interest associated with this chapter.

ACKNOWLEDGEMENTS

We would like to thank Rachel M. West (rmartwest@gmail.com) for the English editing and proofreading of our manuscript.

REFERENCES

[1]   Hansch C, Fujita T. p-σ-π Analysis. A method for the correlation of biological activity and chemical structure. J Am Chem Soc 1964; 86(8): 1616-1626.
[2]   Showalter HDH, Denny WA. A roadmap for drug discovery and its translation to small molecule agents in clinical development for tuberculosis treatment. Tuberculosis (Edinb) 2008; 88(Suppl 1): S3–17.

[3]   Avorn J. The $2.6 billion pill--methodologic and policy considerations. N Engl J Med 2015; 372: 1877–1879.

[4]   Morris GM, Huey R, Lindstrom W, *et al.* AutoDock4 and AutoDockTools4: Automated docking with selective receptor flexibility. J Comput Chem 2009; 30: 2785–2791.

[5]   Trott O, Olson AJ. AutoDock Vina: improving the speed and accuracy of docking with a new scoring function, efficient optimization, and multithreading. J Comput Chem 2010; 31: 455–461.

[6]   Cramer GM, Ford RA, Hall RL. Estimation of toxic hazard--a decision tree approach. Food Cosmet Toxicol 1978; 16: 255–276.

[7]   Patlewicz G, Jeliazkova N, Safford RJ, Worth AP, Aleksiev B. An evaluation of the implementation of the Cramer classification scheme in the Toxtree software. SAR QSAR Environ Res 2008; 19(5-6): 495–524.

[8]   Verhaar HJM, van Leeuwen CJ, Hermens JLM. Classifying environmental pollutants. 1: Structure-activity relationships for prediction of aquatic toxicity. Chemosphere 1992; 25: 471–491.

[9]   Hermens JL. Electrophiles and acute toxicity to fish. Environ Health Perspect 1990; 87: 219–225.

[10]   Verhaar HJ, Solbé J, Speksnijder J, van Leeuwen CJ, Hermens JL. Classifying environmental pollutants: Part 3. External validation of the classification system. Chemosphere 2000; 40: 875–883.

[11]   Enoch SJ, Hewitt M, Cronin MTD, Azam S, Madden JC. Classification of chemicals according to mechanism of aquatic toxicity: an evaluation of the implementation of the Verhaar scheme in Toxtree. Chemosphere 2008; 73(3): 243-248.

[12]   Gerner I, Schlegel K, Walker JD, Hulzebos E. Use of physicochemical property limits to develop rules for identifying chemical substances with no skin irritation or corrosion potential. QSAR Comb Sci 2004; 23: 726–733.

[13]   Enoch SJ, Madden JC, Cronin MTD. Identification of mechanisms of toxic action for skin sensitisation using a SMARTS pattern based approach. SAR QSAR Environ Res 2008; 19: 555–578.

[14]   Enoch SJ, Cronin MTD. A review of the electrophilic reaction chemistry involved in covalent DNA binding. Crit Rev Toxicol 2010; 40: 728–748.

[15]   Rydberg P, Gloriam DE, Zaretzki J, Breneman C, Olsen L. SMARTCyp: A 2D method for prediction of cytochrome P450-mediated drug metabolism. ACS Med Chem Lett 2010; 1: 96–100.

[16]   Enoch SJ, Ellison CM, Schultz TW, Cronin MTD. A review of the electrophilic reaction chemistry involved in covalent protein binding relevant to toxicity. Crit Rev Toxicol. 2011; 41(9): 783–802.

[17]   Mortelmans K, Zeiger E. The Ames Salmonella/microsome mutagenicity assay. Mutat Res. 2000; 455 (1–2): 29–60.

[18]   Debnath AK, Debnath G, Shusterman AJ, Hansch C. A QSAR investigation of the role of hydrophobicity in regulating mutagenicity in the Ames test: 1. Mutagenicity of aromatic and heteroaromatic amines in Salmonella typhimurium TA98 and TA100. Environ Mol Mutagen 1992; 19: 37–52.

[19]   Benigni R, Bossa C, Netzeva T, Rodomonte A, Tsakovska I. Mechanistic QSAR of aromatic amines: new models for discriminating between homocyclic mutagens and nonmutagens, and validation of models for carcinogens. Environ Mol Mutagen 2007; 48: 754–771.

[20]   Speck-Planche A, Cordeiro MNDS. Simultaneous virtual prediction of anti-Escherichia coli activities and ADMET profiles: A chemoinformatic complementary approach for high-throughput screening. ACS Comb Sci 2014; 16: 78–84.

[21]   Speck-Planche A, Cordeiro MNDS. Computer-aided discovery in antimicrobial research: In silico model for virtual screening of potent and safe anti-pseudomonas agents. Comb Chem High Throughput Screen 2015; 18: 305–314.

[22]   Redfern WS, Waldron G, Winter MJ, *et al.* Zebrafish assays as early safety pharmacology screens: paradigm shift or red herring? J Pharmacol Toxicol Methods 2008; 58(2): 110-7.

[23]   Zak O, O'Reilly T. Animal models in the evaluation of antimicrobial agents. Antimicrob Agents Chemother 1991; 35(8): 1527-31.

[24]   Van Meer PJ, Kooijman M, Gispen-de Wied CC, Moors EH, Schellekens H. The ability of animal studies to detect serious post marketing adverse events is limited. Regul Toxicol Pharmacol 2012; 64(3): 345-9.

[25]   Velkov T, Bergen PJ, Lora-Tamayo J, Landersdorfer CB, Li J. PK/PD models in antibacterial development. Curr Opin Microbiol 2013; 16(5): 573-9.

[26] Aung AK, Haas DW, Hulgan T, Phillips EJ. Pharmacogenomics of antimicrobial agents. Pharmacogenomics 2014; 15(15): 1903-30.

[27] Andes D, Craig WA. Animal model pharmacokinetics and pharmacodynamics: a critical review. Int J Antimicrob Agents 2002; 19(4): 261-8.

[28] Tang C, Prueksaritanont T. Use of *in vivo* animal models to assess pharmacokinetic drug-drug interactions. Pharm Res 2010; 27(9): 1772-87.

[29] Ordas A, Raterink RJ, Cunningham F, *et al*. Testing tuberculosis drug efficacy in a zebrafish high-throughput translational medicine screen. Antimicrob Agents Chemother 2015; 59(2): 753-62.

[30] Berghmans S, Butler P, Goldsmith P, *et al*. Zebrafish based assays for the assessment of cardiac, visual and gut function--potential safety screens for early drug discovery. J Pharmacol Toxicol Methods 2008; 58(1): 59-68.

[31] He JH, Guo SY, Zhu F, *et al*. A zebrafish phenotypic assay for assessing drug-induced hepatotoxicity. J Pharmacol Toxicol Methods 2013; 67(1): 25-32.

[32] Li C, Lin WS, McGrath P. Whole zebrafish cytochrome P450 microplate assays for assessing drug metabolism and drug safety. J Pharmacol Toxicol Methods 2009; 60(2): 233.

[33] Zhu JJ, Xu YQ, He JH, *et al*. Human cardiotoxic drugs delivered by soaking and microinjection induce cardiovascular toxicity in zebrafish. J Appl Toxicol 2014; 34(2): 139-48.

[34] McKee RA, Wingert RA. Zebrafish renal pathology: Emerging models of acute kidney injury. Curr Pathobiol Rep 2015; 3(2): 171-181.

[35] Barros TP, Alderton WK, Reynolds HM, Roach AG, Berghmans S. Zebrafish: an emerging technology for in vivo pharmacological assessment to identify potential safety liabilities in early drug discovery. Br J Pharmacol 2008; 154(7): 1400-13.

[36] Hentschel DM, Park KM, Cilenti L, Zervos AS, Drummond I, Bonventre JV. Acute renal failure in zebrafish: a novel system to study a complex disease. Am J Physiol Renal Physiol 2005; 288(5): F923-9.

[37] Legrand N, Ploss A, Balling R, *et al*. Humanized mice for modeling human infectious disease: challenges, progress, and outlook. Cell Host Microbe 2009; 6(1): 5-9.

[38] Peltz G. Can 'humanized' mice improve drug development in the 21st century? Trends Pharmacol Sci 2013; 34(5): 255-60.

[39] Scheer N, Wilson ID. A comparison between genetically humanized and chimeric liver humanized mouse models for studies in drug metabolism and toxicity. Drug Discov Today 2015 Sep 7. pii: S1359-6446(15)00342-6.

[40] Nishimura T, Hu Y, Wu M, *et al*. Using chimeric mice with humanized livers to predict human drug metabolism and a drug-drug interaction. J Pharmacol Exp Ther 2013; 344(2): 388-96.

[41] Hu Y, Wu M, Nishimura T, Zheng M, Peltz G. Human pharmacogenetic analysis in chimeric mice with 'humanized livers'. Pharmacogenet Genomics 2013; 23(2): 78-83.

[42] Brehm MA, Jouvet N, Greiner DL, Shultz LD. Humanized mice for the study of infectious diseases. Curr Opin Immunol 2013; 25(4): 428-35.

[43] Sliva K. Latest animal models for anti-HIV drug discovery. Expert Opin Drug Discov 2015; 10(2): 111-23.

[44] Zhang L, Su L. HIV-1 immunopathogenesis in humanized mouse models. Cell Mol Immunol 2012; 9(3): 237-44.

[45] Bird BH, Spengler JR, Chakrabarti AK, Khristova ML, Sealy TK, Coleman-McCray JD, *et al*. Humanized mouse model of Ebola virus disease mimics immune responses in human disease. J Infect Dis 2015 Nov 17. pii: jiv538.

[46] Frias-Staheli N, Dorner M, Marukian S, Billerbeck E, Labitt RN, Rice CM, Ploss A. Utility of humanized BLT mice for analysis of dengue virus infection and antiviral drug testing. J Virol 2014; 88(4): 2205-18.

[47] Chiba K. Perspective of humanized mouse models for assessing PK/PD and toxic profile of drug candidates in preclinical study. Drug Metab Pharmacokinet 2014; 29(1): 1-2.

[48] Ling LL, Schneider T, Peoples AJ, *et al*. A new antibiotic kills pathogens without detectable resistance. Nature 2015; 517(7535): 455-9.

[49] Campion S, Aubrecht J, Boekelheide K, *et al*. The current status of biomarkers for predicting toxicity. Expert Opin Drug Metab Toxicol 2013; 9(11): 1391-408.

[50]   Castro-Pastrana L, Carleton BC. Improving Pediatric Drug Safety: need for more efficient clinical translation of pharmacovigilance knowledge. J Popul Ther Clin Pharmacol 2011; 18(1): e76-e88.

[51]   Aronson JK. Distinguishing Hazards and Harms, Adverse Drug Effects and Adverse Drug Reactions. Drug Saf 2013; 36(3): 147-153.

[52]   Van der Graaf R, Roes KC, Van Delden JJ. Adaptive trials in clinical research: scientific and ethical issues to consider. JAMA 2012; 307(22): 2379-80.

[53]   Watkins PB, Merz M, Avigan MI, Kaplowitz N, Regev A, Senior JR. The clinical liver safety assessment best practices workshop: rationale, goals, accomplishments and the future. Drug Saf 2014; 37(Suppl 1): S1-7.

[54]   Senior JR. Evolution of the Food and Drug Administration approach to liver safety assessment for new drugs: current status and challenges. Drug Saf 2014; 37(Suppl 1): S9-17.

[55]   FDA [Internet]. Guidance for industry drug-induced liver injury: premarketing clinical evaluation. Rockville, MD: FDA 2009 [cited: 15th Jan 2016]. Available from: http://www.fda.gov/downloads/Drugs/./Guidances/UCM174090.pdf

[56]   Watkins PB, Desai M, Berkowitz SD, *et al*. Evaluation of drug-induced serious hepatotoxicity (eDISH): application of this data organization approach to phase III clinical trials of rivaroxaban after total hip or knee replacement surgery. Drug Saf 2011; 34(3): 243-52.

[57]   Hu Z, Lausted C, Yoo H, *et al*. Quantitative liver-specific protein fingerprint in blood: a signature for hepatotoxicity. Theranostics 2014; 4(2): 215-28.

[58]   Collins SL, Carr DF, Pirmohamed M. Advances in the Pharmacogenomics of Adverse Drug Reactions. Drug Saf 2016; 39(1): 15-27.

[59]   Leone A, Nie A, Brandon Parker J, *et al*. Oxidative stress/reactive metabolite gene expression signature in rat liver detects idiosyncratic hepatotoxicants. Toxicol Appl Pharmacol 2014; 275(3): 189-97.

[60]   Cui Y, Paules RS. Use of transcriptomics in understanding mechanisms of drug-induced toxicity. Pharmacogenomics 2010; 11(4): 573-585.

[61]   Weiler S, Merz M, Kullak-Ublick GA. Drug-induced liver injury: the dawn of biomarkers? F1000Prime Rep. 2015; 7: 34.

[62]   Wallace KB, Hausner E, Herman E, *et al*. Serum troponins as biomarkers of drug-induced cardiac toxicity. Toxicol Pathol 2004; 32(1): 106-21.

[63]   Piccini JP, Whellan DJ, Berridge BR, *et al*. Current challenges in the evaluation of cardiac safety during drug development: translational medicine meets the Critical Path Initiative. Am Heart J 2009; 158(3):317–326.

[64]   Stockbridge N, Morganroth J, Shah RR, Garnett C. Dealing with global safety issues: was the response to QT-liability of non-cardiac drugs well-coordinated? Drug Saf 2013; 36(3): 167-82.

[65]   De Ponti F, Poluzzi E, Cavalli A, Recanatini M, Montanaro N. Safety of non-antiarrhythmic drugs that prolong the QT interval or induce torsade de pointes: an overview. Drug Saf 2002; 25(4): 263-86.

[66]   Raschi E, Poluzzi E, Zuliani C, Muller A, Goossens H, De Ponti F. Exposure to antibacterial agents with QT liability in 14 European countries: trends over an 8-year period. Br J Clin Pharmacol 2009; 67(1): 88-98.

[67]   Poluzzi E, Raschi E, Motola D, Moretti U, De Ponti F. Antimicrobials and the risk of torsades de pointes: the contribution from data mining of the US FDA Adverse Event Reporting System. Drug Saf 2010; 33(4): 303-14.

[68]   European Agency for the Evaluation of Medicinal Products (EMEA) [Internet]. Committee for Proprietary Medicinal Products (CPMP): points to consider: the assessment of the potential for QT interval prolongation by non-cardiovascular medicinal products. CPMP/986/96. London: EMEA 1997 [cited: 15th January 2016]. Available from: http://www.fda.gov/ohrms/dockets/ac/03/briefing/pubs/cpmp.pdf

[69]   Paltoo B, O'Donoghue S, Mousavi MS. Levofloxacin induced polymorphic ventricular tachycardia with normal QT interval. Pacing Clin Electrophysiol 2001; 24: 895–7.

[70]   Scheiber J, Jenkins JL, Sukuru SC, *et al*. Mapping adverse drug reactions in chemical space. J Med Chem 2009; 52(9): 3103-7.

[71]   Bass AS, Darpo B, Breidenbach A, *et al*. International Life Sciences Institute (Health and Environmental Sciences Institute, HESI) initiative on moving towards better predictors of drug-induced torsades de pointes. Br J Pharmacol 2008; 154(7): 1491-501.

[72]   Vilar S, Tatonetti NP, Hripcsak G. 3D pharmacophoric similarity improves multi adverse drug event identification in pharmacovigilance. Sci Rep 2015; 5: 8809.

[73]   Park J, Noh K, Lee HW, *et al*. Pharmacometabolomic approach to predict QT prolongation in guinea pigs. PLoS One 2013; 8(4): e60556.

[74]   Niemeijer MN, van den Berg ME, Eijgelsheim M, Rijnbeek PR, Stricker BH. Pharmacogenetics of Drug-Induced QT Interval Prolongation: An Update. Drug Saf 2015; 38(10): 855-67.

[75]   Owens RC Jr. QT prolongation with antimicrobial agents: understanding the significance. Drugs 2004; 64(10): 1091-124.

[76]   Burt D, Crowell SJ, Ackley DC, Magee TV, Aubrecht J. Application of emerging biomarkers of acute kidney injury in development of kidney-sparing polypeptide-based antibiotics. Drug Chem Toxicol 2014; 37(2): 204-12.

[77]   Davis JW 2nd, Goodsaid FM, Bral CM, *et al*. Quantitative gene expression analysis in a nonhuman primate model of antibiotic-induced nephrotoxicity. Toxicol Appl Pharmacol 2004; 200(1): 16-26.

[78]   McWilliam SJ, Antoine DJ, Sabbisetti V, *et al*. Reference intervals for urinary renal injury biomarkers KIM-1 and NGAL in healthy children. Biomark Med 2014; 8(10): 1189-97.

[79]   Bennett MR, Nehus E, Haffner C, Ma Q, Devarajan P. Pediatric reference ranges for acute kidney injury biomarkers. Pediatr Nephrol 2015; 30(4): 677-85.

[80]   McWilliam SJ, Antoine DJ, Sabbisetti V, *et al*. Mechanism-based urinary biomarkers to identify the potential for aminoglycoside-induced nephrotoxicity inpremature neonates: a proof-of-concept study. PLoS One 2012; 7(8): e43809.

[81]   Davis JW, Kramer JA. Genomic-based biomarkers of drug-induced nephrotoxicity. Expert Opin Drug Metab Toxicol 2006; 2(1): 95-101.

[82]   Velo G, Moretti U. Ecopharmacovigilance for better health. Drug Saf 2010; 33(11): 963-8.

[83]   Oliveira R, McDonough S, Ladewig JC, Soares AM, Nogueira AJ, Domingues I. Effects of oxytetracycline and amoxicillin on development and biomarkers activities of zebrafish (Danio rerio). Environ Toxicol Pharmacol 2013; 36(3): 903-12.

[84]   Bartoskova M, Dobsikova R, Stancova V, *et al*. Norfloxacin--toxicity for Zebrafish (Danio rerio) focused on oxidative stress parameters. Biomed Res Int 2014; 2014: 560235.

[85]   Plhalova L, Zivna D, Bartoskova M, *et al*. The effects of subchronic exposure to ciprofloxacin on zebrafish (Danio rerio). Neuro Endocrinol Lett 2014; 35(Suppl 2): 64-70.

[86]   Dong L, Gao J, Xie X, Zhou Q. DNA damage and biochemical toxicity of antibiotics in soil on the earthworm Eisenia fetida. Chemosphere 2012; 89(1): 44-51.

[87]   Glynn P, Unudurthi SD, Hund TJ. Mathematical modeling of physiological systems: An essential tool for discovery. Life Sci 2014; 111(1-2): 1-5.

[88]   Kane-Gill SL, Wytiaz NP, Thompson LM, *et al*. A real-world, multicenter assessment of drugs requiring weight-based calculations in overweight, adult critically ill patients. Sci World J 2013; 2013: 909135.

[89]   Ghobadi C, Johnson TN, Aarabi M, *et al*. Application of a systems approach to the bottom-up assessment of pharmacokinetics in obese patients: expected variations in clearance. Clin Pharmacokinet 2011; 50(12): 809-22.

[90]   Mahmood I. Prediction of clearance and volume of distribution in the obese from normal weight subjects: an allometric approach. Clin Pharmacokinet 2012; 51(8): 527-42.

[91]   Le J, Capparelli EV, Wahid U, *et al*. Bayesian estimation of vancomycin pharmacokinetics in obese children: matched case-control study. Clin Ther 2015; 37(6): 1340-51.

[92]   Sampson M, Cohen-Wolkowiez M, Benjamin D Jr, Capparelli E, Watt K. Pharmacokinetics of Antimicrobials in Obese Children. GaBI J 2013; 2(2): 76-81.

[93]   Castro-Pastrana LI, Ghannadan R, Rieder MJ, Dahlke E, Hayden M, Carleton B. Cutaneous adverse drug reactions in children: an analysis of reports from the Canadian Pharmacogenomics Network for Drug Safety (CPNDS). J Popul Ther Clin Pharmacol 2011; 18: e106-20.

[94]   Caudle KE, Klein TE, Hoffman JM, *et al*. Incorporation of Pharmacogenomics into Routine Clinical Practice: the Clinical Pharmacogenetics Implementation Consortium (CPIC) Guideline Development Process. Curr Drug Metab 2014; 15: 209-217.

[95]   Pharmgkb.org [Internet]. Dosing Guidelines – CPIC. Stanford, CA: PharmGKB; c2001-2015 [cited: 15th January 2016]. Available from: https://www.pharmgkb.org/view/dosing-guidelines.do?source=CPIC

[96]   Whirl-Carrillo M, McDonagh EM, Hebert JM, *et al.* Pharmacogenomics Knowledge for Personalized Medicine. Clin Pharmacol Ther 2012; 92(4): 414-417.

[97]   Martin MA, Hoffman JM, Freimuth RR, *et al.* Clinical Pharmacogenetics Implementation Consortium Guidelines for HLA-B Genotype and Abacavir Dosing: 2014 update. Clin Pharmacol Ther 2014; 95(5): 499-500.

[98]   Leckband SG, Kelsoe JR, Dunnenberger HM, *et al.* Clinical Pharmacogenetics Implementation Consortium guidelines for HLA-B genotype and carbamazepine dosing. Clin Pharmacol Ther 2013; 94(3): 324-8.

[99]   Amstutz U, Ross CJ, Castro-Pastrana LI, *et al.* HLA-A 31:01 and HLA-B 15:02 as genetic markers for carbamazepine hypersensitivity in children. Clin Pharmacol Ther 2013; 94(1): 142-9.

[100]   Shaw K, Amstutz U, Castro-Pastrana L, *et al.* Pharmacogenomic investigation of adverse drug reactions (ADRs): the ADR prioritization tool, APT. J Popul Ther Clin Pharmacol 2013; 20(2): e110-27.

[101]   Stockmann C, Sherwin CM, Ampofo K, *et al.* Characteristics of antimicrobial studies registered in the USA through ClinicalTrials.Gov. Int J Antimicrob Agents 2013; 42(2): 161-6.

CHAPTER 4

Topical Antimicrobials: Classification and Performance

Daryl S. Paulson[*]

BioScience Laboratories, Inc., Bozeman, Montana, USA

Abstract: Since the discovery by Semmelweis that washing hands with chlorine decreased morbidity and mortality rates, the antimicrobial products market has grown tremendously. This chapter provides a brief introduction to the topical antimicrobial products currently on the market, how they are classified, how they work, and the purposes for which they are best suited. Among the first products used as a surgical scrub was an iodine complex (a tincture of iodine and an aqueous iodophor), which provides excellent immediate antimicrobial action. Another product, Chlorhexidine gluconate, which was first synthesized in 1950, has proved to provide high levels of antimicrobial activity and considerable effectiveness in healthcare personnel handwash applications. Alcohol and alcohol compounds also provide effective immediate effects but little to no residual or persistent activity. As the market has developed and scientific knowledge increased, product manufacturers have greatly improved product formulations, including the development of products containing quaternary ammonium compounds, which are used in household cleaners, disinfections, skin and hair care formulations, sanitizers, sterilizing solutions for medical devices, and even preservatives; parachlorometaxylenol product formulations are used primarily for healthcare personnel handwashes, as they are effective in removing transient microorganisms from the hands and have low skin irritation potential; and triclosan, which has fair immediate and persistent antimicrobial ability, but no residual action, has been formulated for a wide range of applications, including the food industry and consumer product lines. New products are constantly being formulated, tested, and brought to the market, according to the guidelines of the Food and Drug Administration.

Keywords: Alcohol, CHG, healthcare personnel handwash, iodine, PCMX, products, surgical scrubs, topical antimicrobial.

INTRODUCTION

Semmelweis' [1] mandate - that physicians washed their hands with chlorine before they performed patient examinations - decreased morbidity and mortality rates in maternity wards and resulted in many positive changes in the antimicrobial

[*]**Address correspondence to Daryl S. Paulson:** BioScience Laboratories, Inc., 1765 South 19th Avenue, Bozeman, Montana 59715, USA; Tel: 406-587-5735, EXT. 104; Fax: 406-586-7930; E-mail: dpaulson@biosciencelabs.com.

Atta-ur-Rahman (Ed)
All rights reserved-© 2016 Bentham Science Publishers

market in the past twenty-five years. Among the changes, the market has seen many new developments in products and new methods of decontaminating the hand surfaces prior to examining patients or performing surgery [2]. Also, the Food and Drug Administration (FDA) has mandated their own requirements as to how these products must perform [3]. The questions that this chapter will answer include: 1) "What are now the different classifications of antimicrobials?", 2) "How do they work?", and 3) "Which one is best to use?"

The antimicrobial products of primary interest include iodine complexes (aqueous iodophors and tinctures), iodine and alcohol, aqueous formulations of chlorhexidine gluconate (CHG), triclosan, and parachlorometaxylenol (PCMX) alcohol formulations with tinctures of iodine or CHG, as well as quaternary ammonium products and combinations of quaternary ammonium and alcohol. Let us review some general aspects of these topical antimicrobials.

IODINE COMPLEXES

Iodine was one of the first substances used as a surgical scrub, healthcare personnel handwash, and a preoperative skin preparation [4]. In its pure form, iodine is relatively insoluble in water without a solubilizing agent, but it dissolves well in various alcohols to provide an iodine tincture. Tinctures of iodine are used primarily as antiseptics for healthcare personnel handwashes, surgical scrubs and preoperative skin preparations [5].

By far, the most common form of iodine for use as a topical antimicrobial is the iodophor. Iodophors are complexes of elemental iodine (tri-iodine) linked to a carrier having several functions: 1) increased degrees of solubility in aqueous solution for the iodine; 2) provision of a sustained release reservoir of the iodine; and 3) reduced equilibrium concentrations of free iodine. The most commonly used carriers are neutral polymers, polyacrylic acids, polyether glycols, polyamides, polysaccharides and polyalkalines.

The most commonly used iodophor is povidone iodine, a compound of 1-vinyl-2-pyrrolidinone polymer with available iodine ranging between 9% and 12% (United States Pharmacopoeia XXIII) [6].

Range of Action

Iodophors and tinctures of iodine provide excellent immediate antimicrobial action against a broad range of viruses, both Gram-positive and Gram-negative bacteria, fungi (molds and yeasts), and various protozoa [7]. In fact, almost all important human disease-causing microorganisms, including enteric bacteria, enteric viruses, protozoan trophozoites and cysts, mycobacteria, spores of *Bacillus spp.*, and *Clostridium spp.* and many fungal species are susceptible to free iodine [7]. It should be noted, however, that exposure times and concentrations of available iodine required vary.

In topical application to skin surfaces (*e.g.*, hands and body surfaces in the inguinal, abdominal, anterior cubital, subclavian, and femoral regions), iodophors and tinctures of iodine providing at least 1% available iodine demonstrate effective immediate and persistent antimicrobial properties. In general, however, neither provides residual antimicrobial action [8].

Application

Healthcare Personnel Handwashes

This application removes transient microorganisms from the hands of surgical staff members examining a prospective surgical candidate, for healthcare personnel professionals examining patients, and for citizens trying to stay healthy. Its purpose is to kill only transient microorganisms picked up by contact with contaminated hands or surfaces with other surfaces before they can be passed on to other patients, staff members, or citizens [9].

There are several companies making low levels of this product (6-7% concentration) used for this purpose. However, the irritation and staining potential of these products, as well as the slow drying process, has eroded the markets (See PVPI plus Alcohol).

However, certain medical practitioners from the "old school" still recommend this product. It is effective, one can see it on the hand surfaces, and it demonstrates good antimicrobial properties, as it has the ability to kill the vast majority of various microorganisms in relatively high numbers.

Surgical Scrub Formulations

A surgical scrub procedure is more broad-spectrum in its ability than a healthcare personnel handwash. Recall that a healthcare personnel handwash is intended to remove only those bacteria, yeasts, molds, and viruses-those "picked up from other sources"-which are transient. The surgical scrub formulation is intended to remove these transient organisms and the deeper, resident microorganisms that normally reside on the hand surfaces, in skin crevices, and under the fingernails.

The microorganisms normally residing on the hand surfaces are predominantly *Staphylococcus epidermidis*, but there are many other types of bacteria that also reside there, including *Actinobacteria*, *Corynebacteria*, *Propionibacterium*, *Micrococcineae*, and others, such as *Proteobacteria*, which have not been classified. It depends upon the nutrients, the hand surface areas, the environment where the hands have been, the amount of moisture, and the chemicals to which the hands have been subjected.

Iodophors are effective in killing these microorganisms, and they were the drug of choice for many years, containing 5%-10% active ingredient [10]. Their use is gradually being eroded by chlorhexidine gluconates, combinations of CHGs, and alcohols, in addition to other alcohol combinations, to provide more persistent antimicrobial effects. There is also a combination of alcohol and PVPI, which is competing against the alcohol and CHG products [11].

The down-side of PVPI is that it tends to severely stain garments; also, the application time is overly long (taking up to 5-6 minutes) for modern hospital settings [9]. This keeps a surgeon and his staff waiting, and waiting costs money. Additionally, some users are hyper-allergic to iodine complexes.

Preoperative Skin Preparations

When a patient undergoes surgery, her skin is prepared at the proposed incision site with a preoperative skin solution. In these cases, the drug must reduce the bacteria (both resident and transient) considerably and keep those counts below baseline for six hours post-preparation [3].

There are many types of microorganisms at various levels at the sites, so a broad-spectrum drug is necessary, and iodine is broad-spectrum. Most products are marketed in a 5-10% povidone solution. It is not a fast-acting drug, so it requires considerable preparation and drying time. Older surgeons were taught to make their incisions within the stained area; hence, they tend to prefer it, because they can clearly see the dark orange coloration of the prepped area as the application dries.

ALCOHOL AND PVPI

When alcohol was added to the formulations of PVPI, it enhanced the product considerably. It has a both faster application time and drying time, and it now has greater immediate efficacy from the alcohol and increased persistence from the PVPI [12].

The major change with this product has been for the preoperative skin preparation application. Now, it can compete with the other products more successfully. In this study, the FDA requires a three log_{10} reduction at the inguinal site and a two log_{10} reduction at the abdominal site at ten minutes. If alcohol is included in the formulation, it can compete for two minutes.

CHLORHEXIDINE GLUCONATE

Chlorhexidine gluconate (CHG) was first synthesized in 1950 by ICI Pharmaceuticals in England [13]. CHG has high levels of antimicrobial activity, and relatively low levels of toxicity to mammalian cells. Additionally, CHG has a strong affinity for skin and mucous membranes [14]. As a result, CHG has been used as a topical antimicrobial for wounds, skin-prepping, and mucous membranes (especially in dentistry), where it provides, by virtue of its proclivity for binding to the tissues, extended antimicrobial properties [15]. CHG also has value as a product preservative, including ophthalmic solutions, and as a disinfectant of medical instruments and hard surfaces [10].

The antimicrobial activity of CHG is pH-dependent, with an optimal use range of 5.5-7.0, a nice match with the body's usual pH range. The relationship between antimicrobial effectiveness of CHG and pH varies with the microorganism, however. For example, its antimicrobial activity against *Staphylococcus aureus* and *Escherichia coli* increases with an increase in pH, but the reverse is true for *Pseudomonas aeruginosa*.

CHG also works well in the presence of blood and other organic material.

Healthcare Personnel Handwash (HCPHW)

Chlorhexidine gluconate was a very effective product for healthcare personnel handwash applications. It has immediate kill properties, long-term effects, and residual properties. However, for healthcare personnel handwashes, only the immediate effects are important.

There is the potential problem of removing all the normal flora from the hands, and then what would grow back? This has been a problem with the products used on this area.

The solution strength is generally 0.5% to 4.0%.

Surgical Scrubs

For surgical scrub procedures, the 4.0% CHG is a very good formulation, having fairly fast kill rates and long-term or persistent effects. It also has residual effects; that is, as the product is used for several days, it binds to the stratum corneum and provides additional antimicrobial properties. The product kills a wide variety of microorganisms to a large degree.

Preoperative Skin Preparations

For this procedure, the 4.0% CHG is still an excellent product, having fairly fast-acting properties and broad-spectrum effects. It has long-term and persistent effects, which make it more antimicrobial over longer periods of time.

There was a problem with the product when it was first introduced. Recall that it basically competed against PVPI, which left a dark orange color when it dried. The problem was that CHG dried clear following application, without the tinted stain of PVPI, so that healthcare professionals could not see it on the skin. Therefore, they did not use it. Today, CHGs contain a dark-colored stain, making it visible on the skin.

ALCOHOLS

There is much debate concerning alcohol's effectiveness as a skin antiseptic [16, 17]. The antimicrobial efficacy of alcohol is highly dependent upon the concentration used, as well as the moisture level of the microbial environment treated. The short chain, monovalent alcohols - ethanol and isopropanol - are probably the most effective for skin disinfection because they are highly miscible with water, have low toxicity and allergenic potential, are fast-acting and are microbiocidal, as opposed to microbiostatic.

At first, alcohols were very drying to the hands upon repeated use, so they were not used extensively. Eleanor Fendler, of GOJO Industries, Inc., found a way to add emollients to the formula without inactivating the alcohol. Now alcohols have basically taken over this niche market.

The microbiocidal activity of the alcohols is largely a function of their ability to coagulate proteins [18]. The literature suggests, however, that the microbiocidal effects of alcohols are, too, a result of their solubility in lipids [19]. Protein coagulation takes place on the cell wall and the cytoplasmic membrane, as well as among the various plasma proteins [20].

Alcohols generally are inactive against bacterial spores [18]. And, although there is much controversy in the literature concerning the efficacy of alcohols against viruses, there appears to be general agreement that enveloped, lipophilic viruses are more susceptible to inactivation by alcohols than are naked viruses [21-26]. Lastly, the fungicidal properties of alcohols vary among fungal species, but in general, alcohols demonstrate a relatively high degree of mycidal/-static activity [27].

Although alcohols, as topical skin disinfectants, provide excellent immediate antimicrobial activity, they have virtually no persistent or residual properties [28]. Hence, their value as surgical scrubs and preoperative skin preps is seriously limited. Alcohols have been shown to provide adequate results as healthcare personnel handwashes or preinjection skin preps in removing or killing transient and resident microorganisms, but when used at strengths of 70% and greater, they tend to be drying to the skin, resulting in significant irritation [28].

Healthcare Personnel Handwashes

Alcohols are unsurpassed in this area. They are fast-acting and, once they are dry, they have no more antimicrobial effects. They do not have persistent effects, so there is no concern about its use changing the normal resident hand flora.

Alcohols are also used in schools, public places, cruise ships, restaurants, and other places where infections are known to occur.

Surgical Scrubs/Preoperative Skin Preparations

Alcohol products by themselves are not suitable for these applications, because they lack persistent antimicrobial effects.

ALCOHOL PLUS CHLORHEXIDINE GLUCONATE

Currently, there is much interest in alcohol tinctures of CHG. These alcohol/CHG products may prove to be highly effective for use as preoperative skin preparations, surgical scrubs and healthcare personnel handwash formulations. Additionally, tincture of CHG may be useful as both a preinjection and pre-arterial/venous catheterization prep. Preparations of alcohol/CHG combine the excellent immediate antimicrobial properties of alcohol with the persistence properties of CHG to provide a clinical performance superior to either alcohol or CHG alone. They can be used in two minutes instead of waiting ten minutes before making the surgical incision. This has greatly speeded up the surgical process.

These dual formulations also offer two drugs with different antimicrobial profiles that have additional benefits. These benefits will be demonstrated in the following figures.

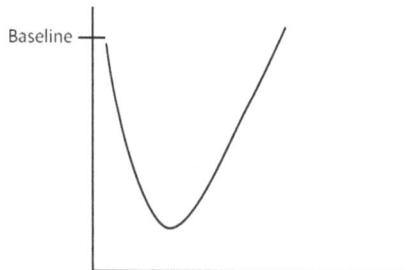

Figure 1: Alcohol Only.

From Fig. **1**, a tremendous reduction in microorganisms immediately after the application is apparent. However, the microbial counts rebound as soon as the product dries, so there is no persistence.

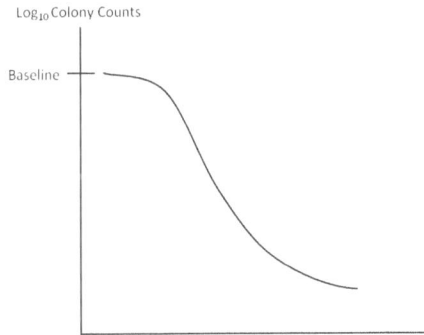

Figure 2: CHG Only.

As shown in Fig. **2**, the effects of the CHG are long-term. It takes about two to three hours for the antimicrobial counts to begin to rebound.

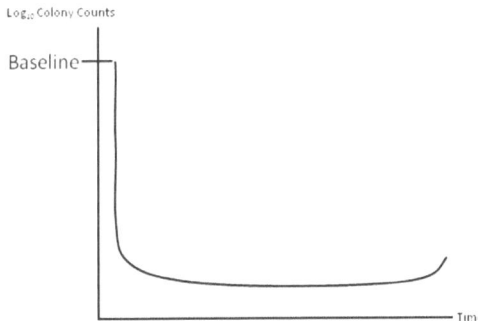

Figure 3: Alcohol Plus CHG.

Fig. **3** demonstrates the tremendously fast-acting effect of the alcohol and the persistence of CHG. There is also more $\log_{10}$ kill of microorganisms, due to the dual action.

Healthcare Personnel Handwashes

These are not used because only the immediate antimicrobial properties are required, so alcohol fits this niche and is more cost-effective. There is also the continued fear of changing the normal flora ecosystem of the hands.

Surgical Scrubs

There is considerable market opportunity for a product such as this. The alcohol cuts down on the dry time, so it is usable right away. The CHG provides persistent and residual activity.

Preoperative Skin Preparation

In this area, the dual action properties of these products have really come into play. It handles the task very effectively. The alcohol removes many microorganisms in the first seconds of the product's contact with the skin. Then the CHG keeps the microorganism count down over the course of the surgery.

OTHER ALCOHOL COMBINATION PRODUCTS

Alcohol combined with other products, like PVPI, are much more appealing. When different products are formulated with alcohol, such as inert ingredients like preservatives, the alcohol seems to work much more effectively.

QUATERNARY AMMONIUM COMPOUNDS

Quaternary ammonium chlorides (QACs) occupy a unique niche in the world of antimicrobial compounds [29]. Rather than being a single, well-defined substance, as is the case for many such active ingredients, QACs are composed of a diverse, eclectic collection of substances that share a common chemical motif, namely a molecular structure containing a positively-charged nitrogen atom covalently bonded to four carbon atoms [30]. This quaternary ammonium group is responsible for the name of these antimicrobial compounds and also plays a dominant role in determining their chemical behavior.

The first reports of quaternary ammonium compounds with biocidal activity appeared in 1916 [31]. Since that time, QACs have grown in popularity and been utilized extensively as active ingredients in many types of products, including household cleaners, institutional disinfectants, skin and hair care formulations, sanitizers, sterilizing solutions for medical instruments, preservatives in eye drops and nasal sprays, mouthwashes, and even in paper processing and wood preservatives [32]. As a group, QACs are effective across a broad spectrum of microorganisms, including bacteria, certain molds and fungis, and viruses [32]. However, the specific activity of QACs is as diverse as their range of chemical structures. QAC antimicrobial effectiveness is highly formulation-and packaging-dependent, since many ingredients affect QAC activity [33]. Some components reduce the QAC efficiency while others may synergise their activity or expand the spectrum of affected microorganisms [34]. This fact led to some confusion and apparent contradiction in the published literature as to the actual effectiveness of QACs in their role as antimicrobials [35].

In addition to their antimicrobial activity, QACs also behave as surfactants, assisting with foam development and cleansing action. They are also attracted to the skin and hair, where small amounts remain bound after rinsing. This contributes to a soft, powdery after feel on skin, unique hair-conditioning effects, and long-lasting, persistent activity against microorganisms. These various attributes and multifunctional roles of QACs appeal to formulators and are responsible for their incorporation into many consumer products.

PARACHLOROMETAXYLENOL (PCMX)

PCMX is one of the oldest antimicrobial compounds in use, dating back to 1913. It has not been widely used as a surgical or presurgical skin preparation because of its relatively low antimicrobial efficacy [36].

Because of the absence of substantive data, the FDA in 1972 did not designate PCMX as a safe and effective antimicrobial, and it was not formulated at the time for medical purposes such as surgical scrubs, preoperative skin preps or healthcare personnel handwashes [3]. The initial evaluations from the FDA listed PCMX as a Category III product, meaning that there were not enough data to recognize it as both safe and effective as a topical antimicrobial [3].

Studies since 1980 have demonstrated PCMX to be safe for human use. After this determination, a number of companies became interested in developing PCMX for use as a topical antimicrobial, and later studies demonstrated PCMX to be an effective antimicrobial compound.

Current over-the-counter formulations demonstrate varying degrees of antimicrobial efficacy, depending upon the formulation. Generally, PCMX products achieve fair to good immediate effects and fair persistent effects, but like iodophors, they provide no residual antimicrobial activity. PCMX products currently are formulated mainly for healthcare personnel handwash applications. These are effective in removing transient (contaminant) microorganisms from the hands and have low skin irritation properties.

TRICLOSAN

Triclosan, like PCMX, provides varying degrees of antimicrobial efficacy, depending upon the specific formulation and the species of organism tested. Triclosan has been formulated for a wide range of applications and is currently used in healthcare personnel handwash formulations, in the food industry to cleanse workers' hands, and in consumer product lines, including hand soaps, shower gels and body cleansers. Triclosan, like PCMX, provides fair immediate and persistent effects, but no residual action.

SUMMARY

This has been a brief discussion of topical antimicrobial products used as surgical scrubs, preoperative skin preparations, and healthcare personnel handwashes. It should be emphasized that these products continue to improve, as science continues to expand its knowledge. Product manufacturers can then utilize that knowledge to develop better products that can be differentiated within the market, resulting in more sales.

CONFLICT OF INTEREST

The author confirms that this chapter content have no conflict of interest.

ACKNOWLEDGEMENTS

Declared None.

REFERENCES

[1]   Semmelweis IP. The etiology, concept, prevention of childbed fever. Am J Obstet Gynecol 1995; 172(1 pt 1): 236-237.

[2]   Paulson DS. Topical antimicrobial testing and evaluation. New York: Marcel Dekker, Inc., 1999.

[3]   Food and Drug Administration (US). Tentative final monograph for health care antiseptic drug products. Federal Register. 21 Code of Federal Regulations, parts 333 and 369; June, 1994; pp. 31402-31452.

[4]   Shelanski, HA, Shelanski, MY. PVP-Iodine: History, toxicity, and therapeutic uses. J Int Coll Surg 1956; 25:727-734.

[5]   Paulson, DS. Developing effective topical antimicrobials. Soap Cosmet Chem Spe Dec., 1997; 50-58.

[6]   The United State Pharmacopeia, 23rd Ed. Whitehouse Station, NJ: Merck & Co., 1996.

[7]   Gottardi, W. Iodine and Iodine Compounds. In: Bloch, SS, Ed. Disinfection, sterilization, and preservation, 5th Ed. Malvern, PA: Lea & Febiger 1991; pp. 152-166.

[8]   Gröeschel, DH, Pruett, TL. Surgical Antisepsis. In Block, SS, Ed. Disinfection, sterilization, and preservation, 4th Ed. Philadelphia, PA: Lea & Febiger 1991, pp 642-654.

[9]   Paulson, DS. Designing a handwash for healthcare workers. Soap Cosmet Chem Spe June, 1996.

[10]   Bruch, MK. Chloroxylenol: An old-new antimicrobial. In Ascenzi, JM, Ed. Handbook of Disinfectants and Antiseptics. New York: Marcel Dekker, Inc., 1996: pp. 265-294.

[11]   Paulson, DS. Comparative evaluation of five surgical scrub formulations. AORN J 1994; 60:2, 246-256.

[12]   Paulson, DS. A broad-based approach to evaluating topical antimicrobial products. In Ascenzi, JM, Ed. Handbook of Disinfectants and Antiseptics. New York: Marcel Dekker, Inc. 1996; pp. 23-42.

[13]   Denton, GW. (1991). Chlorhexidine. In Block, SS, Ed. Disinfection, sterilization, and preservation, 4th Ed. Philadelphia, PA: Lea & Febiger. 1991; pp. 274-289.

[14]   Bloomfield, SF. Chlorhexidine and iodine formulations. In Ascenzi, JM, Ed. Handbook of Disinfectants and Antiseptics. New York: Marcel Dekker, Inc. 1996; pp. 133-158.

[15]   Ranganathan, NS. Chlorhexidine. In Ascenzi, JM, Ed. Handbook of Disinfectants and Antiseptics. New York: Marcel Dekker, Inc. 1996: pp. 235-264.

[16]   Larson, EL, Morton, HE. Alcohols. In Block, SS, Ed. Disinfection, sterilization, and preservation. Malvern, PA: Lea & Febiger 1991; pp. 191-203.

[17]   Rolter, ML. Alcohols for antisepsis of hands and skin. In Ascenzi, JM, Ed. Handbook of Disinfections and Antiseptics. New York: Marcel Dekker, Inc. 1996; pp. 177-233.

[18]   19. Beck, WC. Benefits of alcohol rediscovered. AORN J. 1984; 40:172-176.

[19]   Klein, M, & Deforest, A. Antiviral action of germicides. Soap Chem Special, 1963; 39:70-72.

[20]   Kubo, I, Muroi, H, Kubo, A. (1993). Antibacterial activity of long chain alcohols against *Streptococcus Mutans*. J Agr Food Chem, 1993; 41: 2447-2450.

[21]   Aly, R, Maibach, HI. A comparison of the antimicrobial effect of 0.5% chlorhexidine (Hibistat) and 70% isopropyl alcohol on hands contaminated with *Serratia Marcescens*. Clin Exp Dermatol 1980; 5:197-201.

[22]   Ansar, SA, Sattar, SA, Springthorpe, VS, *et al*. *In vivo* protocol for testing efficacy of hand-washing agents against viruses and bacteria: experiments with rotavirus and *Escherichia Coli*. Appl Environ Microbiol 1989; 55: 3113-3118.

[23]   Kurtz, JB, Lee, TW, Parsons, AJ. (1980). The action of alcohols on rotavirus, astovirus, and enterovirus. J Hosp Infect 1980; 1:321-325.

[24]   Gordon, MU. Studies of the viruses of vaccinia and variola. Privy Council, Medical Research Council, Special Report Series No. 98, London, 1925.

[25]   Groupe, V, Engle, CC, Gaffney, PE, *et al*. Virucidal activity of representative antiinfective agents against influenza A and vaccinia viruses. Appl Microbiol 1955; 3:333-336.

[26]   Bellamy, K. A review of the test methods used to establish virucidal activity. J Hosp Infect 1995; 30 (Suppl): 389-396.

[27]   Ayliffe, GAJ, Bobh, JR, Davis, JG, *et al*. Hand disinfection: a comparison of various agents in laboratory and ward studies. J Hosp Infect 1988; 11: 336-342.

[28]   Paulson, DS, Fendler, EJ, Dolan, MJ, *et al*. A close look at alcohol gel as an antimicrobial sanitizing agent. Am J Infect Control 1999; 27:332-338.

[29]   Ditoro, RD. New generation of biologically active quaternaries. Soap and Chemical Specialties 1969; 47-52, 86-88, 91-92.

[30]   Budavari, S. Ed. The Merck Index. An Encyclopedia of Chemicals, Drugs, and Biologicals, 11th Ed. Rahway, NJ: Merck and Co., Inc, 1989.

[31]   Windholz, M., Ed. The Merck Index. An Encyclopedia of Chemicals, Drugs, and Biologicals, 9th Ed. Rahway, NJ: Merck and Co., Inc., 1976.

[32]   Reybrouck, G. Evaluation of the antibacterial and antifungal activity of disinfectants. In Russell, AD, Huge, B, Ayliffe, GAJ, Eds. Principles and practice of disinfection, preservation and sterilization, 2nd Ed. London: Blackwell Science, 1992; pp. 114-133.

[33]   Furuta, T. Effect of alkaline builders and surfactants on the bactericidal activity of didecyldimethylammonium chloride. J Antibact Antifung Agents 1992; 20(12); 617-622.

[34]   Ahlstrom, B., Chelminska-Bertilsson, M, Thompson, RA, Edebo, L. Long-chain alkanoylcholines: a new category of soft antimicrobial agents that are enzymatically degradable. Antimicrob Agents Chemother 1995; 39(1):50-55.

[35]   Taylor, JH, Rogers, SJ, Holah, JT. A comparison of the bactericidal efficacy of 18 disinfectants used in the food industry against *Escherichia coli* O157:H7 and *Pseudomonas aeruginosa* at 10 and 20 degrees C. J Appl Microbiol 1999; 87(5):718-725.

[36]   Paulson, DS. Research designs for the soaps and cosmetics industry: a basic approach. Soap Cosmet Chem Spe Nov, 1995; pp. 50-58.

Frontiers in Clinical Drug Research: Anti-Infectives, Vol. 2, 2016, 151-203

CHAPTER 5

Identification of Nosocomial Pathogens and Antimicrobials Using Phenotypic Techniques

Marie Horká[1,*], Anna Kubesová[1], Dana Moravcová[1], Jiří Šalplachta[1], Jozef Šesták[1], Marie Tesařová[1] and Filip Růžička[2,3]

[1]Institute of Analytical Chemistry of the Czech Academy of Sciences, v. v. i., Veveří 97, 602 00 Brno, Czech Republic and [2]The Department of Microbiology, Faculty of Medicine, Masaryk University, Brno, Czech Republic and [3]St. Anne's University Hospital, Brno, Pekařská 53, 65691 Brno, Czech Republic

Abstract: Nosocomial infections caused by multidrug-resistant strains increase morbidity and mortality in hospitalized patients, prolong hospitalization, and they have significant negative economic impact. Currently, nosocomial infections are included in a broader concept as healthcare-associated infections. These are caused by a wide variety of pathogens, typically *Staphylococci, Enterococci, Pseudomonas aeruginosa, Klebsiella spp., Escherichia coli,* etc. Certain fungal agents, *e.g.*, yeasts of *Candida* genus and aspergilla, are also associated with these infections. The situation is further complicated by the development of resistance in the gram-positive cocci such as staphylococci or enterococci to second-line antibiotics used for the treatment of gram-negative bacteria and resistant gram-positive bacteria. Pathogenesis of mentioned infections plays a key role in forming biofilms on artificial surfaces.

Rapid detection and identification of etiological agents of nosocomial infections and determination of antibiotic susceptibility of pathogens are required for the optimal therapeutic scheme. Chromatographic methods such as high performance liquid chromatography or liquid chromatography-mass spectrometry are universal techniques widely applied to this purpose. However, only capillary electrophoretic techniques are able to determine both, antibiotics and microorganisms, during a single analysis. Differences in the chemotaxonomic fingerprints of the microorganisms can be utilized by matrix-assisted laser desorption/ionization time-of-flight mass spectrometry. In this chapter, we would like to outline an overview of available analytical techniques capable of rapidly identifying and estimating levels of antibiotics as well as microorganisms in real samples with a focus on nosocomial infections.

Keywords: Antibiotics and antifungals, capillary electrophoretic techniques, liquid chromatography, MALDI-TOF mass spectrometry, microorganisms, Nosocomial infections.

*Corresponding author Marie Horka: Institute of Analytical Chemistry of the Czech Academy of Sciences, v. v. i., Veveří 97, 602 00 Brno, Czech Republic; Tel: +420 532 290 221; Fax: +420 541 212 113; E-mail: horka@iach.cz

Atta-ur-Rahman (Ed)
All rights reserved-© 2016 Bentham Science Publishers

INTRODUCTION

Hospital-Acquired Infections

Nosocomial infections belong to the group of healthcare-associated infections (HAIs) [1] which are not only limited to hospitalization but also include all infections resulting from any interaction associated with the health care. The Council of the European Union considers HAIs as diseases that are "related to the presence of an infectious agent or its products in association with exposure to healthcare facilities or health care procedures or treatments" [2], with a lack of evidence that the infection was present or incubated at the time of entry of patient into the health care setting. Centers for Disease Control and Prevention define HAIs in a similar way [1].

The situation of HAIs is further complicated and aggravated by the increasing incidence of multidrug-resistant bacteria (MDRB) promoted by extensive use of antimicrobials during the last decades. The infections caused by MDRB contrary to those caused by susceptible bacteria are associated with significantly higher mortality, length of hospitalization, and health care costs [3, 4]. The European Centre for Disease Prevention and Control (ECDC) demonstrated that annually, HAIs involve 4.1 million patients in the European Union (EU) Member States and these infections directly result in approximately 37,000 deaths [2].

HAIs are caused by a wide variety of pathogens; namely *Staphylococci, Enterococci, Pseudomonas aeruginosa, Klebsiella spp., Escherichia coli,* etc. Especially, multiresistant strains of methicillin-resistant *Staphylococcus aureus* (MRSA), vancomycin-resistant enterococci (VRE), and extended-spectrum lactamase producing gram-negative bacteria. These are very dangerous and their treatment is complicated [3, 5]. Also, certain fungal agents are commonly associated with HAIs, *e.g.,* yeasts of *Candida* genus and aspergilli [6].

MRSA strains are considered as the most problematic nosocomial pathogens. These bacteria contain genes encoding penicillin-binding protein that differs from other penicillin-binding proteins in a way that its active site does not bind to methicillin or other β-lactam antibiotics [7]. Therefore, MRSA becomes resistant to the beta-lactam antibiotics, including those commonly used to treat ordinary staphylococcal infections. Only in the European Union, 171,200 of HAIs caused by MRSA were recognized in 2008 where 5,400 of extra deaths and 1,050,000 of extra days of hospitalization can be attributed to MRSA infections. The extra in-hospital costs attributable to MRSA were estimated to reach approximately 380 million EUR annually [8]. The development of antibiotic resistance of the gram-positive cocci such as staphylococci or enterococci to second-line antibiotics also complicates the treatment of diseases caused by these bacteria [9, 10].

Next to *S. aureus,* coagulase-negative staphylococci are other agents causing nosocomial infections. These infections are usually associated with indwelling medical devices, *e.g.*, catheter-related sepsis [11]. The pathogenesis of these infections strongly depends on the ability of pathogens to form biofilms on artificial surfaces [12] because the growth in the biofilm form protects the bacterial cells from the attacks of the immune system as well as from the effect of antibiotics. Therefore, it is difficult to eradicate these focuses through a conservative therapy, which results in the chronic character of biofilm infections and in the poor response to the antibiotics [12, 13].

P. aeruginosa is one of the leading gram-negative organisms associated with nosocomial infections, especially in patients with compromised host defense mechanisms. *P. aeruginosa* typically infects the airways, urinary tract, burns, wounds, and also causes blood stream infections [3, 5]. These bacteria show inherent (natural) resistance to a number of antimicrobial agents [14]. *P. aeruginosa* also easily develops resistance to anti-pseudomonas drugs in a hospital environment. One of the most serious types of the resistance is based on the production of broad-spectrum beta-lactamases, which inhibit the activity of many β-lactam antibiotics, and carbapenemases providing the resistance to all beta-lactams including carbapenems [15]. Those strains that exhibit resistance to at least three unrelated classes of antibiotics, especially β-lactams, carbapenems, and aminoglycosides, are considered as MDRB [16].

Enterobacteria belong to the important nosocomial pathogens as well. Particularly, *E. coli* and *Klebsiella* sp., are leading etiological agents of nosocomial urinary tract infection [3]. In addition, these bacteria cause a number of other serious HAIs, *e.g.*, pneumonia, bloodstream infections, and surgical wound site infections [3, 5]. These bacteria often produce extended-spectrum beta-lactamases or carbapenemases [17]. In addition, these strains frequently acquire co-resistance to many other classes of antibiotics in a hospital environment. The fact, that these bacteria show resistance to multiple antibiotics, increases the importance of the problem [18].

Fungal HAIs are less common than the bacterial HAIs, and they are restricted to immunocompromised patients. Difficult therapy and high mortality are characteristic for this type of infection [19]. The most common fungi causing

HAIs are yeasts of the genus *Candida* of which *Candida albicans* is most prevalent. However, the increased incidence of other *Candida* species occurs in recent decades. *Candida parapsilosis* and *Candida tropicalis* are typically associated with the use of catheters or other indwelling medical devices, enabling a biofilm formation [20]. The highest mortality associated with *Candida krusei* and *Candida glabrata*, can be probably related to their resistance to azole antifungals [19, 20]. *Aspergillus fumigatus* represents an example of the filamentous fungi, which is the most common cause of HAIs. It is usually manifested in the form of pulmonary invasive aspergillosis [21].

Identification of the Etiological Agents of Nosocomial Infections

Early identification of the etiological agents of nosocomial infections improves antimicrobial use and clinical outcome, reduces antibiotic resistance and last but not least it also saves money spent for the treatment. Currently, two groups of microbial identification methods, namely phenotyping and genotyping, are used for identification of the microorganisms (MOs) and for the detection of their resistant variants. Traditional phenotyping includes in particular the classical techniques which have been improved by applying molecular biology techniques while modern phenotyping covers analysis of chemotaxonomic fingerprints obtained by matrix-assisted laser desorption/ionization time-of-flight mass spectrometry (MALDI-TOF MS) and organisms are classified on the basis of chemistry of microbial cells and chemical markers [22]. Molecular genotyping includes the determination of plasmid profile, analysis of chromosomal DNA - genome fingerprinting, pulsed-field gel electrophoresis, gene probes, ribotyping, insertion sequence analysis, polymerase chain reaction-based methods, repetitive deoxyribonucleic acid sequence analysis, and deoxyribonucleic acid microarrays [23]. The traditional phenotyping methods can be useful, but they have some limitations that can be solved by molecular genotyping and by modern phenotyping and chemotaxonomic methods. A combination of techniques will be more often of greater value than any single technique. The phenotyping methods based on chemotaxonomy provide a better classification of microorganisms (MOs). They establish degrees of correlation between MOs, trace aspects of their evolution, and identify clinically important organisms [22].

Microbial Susceptibility Testing

The evaluation of antimicrobial susceptibility of the relevant microbial pathogens, *e.g.*, etiological agents of nosocomial infections is an important task of the each clinical microbiological laboratory. The aim of *in vitro* antimicrobial susceptibility testing is to provide a reliable predictor of how an organism is likely to respond to antimicrobial therapy in the infected host [24]. Antimicrobial susceptibility testing is performed by phenotypic or genotypic methods.

The basis of the most phenotypic methods is the assessment of the minimum inhibitory concentration (MIC) of an antimicrobial [25]. *In vitro* antimicrobial susceptibility testing can be performed using a variety of formats, the most common being a disk diffusion, agar dilution, broth macro dilution, broth micro dilution, and a concentration gradient test. All formats are based on the assessment of the inhibitory effect of antibiotics on the tested MOs. The above mentioned methods are able to provide reproducible and repeatable results if all the recommended procedures are correctly followed. Guidelines issued by the Clinical and Laboratory Standards Institute [24] or The European Committee on Antimicrobial Susceptibility Testing guidelines [25] are generally accepted. These methods are not expensive, but they are laborious, time consuming, and they require the use of specific testing conditions.

In special circumstances, other methods should be used for the detection of particularly resistant phenotypes, *e.g.*, detection of extended-spectrum beta-lactamase by double disc synergy test and/or by combination with the disk method [26] or by detection of penicillin-binding protein 2a in MRSA with the use of a latex agglutination test [27]. These methods complement the methods based on MIC assessment and enhance their reliability.

The use of genotypic approaches for detection of the genes responsible for particular types of resistance could increase the speed and accuracy of diagnostics. Numerous DNA-based assays have been developed for this purpose, *e.g.*, PCR methods for detection of MRSA, vancomycin-resistant enterococci, betalactamases, *etc.* [28, 29]. These fast methods enable to predict an antimicrobial resistance of phenotypes, but they do not indicate the real phenotypic expression of genes. Therefore, genotypic methods are usually useful in tandem with traditional phenotypic laboratory methods [28]. Moreover, genotypic methods are laborious and highly expensive in comparison with phenotypic methods [29].

Outlines

As it was mentioned before, rapid and accurate microbial species identification enables to avoid an inappropriate antimicrobial treatment and it is an essential for early and targeted antimicrobial therapy especially in causes of nosocomial infections. We would like to outline the potential of analytical techniques such as capillary zone electrophoresis (CZE) and capillary isoelectric focusing (CIEF) for analysis of MOs. Due to the fact that hyphenated techniques such as high performance liquid chromatography (HPLC) coupled to mass spectrometry become very popular in the field of MOs identification and classification, an application of chromatographic techniques in the analysis of important human pathogens is also reviewed in the following text. Part of this chapter also deals with MALDI-TOF MS analysis of MOs due to its ability to simplify MOs identification and classification through species-specific fingerprints.

Simultaneously, precise and sensitive methods for determination of different classes of antimicrobials/antifungals or their metabolites are required in clinical research. This need arises from the fact that there are only small differences between effective and toxic concentration of the given drug. Therefore, it is important to monitor their levels in human body fluids such as urine, plasma, serum, *etc.*, to ensure the optimal therapeutic dose and to minimize a risk of toxic side effects. Multiple analytical methodologies have been developed and used for antibiotic estimation in different matrices. These include, in particular chromatographic methods such as high performance liquid chromatography (HPLC) or liquid chromatography-mass spectrometry, which are universal techniques widely applied to this purpose. Part of this chapter is dedicated to HPLC analysis of antimicrobials/antifungals in real samples. The application of CZE and CIEF to analysis and determination of antimicrobials/antifungals is also discussed because only these techniques are capable to detect and identify antimicrobials as well as MOs together in a single analysis quickly and directly from real samples, particularly in case of nosocomial infections [30].

CAPILLARY ELECTROPHORETIC TECHNIQUES

The capillary electrophoretic techniques (CE) play an important role in the analysis of various samples due to their versatility, wide variety of detection systems, low consumption of samples, electrolytes, additives, and other reagents. An arrangement of CE setup is shown in Fig. (**1**). Both ends of the separation capillary are immersed into reservoirs containing appropriate buffer solutions and electrodes. The electrodes are connected to the high voltage power supply (3-10 kV) and the charged species in the capillary migrate to the oppositely charged electrode. The sample is introduced into the separation capillary by applying pressure to the inlet or by applying a voltage. The untreated fused silica capillary is usually used for separation which results in the electroosmotic flow generation. Intensity and direction of electroosmotic flow can be suppressed or reversed, e. g., by static or dynamic coating of the inner surface of fused silica capillary. UV-VIS detection, contactless conductivity detection, and electrospray mass spectrometry (ESI-MS) are predominantly used detection techniques. When UV-VIS and contactless conductivity detection are employed, an absorbance or conductivity is measured in a short section of fused silica capillary. UV-VIS detection requires the protective polyimide layer to be removed from the capillary at the point of detection. ESI-MS requires a sophisticated ESI interface to be connected to the end of the separation capillary.

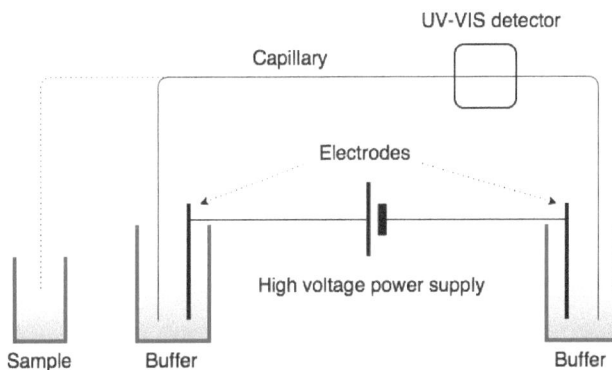

Fig. (1). An arrangement of CE setup.

One of the most important aspects of capillary electrophoretic methods is their ability to separate large molecules with on-line detection in free solution [31]. The second advantage of CE techniques is short separation time compared to conventional microbiological assays which is beneficial for the analyses of MOs.

Microorganisms as an Analyte for Capillary Electrophoretic Techniques

Microbial cells are generally amphoteric [32]. The surface charge depends on the environmental factors [32-34] and it is a result of the dissociation or protonation of carboxyl, phosphate, and amino groups in a three-dimensional surface of the ion-penetrable layer of the microbial cell upon contact with the aqueous phase. The charged surface leads to the formation of electric double layer between the solid surface and the surrounding liquid. This electric double layer is characterized by the electrokinetic potential, ζ (zeta potential) [34].

Separation of MOs by CZE is based on the differences in the electrophoretic mobilities of cells, which characterize the MOs [32]. In CIEF, analytes are separated according to their isoelectric points in a pH gradient generated by carrier ampholytes under the influence of a direct electric field [23, 30, 35]. Isoelectric point, p*I*, responds to the value of the pH when the electrophoretic mobility of analyte is zero. CIEF is used for the separation of amphoteric species such as peptides and proteins [30, 36-43], and even MOs [32, 44]. The pI of the cell surface is determined by the balance between anionic and cationic acid/base groups assuming no specific adsorption [45]. The value of pI for most bacteria was found in the pH range from 1.5 to 4.5 [34, 46, 47]. The pI value is a more suitable parameter for predicting the surface properties of cells than the electrophoretic mobility [45, 48]. The hydrophobicity of the microbial cell surface depends on the cell wall composition, and is a major parameter indicating affinity of cells to the inner surface of separation capillary [49-51]. This parameter differs from one MO to another [52].

Several factors, *e.g.*, amphoteric and aggregation behaviors of MOs, cell lysis [53], ionic strength, presence of oxygen or surfactant, among other considerations [54, 55] have to be solved prior to preparation of microbial sample and selection of the background electrolyte (BGE) in CZE or the catholyte and anolyte in CIEF. Adhesion of microbial cells to the capillary wall and coaggregation between cells during CE separation, *etc.* [54, 55] are results of typical microbial adhesive interactions. Any of these effects can greatly influence the zone broadening and separation efficiency in CE separation. The advantages of CE for the analysis of MOs are described in Refs. [30, 32, 33, 56-60]. Fast, sensitive and cheap determination of pathogenic bacteria is extremely important in many branches, for example, biotechnology, quality control, and antimicrobial therapy.

Application of Capillary Electrophoretic Techniques to MOs Identification and Classification

CIEF of Nosocomial Pathogens

The pIs of various bacterial species were firstly determined using microelectrophoresis in 1952 [61]. Isoelectric focusing in capillary format was introduced more than thirty years later when Hjertén and Zhu modified the device for high-performance electrophoresis to isoelectric focusing [30, 62]. The first analysis of bacterial samples by CIEF described Armstrong *et al.* in 1999 [53] whose separated various bacteria in a capillary coated by methylcellulose. Yeast cells of *Saccharomyces cerevisiae* were separated by Shen *et al.* [63] two years later. In both cases UV detection at 280 nm was used.

Since 2003, Horká and co-workers published several papers dealing with CIEF analysis of various MOs. Mixed cultures of *E. coli, C. albicans, Staphylococcus epidermidis,* and *Enteroccocus faecalis,* important nosocomial pathogens, were analyzed employing a fused silica capillary with the surface modified by a sol-gel technique [64]. Following studies [65-68] dealt with optimization of separation conditions for CIEF analysis of MOs. Capillaries dynamically modified with polyethylene glycol, PEG 4000, were tested in order to minimize adsorption of the bioanalytes to the capillary wall and to decrease an electroosmotic flow. Durability of capillaries modified by this polymer (PEG 4000) was at least 150 runs [30, 66]. All following CIEF studies employed a segmental injection of the samples, spacers, carrier ampholytes, and p*I* markers to achieve a suitable pH gradient [66]. Another study focused on creation of an acidic pH gradient in the pH range 2-5. The linearity of the pH gradients was improved by a combination of the simple ampholytic electrolytes, commercial carrier ampholytes, and other different additives [67]. Mentioned studies were accomplished employing the hydrodynamic mobilization of focused zones and UV-detection.

The concentration of microbial cells in real clinical samples is usually too low for direct analysis and a labelling of cells is often necessary to improve the detection sensitivity of CE methods. The yellow chromophoric non-ionogenic surfactant HOPAB (poly(ethylene glycol) 3-(2-hydroxy-5-n-octylphenylazo)-benzoate) was used for dynamic modification of proteins and MOs, *E. coli*, *S.epidermidis*, *C. albicans*, and *C. parapsilosis* [69]. Proteins and MOs were separated by CIEF in pH gradient in the range 2-5 using a conventional UV detection at 326 nm. The high sensitivity of this method allowed detection of less than 100 microbial cells injected into the separation capillary. Two years later, red non-ionogenic tenside, 1-[[4-(phenylazo)phenyl]azo]-2- hydroxy-3-naphthoic acid polyethylene glycol ester (PAPAN), was successfully tested as labelling agent for UV/VIS detection of proteins and MOs. The study was extended to strains of *C. tropicalis*, *C. krusei*, *S. cerevisiae*, and *S. aureus* [70]. All experiments covering dynamic labelling of microbial cells by non-ionogenic surfactants confirmed that p*I*s of the native and modified proteins as well as MOs do not change after modification.

The fluorescent non-ionogenic tenside polyethylene glycol 4-(1-pyrene) butanoate (PB-PEG) can also extend detection capabilities in analysis of MOs [68]. Dynamic modification of bacterial cells by PB-PEG enabled a fluorometric detection of MOs such as *E.coli* CCM3954, *S.epidermidis* CCM 4418, *Proteus vulgaris*, *E. faecalis* CCM 4224, and *Stenotrophomonas maltophilia*. This fluorescent non-ionogenic tenside is also suitable for labelling of the yeast strains *C. albicans* CCM 8180, *C. krusei*, *C. parapsilosis*, *C. glabrata*, *C. tropicalis*, and *S. cerevisiae* [35, 68]. Fluorescent p*I* markers were used to trace the pH gradient [71]. The p*I* values of both labelled (PB-PEG) and native MOs were the same.

The high sensitivity of the suggested method allowed detection of cell concentration as low as 10 cells injected into the separation capillary [30, 68]. Another article published in 2007 deals with CIEF separation of a mixture of various yeasts dynamically modified with PB-PEG [65] where the fluorescent detection in the acidic pH gradient in the pH range 2.0–5.5 was used. The influence of various inactivation procedures on p*I* values of *E. coli, S. epidermidis*, and *C. albicans* were also investigated by CIEF with both UV and fluorescent detection (PB-PEG modification). No differences were found between p*I* values of native and inactivated forms of tested MOs except cells of *C. albicans*, which showed the higher p*I* value after thermal inactivation or after inactivation by ethanol [58].

Another way how to simplify the CE analysis of real samples containing low concentration of bacterial cells is introducing of large amount of sample into the separation capillary. Thus, separation capillary with sufficient volume is needed for CIEF separation. Such capillary can be prepared by etching of fused silica capillary with supercritical water (SCW) as a single-piece combination of the tapered separation space with a cylindrical connection of the detection window to the electrode vial. The SCW treated capillary was applied to CIEF separation of MRSA and methicillin-susceptible *S. aureus* (MSSA), agar-cultivated and blood-incubated. Results confirmed that p*I*s of individual focused cells are not affected by the origin of the cells (agar-cultivated and blood-incubated) and higher resolutions of corresponding peak pairs can be achieved in SCW etched capillary when compared to untreated one [72]. The typical electropherogram is shown in Fig. (**2**).

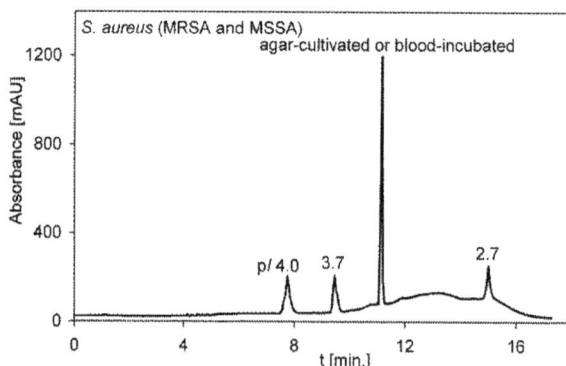

Fig. (2). CIEF with UV detection (280 nm) of 10^8 cell mL^{-1} of *S. aureus* (MRSA and MSSA cells both, agar-cultivated and blood-incubated) in the pH gradient in the range 2.7-4.0 on the fused silica capillary etched by supercritical water.

Another study investigated CIEF separation of important human pathogens, the biofilm-positive and the biofilm-negative *S. epidermidis* strains [56]. Overall, 73 bacterial strains were isolated from the blood cultures and cultivated. All strains were tested by standard phenotypic and genotypic methods. After the classification of individual strains into the biofilm-positive or biofilm-negative group, p*I* values of all characterized strains were estimated by CIEF. The p*I* values of biofilm-negative strains were close to 2.3 while the p*I* values for the biofilm-positive strains were found close to 2.6. The authors confirmed an assumption that the extracellular polysaccharide substance produced by biofilm-positive strains influence the charge of bacterial surface; thus, determined p*I* values of the biofilm-negative strains differ from p*I* values of the biofilm-positive strains [56].

A potential of CIEF technique to distinguish closely related yeast species was also investigated. Yeasts belonging to *Candida* genus are opportunistic human pathogens covering phenotypically similar strains *C. albicans*, *C. dubliniensis*, *C. parapsilosis*, and *C. tropicalis*. CIEF separation was performed in the pH gradients in the range 2.0-3.3 and 2.7-4.7 with UV detection. Individual yeast strains showed different values of p*I*. Besides CIEF analysis, gel IEF analysis was also performed. Fast and simple lysis procedure was used to obtain proteins providing characteristic gel IEF fingerprints for the examined yeast strains [73]. 39 strains of *C. parapsilosis* were characterized by CIEF in the pH gradient in the range 3.3-3.9 with UV detection. It was confirmed again that p*I* values of biofilm-negative and biofilm-positive strains of *C. parapsilosis* are different (see Fig. **3**). Value of p*I* for biofilm-negative *C. parapsilosis* strains was determined as 3.8 and for biofilm-positive strains as 3.6. [74]. A similar study was performed for phenotypically identical *Candida* species, *C. orthopsilosis*, *C. metapsilosis*, and *C. parapsilosis*. All strains were successfully separated under optimized CIEF conditions, including their biofilm-negative and biofilm-positive forms [75].

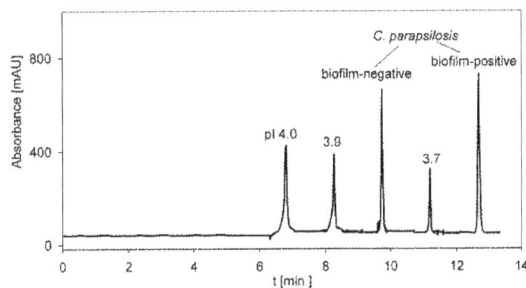

Fig. (3). CIEF with UV detection (280 nm) of both, biofilm-positive and biofilm-negative species of *C. parapsilosis* (10^8 cell mL^{-1}) in the pH gradient in the pH range 3.6-4.0.

It should be noted that CIEF technique is also suitable for separation of filamentous fungi, including *Penicillium* sp., *Aspergillus* sp., and *Fusarium* sp. The p*I*s of relevant native (see Fig. **4**) and PB-PEG labelled conidia were determined by CIEF. Suggested method allowed detection of concentration as low as 10 dynamically labelled conidia injected into the separation capillary [76].

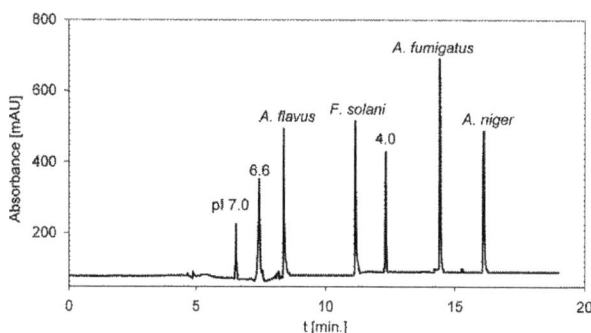

Fig. (4). CIEF of the conidia of filamentous fungi in the pH gradient in pH range 2.0-8.0 with UV detection, 280 nm; sample composition, UV-detectable pI markers p*I* 4.0, 6.6, and 7.0, conidia of *A. niger* CCM 8222, *A. fumigatus* CCM 3960, *F.solani* CCM 8014, and *A. flavus* CCM F-449 (10^8 conidia mL^{-1}).

CZE of Nosocomial Pathogens

As it was mentioned above, CZE separation of MOs when subjected to electric field depends on their different mobilities in the electrophoretic media. The concept of bacteria cell transportation in CE introduced Hjertén in 1987 [77]; however, first results covering separation of bacteria by CZE report Ebersole and McCormick [78]. Pfetsch and Welsch determined the electrophoretic mobility of bacteria using unmodified 1-3m long fused silica capillaries with internal diameter of 250 μm [79].

The most frequent species occurring in human infections are *S. aureus* and *E. coli*. Therefore, these bacteria are considered as etiological agents responsible for many nosocomial infections. Sonohara *et al.* [80] proved that electrophoresis can be used to detect the difference between the surface layer of gram-positive and gram-negative bacteria. In this study, *E. coli* and *S. aureus* were measured in the media at various pH values and ionic strengths. Later, Armstrong *et al.* published the high-efficiency CZE separation of the mixture of MOs, *E. coli* and *S. saprophyticus*, in urine matrix [73, 81]. Sharp peaks of bacteria were detected and their migration times were modified by changing the concentration of the additive, polyethylene glycol, in presented study. The brief sonication before separation was recommended as the prevention of the cluster aggregation. A linear relationship between the electrophoretic mobility and the number of cells in the aggregates was found [53, 82, 83]. In Ref. [84], CE methods employing a different modification of inner capillary wall and polystyrene-divinylbenzene monolithic bed were tested for determination of *E. coli* and *S. aureus* in clinical samples. Another study explored an application of dynamically modified capillary with PEG 600 in order to minimize adsorption of the *E. coli*, *P. vulgaris*, and *S. aureus* cells to the capillary wall. These bacteria were also separated from infected urine without any pretreatment [85]. The same biological matrix has been used by Song *et al.* in another study where the most common species of pathogens included *E. coli*, *K. pneumoniae*, *P. aeruginosa*, *S. aureus*, and *S. epidermidis* were separated by CZE. It was confirmed that bacteria in urine samples can be effectively detected by the "three-plug-injection" method [86].

The selective detection of *S. aureus* using monoclonal antibody-coated latex particles to enrich of *S. aureus* in the presence of other MOs, *E. coli*, *P. aeruginosa*, and *K. pneumonia*, was reported by Gao *et al.* [59]. CZE was also successfully used to differentiate between MRSA and MSSA strains. Analysis was carried out in modified fused silica capillaries etched by supercritical water [72]. Fig. (**5**) shows CZE separation of MRSA strains cultivated from agar and blood. The possibility to apply CZE as a fast and low-cost method for distinguishing between the blood-incubated MRSA or MSSA cells has been tested in Ref. [87]. Low concentrations of bacteria ($\sim 10^2$ cell mL^{-1}) close to levels presented in clinical samples were detected. The migration times of the purified blood-incubated cells and the agar-cultivated cells differed from each other [72, 87]. Three strains of *S. aureus* were tested by independent methods, such as CZE, PCR, and physiological tests in a next study. The results obtained from measurements of electrophoretic method and molecular analyses were compared [88].

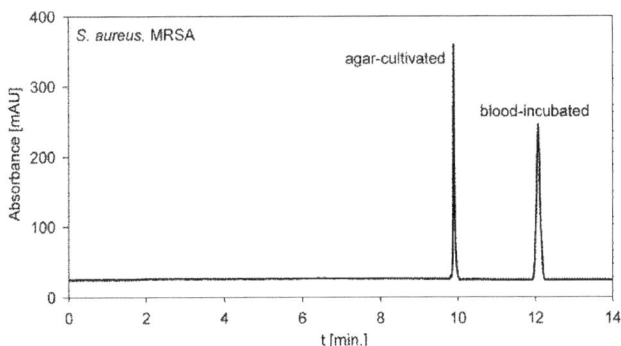

Fig. (5). CZE (UV detection, 280 nm) of the 10^8 cell mL^{-1} of *S. aureus* (MRSA), agar-cultivated and blood-incubated, on the fused silica capillary etched with supercritical water.

The dynamic labelling of bacterial cells was also applied for CZE separations to improve detection sensitivity and to lower the detection limits. Fluorescent non-ionogenic tenside PB-PEG was suggested as a buffer additive for the dynamic modification of the cells *E. coli, C. albicans, E. faecalis,* and *S. epidermidis* [89]. The cells were concentrated and separated by CZE using UV excitation for the on-column fluorometric detection. Detection sensitivity was achieved in order of one to tens of injected cells. PB-PEG can also be used for a dynamic modification of the following yeast cells: *C. albicans, C. glabrata, C. kefyr, C. krusei, C. lusitaniae, C. parapsilosis, C. tropicalis, C. zeylanoides, Geotrichum candidum, S. cerevisiae, Trichosporon asahii,* and *Yarrowia lipolytica* as well [65]. This dye plays a dual role in the separation. It acts as a dynamic coating of fused silica capillary and as a fluorescent reagent at the same time making possible to detect down to ten cells. The rapid separation and detection of the conidia of filamentous fungi appears to be very useful for the purpose of the clinical medicine in the case of fungal infections. The hydrophobic native conidia and conidia dynamically modified by PB-PEG of the filamentous fungi were separated by CZE with UV detection (see Fig. **6**) or fluorometric detection [76]. The detection limit was less than 10 labeled conidia of *A. niger* and other different strains injected to the separation capillary.

In Ref. [75] the narrow peak zones of the cells of *Candida* species, *C. orthopsilosis, C. metapsilosis,* and *C. parapsilosis,* with sufficient resolution were detected after CZE separation. Biofilm-negative and biofilm-positive forms of *C. metapsilosis* and *C. parapsilosis* were distinguished. The migration times of the examined species did not depend on the origin of the tested strains.

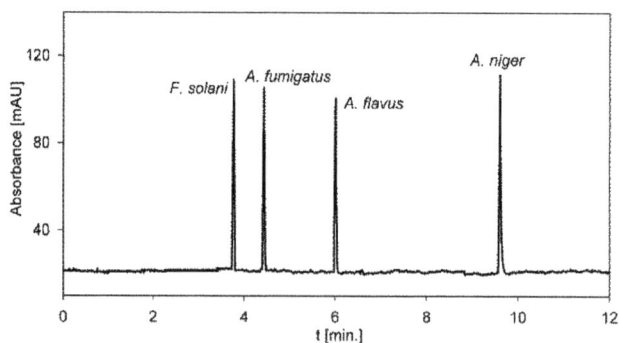

Fig. (6). CZE of the native filamentous fungi conidia (10^8 conidia mL^{-1}) with UV detection, 280 nm.

Another fluorescent dye, Baclight™ Green bacterial stain, was used for CZE analysis of *C. albicans*. This dye interacts with proteins and peptides of the blood plasma and it can reduce the effect of interfering peaks prior to CZE analysis. The cetyltrimethylammonium bromide additive at the concentration of 1 mg mL^{-1} has been used by authors in Ref. [90] to prevent cell lysis and cell aggregation. Cells of *C. albicans* were detected at 516 nm. This procedure enables detection of cell concentration as low as 5 cells per injection. Another procedure allowing the detection of the yeast *C. albicans* directly from the blood utilizes a combination of CZE with whole-cell molecular labeling *via* fluorescence *in situ* hybridization [91]. Also colored chromophoric non-ionogenic surfactant, HOPAB, has been used as a buffer additive for the dynamic modification of MOs such as *E. coli, S. epidermidis*, and the yeasts [69]. MOs were successfully separated and detected by UV detection at 326 nm. Red non-ionogenic surfactant PAPAN 1000 has been prepared for detection in visible spectrum. This buffer additive was used for the dynamic labeling of yeasts, *E. coli* and biofilm-positive and biofilm-negative *S. epidermidis*. It was found, that biofilm-negative *C. parapsilosis* and *C. albicans* migrate in CZE much slower than the other examined MOs [70].

E. coli K-12 was determined by CZE at different pHs and at various ionic strengths of background buffer [79, 92]. Broad bands for MOs were observed which can be attributed to the cell aggregation [32, 79, 92, 93].

As it is apparent from the research, the capillary electrophoretic techniques offer great potential for rapid and sensitive detection of etiological agents of nosocomial infections in clinical samples.

LIQUID CHROMATOGRAPHY

Application of Chromatographic Techniques to MOs Identification and Classification

Liquid chromatography is a highly specific separation technique enabling not only isolation of individual components of the sample mixture, but also sensitive qualitative and quantitative analyses of the complex sample mixtures, especially, if mass spectrometric detection is available. It is an effective tool for processing large numbers of samples in a short period of time. Thus, it has an indispensable role in laboratories where biological samples are being processed and analyzed. In the context of detection and identification of etiological agents of nosocomial infections, mass spectrometry detection is becoming a commonplace while UV-detection is preferred for applications where well known compounds, *e.g.*, antibiotics, their residues, and metabolites, having chromophore groups, are analyzed.

Frequently used reversed-phase chromatography (RP-LC) is not efficient enough to process complex biological samples; thus, multidimensional chromatographic approach has to be applied in both offline as well as online configuration. Moreover, polar and hydrophilic compounds are poorly retained under RP-LC conditions. Ion-pairing chromatography or hydrophilic interaction chromate-graphy removes these obstacles.

Only a few published studies focus on the analysis of different bacterial species or on distinguishing among individual bacterial strains. For example, Lo *et al.* [94] performed LC-MS/MS analyses of the proteolytic digests of cell extracts and described identification up to eight individual bacterial species (*E. faecalis, E. coli, P. aeruginosa, Vibrio parahaemolyticus, S. aureus, Streptococcus agalactiae, S. epidermidis,* and *Streptococcus pyogenes*). A multidimensional chromatographic method combining chromatofocusing of proteins as a first dimension and reversed-phase high-performance liquid chromatography (RP-HPLC) in the second dimension applied Zheng *et al.* [95] for the differential analysis of proteins originating from virulent (O157:H7) or non-virulent strains of *E. coli*. They identified several proteins as potential markers for distinguishing between virulent and nonvirulent strains. Gatlin *et al.* [96] compared the composition of total protein and membrane protein extracts for two isogenic vancomycin-intermediate *S. aureus* strains, (HIP5827 and VP32). They identified 144 proteins using 2-DE and SDS-PAGE combined with micro-capillary LC-MALDI-MS/MS, and multidimensional liquid chromatography [96]. Hewelt-Belka *et al.* [97] describe changes in lipid content of *S. aureus* cells for strains with various sensitivities toward antibiotics using RP-HPLC coupled with quadrupole time-of-flight mass spectrometry.

Another etiological agent of nosocomial infections, which was subjected to comprehensive proteomic analysis is *P. aeruginosa*. Liquid chromatography coupled online with tandem mass spectrometry was managed by Blonder *et al.* [98]. They identify up to 786 proteins when an affinity labelling technique was used to improve the detection of lower abundance membrane proteins. Changes in *P. aeruginosa* subcellular protein compartmentalization due to stress conditions were also studied. Digests of whole cells and membrane proteins labelled with isotope-coded affinity tag reagents were separated by two-dimensional liquid chromatography prior to analysis by electrospray ionization-tandem mass spectrometry [99].

Most published papers deal with the characterization of single species at the level of whole cell proteins, cell membrane proteins, or secreted metabolites. Proteins secreted by methicillin-resistant *S. aureus COL* were characterized by two-dimensional LC combined with whole protein and peptide mass spectrometry

[100]. This research group identified 127 proteins comprising of 59 secreted proteins, seven cell wall anchored proteins, four lipoproteins, four membrane proteins, and 53 cytoplasmic proteins [100]. Also, changes in metabolite secretion of *S. aureus* after exposition to different antibiotics, *e.g.*, fosfomycin and vancomycin, were evaluated. An ion-pairing liquid chromatography–tandem mass spectrometry method was developed for quantification of uridine diphosphate-linked peptidoglycan intermediates in *S. aureus*. [101]. Schallenberger *et al.* investigated the relationship between the secretion and accumulation of proteins in *S. aureus* strains sensitized to arylomycin after arylomycin treatment using multidimensional protein identification technology mass spectrometry [102].

Targeted and untargeted profiling of metabolites involved in biofilm and planktonic growth of *C. albicans* was accomplished by employing of an ion-pairing chromatography-porous graphitic carbon column coupled with a time-of-flight mass spectrometry. The results confirmed changes in amino acid metabolism during *C. albicans* biofilm formation. Suggested method can be applied for screening of novel biomarkers from the microbial metabolome [103]. The same research group characterized nucleotide metabolic profiles of biofilm and planktonic form of *C. albicans*. The effect of treatment with drugs such as 5-fluoropyrimidine, baicalein, and sodium houttuyfonate, on nucleotide metabolism of biofilm form of *C. albicans* was also investigated [104].

Molds are really dangerous pathogens; however, some of them secrete compounds with special properties, *e.g.*, antibacterial or even anticancer activity. Secondary metabolites of eight species from the genus *Aspergillus* (*A. lentulus*, *A. fumigatus*, *A. fennelliae*, *A. niger*, *A. kawachii*, *A. flavus*, *A. oryzae*, and *A. sojae*) were analyzed by liquid chromatography ion-trap mass spectrometry and multivariate statistical analysis. Suggested secondary metabolite profile-based chemotaxonomic classification technique successfully distinguished individual *Aspergillus spp.* The neosartorin was identified as an *Aspergillus lentulus*-specific compound that showed anticancer activity, as well as antibacterial effects on *S. epidermidis* [105].

Ability to efficiently quantify a large number of known cellular metabolites originating from *E. coli* by application of an amino column in a HILIC-ESI-MS/MS method for reliable measurement of 141 metabolites was proved by Bajad *et al.* [106]. The differences between the metabolomes of extracts of *E. coli* grown exponentially in minimal media containing either unlabeled [12C] or isotope-labeled [13C] glucose were investigated. The suggested method reveals appropriate 12C- and 13C-peaks for 79 different metabolites.

New chromatographic approach so-called denaturing HPLC was introduced by Jury *et al.* [107] to subtype bacterial strains of MRSA where the variability within the staphylococcal protein A gene-repeat region is used as a marker of short- and long-term genetic variation.

MATRIX-ASSISTED LASER DESORPTION/IONIZATION TIME-OF-FLIGHT MASS SPECTROMETRY

Since the introduction of soft ionization techniques like matrix-assisted laser desorption/ionization (MALDI) and electrospray ionization (ESI), mass spectrometry has been adopted as a standard method for characterization of large biomolecules. MALDI-TOF MS has been widely used in the analysis of complex protein mixtures including intact microbial cells or cell lysates [108]. In recent years, MALDI-TOF MS has become a powerful and rapid analytical tool for the classification and identification of MOs based on species-specific fingerprints [109-117]. The identification is based on specific mass/charge (m/z) fingerprints of cell components, mainly peptides and proteins, which are characteristic of individual microbial species. Microbial fingerprinting by MALDI-TOF MS is a rapid, accurate, cost-effective, and simple method providing reliable microbial identification at the species or subspecies level [118-121]. In this respect, sample preparation represents a crucial step. The vast majority of recent studies regarding microbial characterization by MALDI-TOF MS deals with intact cells as they require simple and fast sample preparation compared to the analysis of cell lysates [109, 119, 122]. The observable molecular mass range is usually between 2 and 20 kDa where very few metabolites appear [123, 124], which is an advantage because these masses can be easily used as biomarkers. MALDI-TOF MS has important advantages over PCR methods. The technique is rapid and straightforward since it requires the minimum sample handling. Caution is required to avoid contaminants and interferences like salts, *etc.* [125].

Three commercial MALDI systems, developed in the recent years, are routinely used in biological research as well as in clinical medicine, biotechnology, and industry. These systems are mainly used for identification of bacteria and, to a lesser extent, yeast. Currently, there are three commercial systems based on MALDI typing, Andromas (Andromas SAS, Paris, France), BioTyper (Bruker Daltonics, Bremen, Germany), and Vitek-MS with SARAMIS database (bioMérieux, Marcy L'Etoile, France) [126]. Although these systems are technically very similar, each system uses its own databases, algorithms, software, and interpretive criteria for microbial identification [126, 127]. Non-identifications are usually caused by the absence of reference spectra in the database. Nevertheless, microbial databases are updated and the number of included species increases. Moreover, there is a possibility to add new data and create custom databases or expand the current databases [126-129]. Workflow for microbial identification is simple and time-saving.

Since MALDI-TOF MS is a suitable technique for routine microbial identification, it was used for identification of microbial species in clinical microbiology, *e.g.*, rapid diagnosis of bloodstream infections, in recent years [129-138]. The possibility to identify pathogens from clinical samples such as urine or positive blood culture is of high interest. However, there is a problem with the presence of interfering peptides and proteins in the clinical samples. In this respect, several protocols for extraction of microbial components and removal of substances that may interfere in MALDI-TOF MS analysis were developed by different research groups [139-142]. With respect to clinical microbiology, MALDI-TOF MS was applied to the identification of various MOs from cultures, direct microbial identification in blood cultures, urine, and cerebro-spinal fluid.

There are very few applications of MALDI-TOF MS for identification of pathogens in cerebro-spinal fluid for the diagnosis of disease. Several authors described the application of MALDI-TOF MS for the direct detection of MOs in cerebro-spinal fluid causing bacterial meningitis [126, 128, 143, 144]. Bacterial meningitis is usually severe disease and it is one of the most serious manifestations of bacterial infection. In this particular case, the fast and accurate identification of bacterial pathogen is necessary for rapid initiation of antibiotic exposure prophylaxis. From a practical point of view, low bacterial concentration together with limited volume of sample available limits the use of the MS-based method. Moreover, polymicrobial infection can also be an issue. Similar to cerebro-spinal fluid, MALDI-TOF MS was used to directly identify pathogens in urine samples [126, 128, 145-149]. The proposed methods include washing and centrifugation steps to remove leukocytes, erythrocytes, and other interfering components. However, it is likely that more than one bacterial species are present in a urine sample, which makes pathogen identification using direct MALDI-TOF MS analysis difficult. In addition, the presence of host proteins found in urine can negatively affect MALDI-TOF MS identification due to overlaying mass signals [146]. In order to improve reliability of MALDI-TOF MS identification of pathogens in urine samples, MALDI-TOF MS was combined with urine flow cytometry or Gram staining [150, 151]. Another application of MALDI-TOF MS in clinical microbiology is direct identification of MOs from blood culture bottle broth. A number of studies reported successful identification of microbial species from positive blood cultures [136, 152-156]. Sample preparation is a crucial step including the use of serum separators, differential centrifugation, and chemical or detergent lysis. In this respect, a variety of different sample processing protocols were developed including commercial kits [129, 139, 147, 154, 157-163].

In addition to rapid and accurate identification of various MOs in clinical microbiological laboratory, MALDI-TOF MS was used for determination of antimicrobial resistance, especially antibacterial resistance [126-128, 164, 165]. The ability of MALDI-TOF MS to discriminate between resistant and susceptible strains of bacteria was demonstrated by recent studies. There are two strategies for the determination of antibiotic resistance using MALDI-TOF MS. The simplest application of MALDI-TOF MS in antibiotic resistance is to find characteristic differences of protein patterns of susceptible and resistant strains within a species. Monitoring of β-lactamase activity by means of MALDI-TOF MS was described in recent studies [164-170]. β-lactam antibiotics are a broad class of antibiotics containing a β-lactam ring in their molecular structures. This includes penicillin derivatives (penams), cephalosporins (cephems), monobactams, and carbapenems. β-lactam antibiotics inhibit biosynthesis of the peptidoglycan layer of the cell walls of Gram-positive bacteria (broad-spectrum β-lactam antibiotics acting against Gram-negative bacteria are being developed) and these are the most widely used group of antibiotics. Beta-lactam antibiotics are hydrolyzed (inactivated) by beta-lactamases synthesized by resistant MOs [128, 164, 165]. This degradation results in certain changes in the mass profile. Typically, cleavage of the β-lactam ring is characterized by the disappearance of the original ion of antibiotic, which is caused by the addition of a water residue, resulting in an increase of the molecular weight of the antibiotic by 18 *m/z* units. A further mass shift of -44 *m/z* units is usually detected in the mass spectrum as a result of decarboxylation of the β-lactam after hydrolysis. In this application, the bacterial isolates of interest are incubated for a short time with the antibiotic and changes in mass profiles are monitored by MALDI-TOF MS. Another and more complex approach for determination of antibiotic resistance using MALDI-TOF MS is based on the use of isotope-labeled amino acids [128, 164, 165, 171]. In this method, MOs are grown in both drug-containing stable isotope-labeled media and non-labeled media without the drug. Antimicrobial resistance is detected by characteristic mass shifts of one or more peaks in the acquired mass spectra.

DETERMINATION OF ANTIMICROBIALS IN BODY FLUIDS

Antibiotics and antifungals are commonly used drugs in veterinary and human medicine for treatment and prevention of microbial and fungal infections. They can be classified into several groups according to their therapeutic effects and structural characteristics. The most important antibiotics used for the treatment of nosocomial infections belong to the group of β-lactam antibiotics such as penicillins (ampicillin, oxacillin, methicillin), cephalosporins, carbapenems, and tazobactam. Also, drugs from the group of aminoglycosides (amikacin, gentamycin), fluoroquinolones (ciprofloxacin), glycopeptides (vancomycin), linkosamides (clindamycin), and polypeptides (polymixin E = colistion) are frequently used to treat bacterial infections. Amphotericin B, echinocandins, and triazoles (fluconazole, voriconazole, posaconazole) are representatives of antifungals for which it is necessary to monitor their level in biological fluids.

Application of Chromatographic Techniques to Estimate Levels of Antimicrobials in Body Fluids

Combination of LC with UV-detection is a routine technique frequently used to determine concentrations of antimicrobials, due to the fact that these compounds usually contain chromophore group in their molecules. Nowadays, coupling of liquid chromatography to mass spectrometry is obvious extension which offers improved sensitivity and selectivity. Especially, selected reaction monitoring provides unique potential for reliable quantification of low abundant analytes in complex sample mixtures such as biological fluids. Comprehensive outlines of therapeutic drug monitoring and LC-MS/MS are included, *e.g.*, in reviews from Adaway *et al.* [172] or from Pickering *et al.* [173].

Due to the large number of published original works and excellent reviews [174-176] in this field, Tables **1** and **2** summarize papers dealing with determination and quantification of the above mentioned drugs in body fluids by liquid chromatography only over the period from the year 2000 to present.

Table 1. Antibiotics in body fluids determined and quantified by liquid chromatography.

	Matrix	Sample Preparation and Analysis	LOQ (LOD)	notes
Beta-lactam				
Simultaneous determinations	Human plasma	Protein precipitation with acetonitrile; dilution of supernatant in water; C18 column; elution by water-acetonitrile gradient, ESI-MS/MS; run time 7 min	0.1-0.25 mg/L	Piperacillin, benzylpenicillin, flucloxacillin, meropenem, ertapenem, cephazolin and ceftazimide [177]
		Mixed mode solid phase extraction; C18 column, elution by acetate buffer-acetonitrile gradient; ESI-	0.05 – 0.76 mg/L	Amoxicillin, ampicillin, phenoxymethylpenicillin, piperacillin, cefuroxime,

Table 1: contd...

		MS/MS; run time 4 min		cefadroxil, flucloxacillin, meropenem, cefepime, ceftazidime, tazobactam, linezolid and cefazolin [178]
		30,000 molecular weight cut-off centrifugal filter; C18 column; phosphate buffer-acetonitrile isocratic elution depending on the analyte group; UV-VIS 210, 260, 304 nm; run time 5-8 min	0.1 mg/L	Ceftriaxone, cephazolin, cephalotin, meropenem, ertapenem, ampicillin, piperacillin, benzylpenicillin, flucloxacillin, dicloxacillin [179]
	Human serum	Solid phase extraction; C18 column; elution by ammonium formate-methanol gradient; ESI-MS/MS; run time 13 min	0.005-0.5 mg/L	Ampicillin, cefazolin, cefepime, cefmetazole, cefotaxime, doripenem, meropenem, and piperacillin [180]
		Protein precipitation; PFP column; elution by phosphate buffer-methanol gradient; UV 295 nm; run time 7 min	0.5 mg/L	Imipenem, doripenem, meropenem and ertapenem [181]
Meropenem	Human plasma, Filtrate-dialysate, urine	Centrifugation and dilution of supernatant; C18 column; elution by water-acetonitrile gradient; ESI-MS/MS; run time 3 min	0.24-1.22 mg/L	MEM monitoring in critically ill patients with acute kidney injury with sepsis and receiving continuous renal replacement therapy [182]
	Human plasma	Protein precipitation, supernatant evaporation, residue dilution; C18 column; elution by phosphate buffer (87%)-methanol (13%); UV-VIS 295 nm; run time 13 min	0.5 mg/L	Measurement of drug level in critically ill patients a 0, 2, 4 and 8 h after infusion [183]
	Peritoneal fluid, bile	stabilization by 3-morpholinopropanesulfonic acid and ultrafiltration; elution by phosphate buffer-acetonitrile (100:10, v/v); UV-VIS 300 nm; run time 10 min	0.05 mg/L in peritoneal fluid; 0.1 mg/L in bile	Application to Comparative Pharmacokinetic Investigations [184]
Ertapenem	Dried blood spots	Spots on filter paper extracted with 30/70 (%v/v) water/methanol; C18 column; elution by water-acetonitrile gradient; ESI-MS/MS; run time 2.2 min	0.2 mg/L	For blood obtained from finger pricks sampling [185]
	Human plasma, bronco-alveolar lavage fluid	Protein precipitation, liquid-liquid extraction by dichloromethane; aqueous phase analysis; C18 column; elution by ammonium acetate-methanol gradient; UV-VIS 300 nm; run time 25-30 min	0.04 mg/L in plasma and lung tissue, 0.02 mg/L in BAL	No need for pre-concentrating step [186]

Table 1: contd…

Aminoglycosides				
Simultaneous determination	Human plasma	Protein precipitation with acetonitrile; C18 column; elution by water-acetonitrile gradient; ESI-MS; run time < 12 min	0.63-2.34 mg/L,	Daptomycin, amikacin, gentamicin, and rifampicin [187]
	serum	SPE; ZIC-HILIC column; elution by 95-90% acetonitrile gradient; ESI-MS/MS; run time 10 min	0.1 mg/L	Amikacin, gentamicin, kanamycin, neomycin, paromomycin, and tobramycin [188]
Amikacin	Cerebrospinal fluid (CSF)	CSF centrifugation; Mobile phase: 1.8 g/l sodium 1-octanesulphonate, 14 ml/l tetrahydrofuran, 50 ml/l of phosphate buffer and sodium sulphate 20 g/l [189]; pulsed electrochemical detection; run time 20 min	0.06 mg/L	Study of CSF pharmacokinetics of amikacin in neonates [190]
	Human plasma, urine	Dilution with ethanol-sodium carbonate buffer mixture; centrifugation; supernatant analysis; C18 column, elution by phthalate buffer-acetonitrile gradient; chemiluminescent (CL) detection; run time 20 min	0.05 mg/L	Method uses the inhibitory effect of complex of aminoglycoside with Cu(II) on the CL signal provided by the luminol–hydrogen peroxide system [191]
Tobramycin	human drainage tissue fluid	Protein precipitation, liquid-liquid extraction by dichloromethane; aqueous phase analysis; C18 column; elution by water-acetonitrile gradient; ESI-MS/MS; run time < 10 min	1.25 mg/L	Evaluation in four calcaneal osteomyelitis patients [192]
Gentamicin	Plasma, urine	Derivatization in the solid-phase extraction cartridge with 1-fluoro-2,4-dinitrobenzene; C18 column; elution by tris buffer-acetonitrile 68/32 (%v/v); UV-VIS 365 nm; run time 12 min	0.07 mg/L for gentamicin C1, 0.1 mg/L for gentamicins C2 and C1a	Study describes the individual pharmacokinetics of the three gentamicin components C1, C1a and C2 [193]
Cephalosporins				
Simultaneous determination	Plasma, amniotic fluid	Solid phase extraction; C18 column; elution by phosphate buffer-methanol 18/82 (%v/v); UV-VIS 285, 260 nm; run time 30 min	0.035-0.08 mg/L	Cefepime, cefixime and cefoperazone [194]
	Human blood serum, urine	Solid phase extraction; C18 column; acetate buffer-methanol 78:22 (v/v); UV-VIS 265 nm; run time 7 min	0.015-0.03 mg/L	cephalexin and cefadroxil, cefaclor and cefataxim [195]
Fluoroquinolones				
Simultaneous determination	Human plasma	Protein precipitation with 20% trichloroacetic acid, centrifugation,	0.02 mg/L	Norfloxacin, lomefloxacin and

Table 1: contd…

		supernatant analysis; C18 column; elution by 0.1% formic acid–methanol 82:18 (v/v); fluorescent detection 278/450 nm (excitation/emission); run time 7 min		ciprofloxacin [196]
	Human serum	Protein precipitation with perchloric acid and methanol, centrifugation; C8 column; elution by 1%triethylamine-acetonitrile (86/14, v/v); fluorescent detection 278/450 nm (excitation/emission); run time 18 min	0.1 mg/L	Pazufloxacin, ciprofloxacin, and levofloxacin [197]
	Blood serum	Protein precipitation with acetonitrile, evaporation and dilution in water; C8 column, elution by acetonitrile-methanol-citric acid (7:15:78 %, v/v/v); UV-VIS 275 nm; run time 9 min	0.03-0.06 mg/L	Enoxacin, norfloxacin, ofloxacin, and ciprofloxacin [198]
	Urine	Dilution (1:50) with 10mM citric buffer; C18 column, elution by citrate buffer-acetonitrile gradient; UV–VIS at 280 nm and fluorescent detection 280/495 nm (excitation/emission); run time 26 min	0.0008-0.061 mg/L	Pipemidic acid, marbofloxacin, enoxacin, ofloxacin, norfloxacin, ciprofloxacin, danofloxacin, lomefloxacin, enrofloxacin, sarafloxacin, difloxacin, oxolinic acid, nalidixic acid, flumequine and piromidic acid [199]
Ciprofloxacin	Human plasma	Protein precipitation with acetonitrile, evaporation and dilution in mobile phase; C18 column, elution by orthophosphoric acid-methanol-acetonitrile (75/13/12%, v/v/v); fluorescent detection 278/450 nm (excitation/emission); run time 8 min	0.02 mg/L	Application to a population pharmacokinetics study in children with severe malnutrition [200]
		Protein precipitation with acetonitrile, evaporation and dilution in 0.1% formic acid; C18 column, elution by formic acid 0.1%-acetonitrile (92:8 v/v); ESI-MS; run time 16 min	0.025 mg/L	Method adapted for neonates [201]
		Protein precipitation with acetonitrile, centrifugation, analysis of supernatant; C18 column, elution by acetonitrile–2% acetic acid (16:84, v/v); UV-VIS 280 nm; run time 15 min	LOD 0.083 mg/L	Method applied in a pharmacokinetic study of a volunteer who receives a 500 mg ciprofloxacin tablet [202]

Table 1: contd...

Nitroimidazoles				
Simultaneous quantification	Human saliva and gingival crevicular fluid	Dilution with methanol, centrifugation, supernatant analysis; C18 column, elution by phosphate buffer and acetonitrile and methanol (55:15:30, v/v/v); UV-VIS 318 nm; run time 7 min	LOD 0.006-0.011 mg/L	Metronidazole, tinidazole, ornidazole and morinidazole [203]
Metronidazole	Dried blood spots	Extraction of spots with water; C18 column, elution by acetonitrile-0.01M phosphate solution (15:85, v/v); UV-VIS 317 nm; run time 6.5 min	1.8 mg/L	Method was applied to the analysis of 203 samples from neonatal patients for a phamacokinetic/ pharmacodynamic study [204]
	Human plasma	Extraction by ethyl acetate, centrifugation, freeze of aqueous layer, organic phase evaporation and dilution in mobile phase; C18 columns, elution by acetonitrile and 10 mM ammonium acetate (80:20, v/v); ESI-MS/MS; run time 5 min	0.05 mg/L	Method was applied to a pilot bioequivalence study of metronidazole in healthy volunteers [205]
Polypeptides				
Colistin	Human plasma	protein precipitation with trichloroacetic acid and methanol, followed by in-solid phase extraction derivatization with 9-fluorenylmethyl chloroformate; C18 column, elution by acetonitrile, tetrahydrofuran and deionized water (82%, 2%, 16%, v/v/v); fluorescent detection 260/315 nm (excitation/emission); run time 22 min	LOD 0.1 mg/L	Improved selectivity resulted in increased quantification accuracy [206]
	Plasma and urine	SPE; C18 column, elution by acetonitrile–water (20:80, v/v); API-MS/MS; run time 3.8 min	0.01-0.024 mg/L in plasma 0.02-0.058 mg/L in urine	Assay for the quantification of colistins A and B and their prodrugs, colistin methanesulfonate CMS A and CMS B [207]
Glycopeptides				
Vancomycin	Human drainage tissue fluid	Protein precipitation, liquid-liquid extraction by dichloromethane, aqueous phase analysis; C18 column, elution by water-acetonitrile gradient; ESI-MS/MS; run time < 10 min	0.5 mg/L	Evaluation in four calcaneal osteomyelitis patients [192]
	Human plasma, bronchoalveolar lavage fluid	Protein precipitation with acetonitrile, evaporation and dilution in mobile phase; C18 column; elution by phosphate	1 mg/L	Study contains the comparison of HPLC to RIA [208]

Table 1: contd…

		buffer-acetonitrile (89:19 v/v); UV 240 nm; run time 20 min		
	Human plasma	Protein precipitation with acetonitrile, centrifugation, evaporation of supernatant and dilution in methanol; C18 column, elution by phosphate buffer-methanol gradient; fluorescent detection 225/258 nm (excitation/emission); run time 30 min	0.005 mg/L	Linear calibration curve over the range from 0.005 to 1 mg/L [209]
	Serum	Strong cation exchange solid phase extraction; C8 column, elution by 0.1% (v/v) formic acid and acetonitrile (9:1 v/v); ESI-MS; run time 5 min	0.005 mg/L	Method was used to determine levels in patients during perioperative infusion of the drug [210]
Lincosamides				
Clindamycin	Plasma and saliva	Addition of methanol, centrifugation, analysis of supernatant; C18 column, elution by methanol–trifluoroacetic acid 0.01% (40:60, v/v); ESI-MS/MS; run time 3 min	0.01 mg/L	Measurement of clindamycin in samples taken up to 6h after oral and intravenous administration of this drug in infectious patients [211]
	Human plasma	Protein precipitation with 50% trichloroacetic acid, centrifugation and analysis of supernatant; CN column, elution by acetonitrile–distilled water–tetramethylammonium chloride (60:40:0.075, v/v/v); UV-VIS 204 nm; run time 25 min	0.2 mg/L	Analysis of samples taken up to 12 h after a single oral administration of clindamycin in healthy volunteers [212]

Table 2. Antifungals in body fluids determined and quantified by liquid chromatography.

	Matrix	Sample Preparation and Analysis	LOQ (LOD)	Notes
Simultaneous determination	Human plasma	C18 column, gradient ammonium formate or ammonium acetate buffer – acetonitrile or methanol.	0.01-0.1 µg/L	Comparison between a high-resolution single-stage Orbitrap and a triple quadrupole mass spectrometer; anidulafungin, caspofungin, fluconazole, itraconazole, hydroxyitraconazole, posaconazole, voriconazole,

Table 2: contd...

				voriconazole-N-oxide [213]
		LC-MS/MS, C4 column, gradient water with 0.1% formic acid/acetonitrile, run time 8 min.	1.4 – 97.7 µg/L	Determination of anidulafungin, caspofungin, isavuconazole, micafungin, posaconazole, voriconazole in plasma, peripheral blood mononuclear cells, and polymorphonuclear leukocytes [214]
		UPLC-MS/MS; C18 column, gradient ammonium formate buffer – acetonitrile, run time 4.3 min.	0.01-0.02 mg/L	Fluconazole, itraconazole, posaconazole, voriconazole, anidulafungin, caspofungin [215]
		Turbulent flow LC-MS/MS, C18 column, gradient water –methanol, run time 12 min.	0.01 mg/L	Itraconazole, hydroxyitraconazole, posaconazole, voriconazole, fluconazole [216]
		Protein precipitation - methanol/ZnSO$_4$, solid-phase extraction, on-line SPE–HPLC–MS/MS, Allure PFP Propyl column, run time 3 min.	14 ng/mL	Fluconazole, itraconazole, posaconazole, voriconazole [217]
		Extraction by hexane– methylene chloride (70:30, v/v), centrifugation, supernatant evaporation, dilution in mobile phase; C8 column, elution by phosphate buffer-acetonitrile-water (45:52.5:2.5, v/v/v); UV-VIS 255 nm; run time 20 min	0.2 mg/L voriconazole, 0.05 mg/L posaconazole	Voriconazole and posaconazole [218]
	Human serum	Turbulent flow LC-MS/MS, C18 column, gradient water –methanol, run time 12 min.	0.01 mg/L	Itraconazole, hydroxyitraconazole, posaconazole, voriconazole, fluconazole [216]
		Protein precipitation – methanol/acetonitrile (4:21, v/v); LC/MS/MS detection; C18 column; gradient	fluconazole 0.5 mg/L; others 0.1 mg/l	Voriconazole, fluconazole, itraconazole, posaconazole [219]

Table 2: contd…

		elution - acetate buffer with acetonitrile; LC–MS/MS; run time 3.4 min.		
		HPLC-UV, isocratic separation, column C18, 50 mM phosphate buffer, pH 6.0, acetonitrile, and methanol (35:45:20 v/v %), UV 255 nm.	0.03 µg/ml	Voriconazole, itraconazole [220]
		Liquid-liquid extraction by heptane-isoamyl alcohol (90:10, v/v), centrifugation, supernatant evaporation, dilution in mobile phase; C18 column, elution by phosphate buffer-acetonitrile-methanol (35:45:20, v/v/v); UV-VIS 255 nm; run time 20 min	0.1 mg/L	Voriconazole and Itraconazole [220]
	In vitro model of the human alveolus	C18 column, elution by water-acetonitrile gradient; UV-VIS 254 nm + fluorescent detection 273/464 nm (excitation/emission); run time 13 min	LOD 0.0625 mg/L variconazole 0.006 mg/L anidulafungin	Investigation of combination of Voriconazole and Anidulafungin for treatment of Triazole-resistant aspergillus fumigatus in an *in vitro* model of invasive pulmonary aspergillosis [221]
Amphotericin B	Human plasma	SPE; C18 column, elution by acetonitrile-disodium edetate (45:55, v/v); UV-VIS 407 nm; run time < 10 min	LOD 0.005 mg/L	Samples from two healthy human volunteers and from two cancer patients on antifungal therapy [222]
		Protein precipitation using 2% dimethylsulfoxide in acetonitrile; C18 column, elution by ammonium acetate, methanol and acetonitrile gradient; ESI-MS/MS; run time 6.5 min	0.25 mg/L free 1 mg/L liposomal	Determination of free and liposomal Amphotericin B [223]
Anidulafungin	Human plasma	Extraction with methanol solution, centrifugation, supernatant dilution in ammonium acetate solution; C8 column, elution by water-acetonitrile gradient;	0.05 mg/L	Method separates the isobaric openring form of anidulafungin (D1) from anidulafungin [224]

Table 2: contd…

		ESI-MS/MS		
		Protein precipitation with 80:20 MeOH–0.2M ZnSO$_4$ (v/v), online SPE; C18 column, elution by methanol-water (97:3 v/v); ESI-MS/MS; run time 4.5 min	0.04 mg/L	[225]
Fluconazole	Urine	SPE; C18 column, elution by methanol-water (70:30, v/v); UV-VIS 254 nm; run time 3 min	1.28 mg/L	[226]
Iodiconazole	Human plasma	Liquid–liquid extraction with n-hexane; C18 column, elution by methanol–water–formic acid (50:50:0.05, v/v/v); ESI-MS/MS; run time 3.5 min	0.10 µg/L	Determination of the concentration of iodiconazole in human plasma following dermal administration [227]
Itraconazole	Serum	Protein precipitation with acetonitrile, centrifugation, supernatant analysis; C18 column, elution by acetonitrile-water (70:30, v/v); UV-VIS 262 nm; run time 10 min	0.25 mg/L	Simultaneous determination of itraconazole and its major metabolite, hydroxy itraconazole [228]
	Human plasma	Liquid-phase extraction using a hexane-dichloromethane (70:30, v/v); C18 column, elution by orthophosphoric acid–acetonitrile (46:54)–isopropanol (90:10, v/v); fluorescent detection 264/380 nm (excitation/emission); run time 22 min	5 µg/L	Simultaneous determination of itraconazole and its major metabolite, hydroxy itraconazole [229]
Micafungin	Human plasma	Column switching with on-line extraction; C18 column, elution by 0.02 M KH2PO4–acetonitrile (56:44, v/v); fluorescent detection 273/464 nm (excitation/emission); run time 20 min	LOD 0.03 mg/L	Does not require a lengthy pre-purification procedure [230]
Posaconazole	Serum	Column switching with on-line extraction; C18 column, elution by water-acetonitrile (55:45, v/v);	0.1 mg/L	[231]

Table 2: contd...

		fluorescent detection 261/357 nm (excitation/emission); run time 15 min		
		Protein precipitation with acetonitrile, centrifugation, supernatant analysis;; C18 column, elution by acetonitrile-water (60:40, v/v); UV-VIS 262 nm; run time 11 min	0.125 mg/L	Comparison of HPLC and a bioassay, for posaconazole quantification from clinical samples [232]
	Human plasma	A mixed-mode cation exchange SPE; C18 column, elution by water-acetonitrile gradient; ESI-MS/MS; run time 1 min	5 µg/L	[233]
Voriconazole	Plasma	SPE; C18 column, elution by 0.01 M TEMED phosphate buffer-acetonitrile (55:45, v/v); UV-VIS 254 nm; run time 12 min	0.2 mg/L	Validation of assay [234]; long-term drug monitoring in haematological patients [235]
		Protein precipitation by 0.2M ZnSO4-methanol – acetonitrile (150:30:75, v/v/v); C18 pre-column, elution by water-methanol gradient; ESI-MS/MS; run time 2 min	0.13 mg/L	The possibility of omitting calibration to each run was evaluated [236]
	Serum Plasma	Liquid-liquid extraction by methanol-sodium hydroxide; C18 column, elution by 0.01mol/L potassiumphosphate-acetonitrile gradient; UV-VIS 254 nm; run time 10 min	0.1 mg/L	[237]
	Serum	Protein precipitation with acetonitrile, centrifugation, supernatant analysis; C18 column, elution by 2 mM ammonium acetate-methanol gradient; ESI-MS/MS; run time 4 min	0.1 mg/L	Comparison with HPLC-UV assay at a reference laboratory [238]

CIEF and CZE as Tool for Analysis of Antimicrobials in Body Fluids

To determine the effect of antimicrobial therapy, the analysis of biological matrix is required [35, 239, 240]. Biological samples are complex and many components in the matrix can complicate the analysis. Thus, the sample pretreatment is often a necessary step before the CE separation [35, 241]. The topic of separation and determination of antibiotics by CZE was reviewed in Refs. [35, 242-245]. The UV detection or laser-induced fluorescent detection (LIF) is mostly used detection techniques. They are suitable for both, antimicrobials and microbial cells detection. However, there are many other detection systems that have been applied in the analysis of antibiotics by CE such as electrochemiluminescence, electrochemical detection, conductivity detection, MS, *etc.* [242]. The analysis of antibiotic residues in the biological samples requires a pretreatment step [35]. These samples are in most cases pre-treated employing solid phase extraction [246-252], liquid–liquid extraction [253, 254], solid–liquid extraction [255], solvent extraction [256], matrix solid-phase dispersion [257], magnetic solid-phase extraction [258], dispersive liquid–liquid microextraction [259] or liquid–liquid–liquid microextraction [243, 260], dispersive solid–phase extraction, and the extraction with oxidized multi-walled carbon nanotubes [261]. We offer to reader a short overview of the applications of CE techniques used for fast separation and detection of antibiotics/antifungals in biological matrices. Antimicrobials were selected in relation to discussed pathogens.

CIEF of Antibiotics

Antibiotics show acidic, basic, or amphoteric behaviors which depend on the combination of functional groups in their molecules. They represent very suitable analyte for separation by CIEF, *e.g.*, a study covering an optimization of CIEF separation conditions in various pH gradients and determination of the p*I*s of selected antibiotics was published in 2014 [262]. The following p*I* values for selected antibiotics were determined; ampicillin 4.9, ciprofloxacin 7.4, ofloxacin 7.1, tetracycline 5.4, tigecycline 9.7, and vancomycin 8.1. Simultaneously, antibiotics were analyzed in real samples such as culture medium or human body fluids. The electropherogram obtained for vancomycin solubilized in human blood is shown in Fig. (**7**). The second part of the study dealt with the effect of different concentrations of tetracycline on the value of p*I* of bacteria *S. epidermidis*. The authors also presented the simultaneous detection of both, ampholytic antibiotics and bacteria *S. epidermidis*, from culture medium or whole human blood.

CZE of Antibiotics

During last years, CZE has confirmed its position as a useful analytical technique for many biological applications. An analysis of fluoroquinolone antibiotics is a good example. Fluoroquinolones are synthetic antibacterial compounds used in human and veterinary medicine for the treatment of various bacterial infections.

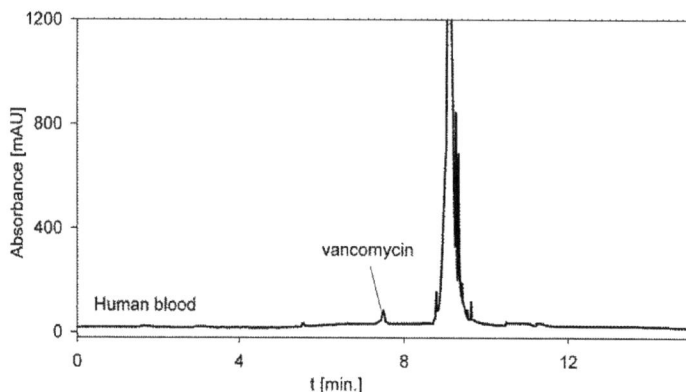

Fig. (7). CIEF (UV detection, 280 nm) of the spiked human blood with vancomycin (1.0 μg mL^{-1}) in the pH gradient in pH range 2.0–9.6.

Although CZE can offer satisfactory separation of quinolone residues, this technique has low concentration sensitivity. Thus, efforts are made in both, the use off-column and on-column pre-concentration in order to achieve low limits of detection (LODs). A methodology combining CZE with UV detection and an off-column single drop liquid–liquid–liquid microextraction was developed for the determination of six fluoroquinolones (gatifloxacin, lomefloxacin, enoxacin, ciprofloxacin, ofloxacin, and pefloxacin) [243, 260]. The extraction and pre-concentration procedures were used in order to increase the sensitivity of the method and to purify real samples before analysis. Using this methodology, good values of recovery (81.8–104.9%) and LODs from 7.4 to 31.5 ng mL^{-1} were obtained. The method was applied also for the simultaneous determination of fluroquinolones in spiked human urine samples. CZE-UV method for determination of fluoroquinolones in biological samples was reported in Refs. [263, 264]. A separation efficiency of seven fluoroquinolones was enhanced when silica nanoparticles (SiNPs) were added into the background buffer [263]. SiNPs acting as pseudostationary phase affected electrophoretic mobilities of analytes and also selectivity of separation. LODs from 2.0 to 7.0 μg mL^{-1} were achieved. The recoveries obtained for the seven quinolones were in the range from 89.2 to 99.5%, what indicates that the method can be applied to the analysis of real samples [263]. An enantioselective CZE method based on electrokinetic chromatography with cyclodextrins (CD-EKC) with UV detection enabled the determination of pazufloxacin enantiomers (a fluoroquinolone broad-spectrum antibiotic) in spiked human urine without a clean-up procedure. Hydroxypropyl-beta-cyclodextrin was used as the chiral selector and LODs of 7.0 μg mL^{-1} for both pazufloxacin enantiomers were reached [265].

The antibiotic fleroxacin (trifluorinated 4-quinolone) and the amino acid proline in human urine were analyzed using a combination of CZE with electrochemiluminescence [266]. $[Ru(bpy)_3]^{2+}$ in phosphate buffer solution was used for the electrochemiluminescent detection and this detection system was then utilized for clinical and biochemical analyses [245, 267]. Suggested method was employed for determination of fleroxacin in human urine after its deproteinization. The separation time around 7 min and low value of LOD for fleroxacin (0.3 ng mL^{-1}) demonstrate a big potential of method for a routine determination of the mentioned antibiotic. The same authors also reported a similar method for the determination of pipemidic acid in the presence of proline in human urine [268]. Pipemidic acid is an antibacterial agent active against *P. aeruginosa*. The developed method was fast (less than 3 min for pipemidic acid), sensitive (LOD, 20 ng mL^{-1}), and it was successfully applied to the determination of this compound in human urine of volunteers treated with pipemidic acid administered orally. In another study of this group, the CZE-electrochemilu-minescent method for the determination of enoxacin in the presence of proline and the drug tetracaine in human urine was developed [269]. Using this methodology, the separation of enoxacin was performed in less than 10 min and LOD was estimated in urine as 20 ng mL^{-1}. The combination of CZE with electrochemiluminescent detection was also used to determine gatifloxacin in biological fluids after sample clean-up using SPE C18 cartridges [270]. The recoveries obtained using this method were 72 % for blood as well as for urine samples. The method showed LOD of 20 ng mL^{-1} which allowed determination of gatifloxacin in urine and blood samples originating from volunteers after oral dosing of gatifloxacin. Enoxacin and ofloxacin were also determined by CZE-electrochemiluminescent method and their LODs were 2.88 and 58 ng mL^{-1}, respectively. The developed method was employed for the determination of enoxacin and ofloxacin in human urine and human serum after deproteinization [243, 271]. Norfloxacin and levofloxacin were determined in urine samples [272] employing a CZE method with the same detection system as in Ref. [267]. Both fluoroquinolones were separated in 9 min. LODs for norfloxacin and levofloxacin ranged from 0.48 to 0.64 mM and recoveries ranged from 84.4 to 90.1% and from 86.1 to 92.3%, respectively. Oxidized multi-walled carbon nanotubes were used as stationary phase for the pre-concentration of fluoroquinolones from human plasma [273]. The CZE-chemiluminescent detection has also been used for ultrasensitive determination of norfloxacin and ciprofloxacin in human urine without any pretreatment step [243, 274]. LODs of 90 and 0.3 pg mL^{-1} for norfloxacin and ciprofloxacin were obtained.

Representatives of β-lactam antibiotics were also successfully determined by CZE. CZE with UV detection was used for separation and determination of penicillin G in urine, blood, and amniotic fluid samples. This analyte was detected in less than 12 min and LOD was 0.5 mM. Although the lower LOD (0.1 mM) was achieved by HPLC method, CZE offers better separation efficiency at lower costs over the HPLC [245, 275]. The simultaneous separation of eight cephalosporins was demonstrated in Ref. [276]. These were separated in 11 min and detected at 214 nm. LODs ranging from 0.5 to 5 µg mL^{-1} and high reproducibility with inter- and intra-day variation within the ranges 0.6–1.6% RSD and 0.5–1.8% RSD, respectively, were reached. The method was applied to the analysis of urine samples from volunteers after taking cefradine and cefuroxime. Cefazolin, which belongs to the cephalosporins, was determined in serum [242, 277], contents of wound drains, and cerebro-spinal fluid in a 24-h postoperative period after the administration of 1 g of the antibiotic. Cefazolin was then separated by CZE with UV-detection at 270 nm.

The antibiotics from the groups of fluoroquinolones and β-lactams were simultaneously determined by CZE with UV detection in Refs. [239, 240]. The cephalosporins, cefazolin, cefminox, and one fluoroquinolone (gatifloxacin) were simultaneously analyzed in urine samples [239]. Rapid and simple methodology was developed for the simultaneous separation of ciprofloxacin, a fluoroquinolone antibiotic from other coadministered drugs (paracetamol and diclofenac) by CZE with UV detection. The method was applied to the analysis of urine samples. LODs of 1 µg mL^{-1} were reached. These results were compared to those obtained by the HPLC method and good agreement was found [278].

Sulfamethoxazole is a sulfonamide bacteriostatic antibiotic frequently used as a part of a synergistic combination with trimethoprim. Micellar electrokinetic chromatography (MEKC) with UV detection was used to determine sulfamethoxazole, trimethoprim, and their main metabolites in spiked human serum. Prior to separation, the sample was deproteinized and preconcentrated (ten times) by evaporation [244, 279]. This pretreatment improved the LODs which ranged from 40 to 60 ng mL^{-1}. MEKC with UV detection was also applied to the analysis of ceftriaxone in human serum and in cerebro-spinal fluid. In this case, both biological samples could be directly injected without any sample pretreatment [244, 280]. However, the same method applied to the analysis of ceftriaxone, cefazolin, cefamandol, cefuroxim, ceftazidim, and cefepime in bronchial secretions provided irreproducible results. The analysis required additional lyophilization and dissolution of the sputum samples to become reproducible [280].

Doxycycline is tetracycline antibiotic. It was determined in human urine by MEKC with UV detection [281]. The method can be used for the analysis of human urine samples without pretreatment [282].

Fosfomycin is most often indicated drug in the treatment of urinary tract infections. CZE with UV detection was also applied to the quantitative determination of fosfomycin in pus from patients. The LOD was obtained as 4.5 $\mu g\ mL^{-1}$ [283]. In Ref. [284] human plasma and microdialysis samples containing fosfomycin were collected from patients. Proteins in plasma samples were precipitated by methanol and supernatant was injected into the CZE system equipped with indirect UV detection (254 nm) or contactless conductivity detection. LODs ranged from 0.6 to 2 $\mu g\ mL^{-1}$.

CZE combined with LIF detection with argon-ion laser was used for the separation of aminoglycoside bacteriocidal antibiotics, bekanamycin, kanamycin, paromomycin, and tobramycin in human plasma. The method enabled the determination of these antibiotics in less than 9 min. A simple clean-up procedure, deproteinization with acetonitrile, was used for the sample treatment. After derivatization of analytes by 6-carboxyfluorescein succinimidyl ester, LODs ranging from 3.9 to 8.2 nM for standards and from 14.4 to 24.0 nM for plasma samples were obtained [285]. CZE with conductivity detection was employed for the determination of tobramycin spiked in human serum using kanamycin B as internal standard. This method enabled the direct quantification of the non-UV-absorbing species [244, 286]. The determination of aminoglycoside gentamicin components (C1, C1a, C2a, and C2) in human serum was performed after SPE and sample derivatization by CZE-UV detection at 230 nm. SPE recoveries were found from 78 to 93% and LODs about 0.3 $\mu g\ mL^{-1}$ were achieved for all gentamicin components [287]. The determination of clarithromycin in biological fluids was proposed by Peng *et al.* [288]. This antibiotic was modified after CZE separation by tris (2,2-bipyridyl)ruthenium (II) ($[Ru(bpy)_3]^{2+}$) and product of the reaction was monitored by electrochemiluminescent detection. Compared to an HPLC method, the developed CZE method was faster, simpler, and more sensitive (LOD 30 nM). It was successfully applied to the determination of clarithromycin in spiked plasma and urine samples, where the recoveries ranged from 83.3 to 94.6% and from 90 to 95%, respectively.

Macrolide antibiotics are lipophilic compounds with a central lactone ring to which several amino groups and/or neutral sugars are bonded [243, 289]. Macrolide antibiotics are used to treat infections caused by gram-positive bacteria, *Streptococcus pneumoniae*, and *Haemophilus influenzae*, and infections such as respiratory tract and soft tissue infections. They are a good alternative for patients showing penicillin sensitivity or allergy. The macrolide antibiotics were determined by CZE with electrochemiluminescent detection [289-291]. Azithromycin, roxithromycin, and erythromycin which belong to the macrolide antibiotics were separated together and determined in human urine and plasma [243, 291] within 6 min. The detection was based on the enhancement effect of these compounds on the electrochemiluminescence of $[Ru (bpy)_3]^{2+}$. LODs were from 74.9 to 293.57 ng mL^{-1} and this method was successfully applied to the determination of these compounds in human urine and plasma. In Ref. [289], azithromycin, acetylspiramycin, erythromycin, and josemycin were simultaneously determined in human urine and tablets. The samples were directly injected into the separation capillary after the dilution. The total analysis time was 6 min. The reported LODs ranged from 61.4 to 993.6 ng mL^{-1}.

Vancomycin belongs to glycopeptide antibiotics. Monitoring of its concentration in serum is essential to obtain a sufficient efficacy of the treatment as well as to prevent adverse side effects [292-294]. Vancomycin has a bacteriostatic effect on gram-positive bacteria such as MRSA. The micellar electrokinetic chromatography with UV detection at 210 nm was used for the measurement of vancomycin concentration in human serum using direct injection. The limit of detection was 1.0 µg mL^{-1} [294]. Telavancin is a novel lipoglycopeptide antibiotic in late-stage of clinical development designed for the treatment of serious infections caused by gram-positive bacteria. The ability of telavancin to inhibit peptidoglycan synthesis and polymerization of peptidoglycan in intact MRSA cells was evaluated by affinity capillary electrophoresis in conjunction with ESI-MS [295].

Antifungals

Invasive fungal infections are often severe diseases, rapidly progressive, and connected with difficult diagnosis or treatment. Especially, the treatment of immunocompromised patients is long and complex. Posaconazole belonging to antifungals called triazoles has been proven as an effective drug for fungal infection treatment. It is a novel agent with strong antifungal activity and low toxicity. The success of therapy strongly depends on the precise control of drug concentration in the blood. CZE method with field-amplified sample stacking

(FASS) was used for the analysis of posaconazole in the plasma of patients. Combination of SPE and FASS improves the sensitivity of CZE, reduces the matrix effect, and it can be applied to real sample analysis in clinical practice. Time of the analysis less than 5 min and the LOD of 10 ng mL^{-1} were achieved [296]. SPE procedure was also used as a pre-concentration technique for the analysis of ketoconazole, clotrimazole, itraconazole, fluconazole, and voriconazole after their incubation with human liver microsomes. Stability of these compounds was controlled *in vitro* by CZE method. Combination of SPE with CZE method is suitable for the separation and detection of basic drugs *in vitro* [297]. SPE in conjunction with sweeping-MEKC, was applied to determination of voriconazole in plasma. SPE reduces interference from the sample and allows sensitive and selective voriconazole determination. The voriconazole was separated within 10.5 min and the LOD 0.075 µg mL^{-1} was achieved [298]. In the next paper, voriconazole in human plasma and serum was determined by MEKC. UK 115794 was used as an internal standard. The sample was purified by liquid-liquid extraction using a mixture of ethylacetate and dichloromethane. The method was validated and the data from the set of 91 samples from patients treated with voriconazole were compared with results obtained using HPLC. Data obtained from both methods provided excellent agreement. The LODs of 1-6 µg mL^{-1} were determined for voriconazole in human plasma and serum samples [299]. Another study dealt with the development of the separation method for three most widely used triazole antifungal drugs (voriconazole, itraconazole, and posaconazole). Similarly as in the previous articles, SPE before sweeping-MEKC was performed. The developed method was validated and successfully applied to the analysis of clinical samples [300]. The group of fungicides called triazoles also includes drug fluconazole showing low toxicity. Fluconazole was separated by MEKC and obtained data were compared with HPLC data available in the literature. MEKC provided a higher separation efficiency than HPLC. Prior to the analysis, the authors used three different procedures for sample pretreatment (direct sample injection after protein precipitation with acetonitrile, liquid-liquid extraction with dichloromethane, and SPE using C-18 cartridges). The detection limits were as follows: 100 ng mL^{-1} using SPE, 1 µg mL^{-1} using liquid-liquid extraction, and 5 µg mL^{-1} using direct sample injection [301]. Another group of drugs, namely imidazoles, was determined using CD-MEKC. Enantioseparation of tioconazole, isoconazole, and fenticonazole was achieved by CD-MEKC from urine samples which were treated by SPE. All imidazoles were determined within 15 min and the LODs ranged from 2.7 to 7.7 mg L^{-1}[302]. In Ref. [303] levels of flucytosine in human serum of 60 patients were determined by MEKC with UV detection. Flucytosine (80 µg mL^{-1}) was also well separated from another frequently occurring antimycotic drug, amphotericin B. Intraday and interday reproducibility were between 4.5 and 7 %, respectively [303]. CZE analysis of seven antifungal drugs (ketoconazole, clotrimazole, terbinafine, itraconazole, fluconazole, voriconazole, and one GlaxoWellcome product under development) in fused silica capillary with and without additives in the running electrolyte was also studied. The effects of the concentration and type of the running electrolyte on the separation were investigated. The obtained separation times were less than 10 min for all antifungals. The best LOD was lower than 1 µg mL^{-1} for all analyzed antifungal drugs. For some analytes, additives in the electrolyte can improve the selectivity and sensitivity of measurement; however, at the cost of the increase in separation time [304]. CZE was also applied to the determination of echinocandin antifungal agent micafungin. Micafungin was monitored in patients with clinically important deep mycoses. Deproteinization by acetonitrile was necessary for sample pretreatment prior to direct injection into the separation capillary. Time of analysis for micafungin was obtained less than 9 min and LOD was 0.5 mg L^{-1} [305].

CONCLUDING REMARKS

Advanced phenotyping techniques such as CZE, CIEF, LC, and mass spectrometry, can partially solve the critical problems of current medicine arising in the area of healthcare-associated infections. While the separation and identification of antimicrobials and their metabolites belong now almost into the area of application research or into the area of commercial laboratories, the situation in the field of identification of etiological agents of nosocomial infections in the body fluids, in particular blood, is much more complicated. The capillary electrophoretic techniques significantly accelerate the overall time of separation, detection, and identification of MOs, but they are not self-supporting. In the future, a combination of electrophoretic techniques with off-line MALDI-TOF MS detection could improve and simplify an identification of microbial cells. However, the accomplishment of the hard time criteria of MOs analysis requires still a lot of effort based on the fundamental research not only in the field of capillary electrophoretic techniques, but also in the field of MALDI-TOF MS.

ACKNOWLEDGEMENTS

This study was supported by the Ministry of the Interior of the Czech Republic by grants VG20112015021, VG20102015023 and by the Ministry of Education,

Youth and Sports of the Czech Republic (INGOII, No. LG13011) and received institutional support RVO:68081715.

CONFLICT OF INTEREST

The authors confirm that this chapter content has no conflict of interest.

REFFERENCES

[1]   Horan TC, Andrus M, Dudeck MA. Cdc/nhsn surveillance definition of health care-associated infection and criteria for specific types of infections in the acute care setting. Am J Infect Control 2008; 36(5): 309-32.

[2]   European commission [http://ec.Europa.Eu/]. Luxembourg: Council recommendation of 9 june 2009 on patient safety, including the prevention and control of healthcare-associated infections (2009/c151/01) [cited: 9th july 2015]. Council of the European Union. Available from: http://ec.europa.eu/health/patient_safety/docs/council_2009_en.pdf

[3]   Tacconelli E, Cataldo MA, Dancer SJ, et al. Escmid guidelines for the management of the infection control measures to reduce transmission of multidrug-resistant gram-negative bacteria in hospitalized patients. Clin Microbiol Infect 2014; 20: 1-55.

[4]   Cornejo-Juarez P, Vilar-Compte D, Perez-Jimenez C, Namendys-Silva SA, Sandoval-Hernandez S, Volkow-Fernandez P. The impact of hospital-acquired infections with multidrug-resistant bacteria in an oncology intensive care unit. Int J Infect Dis 2015; 31: 31-4.

[5]   Sievert DM, Ricks P, Edwards JR, et al. Antimicrobial-resistant pathogens associated with healthcare-associated infections: Summary of data reported to the national healthcare safety network at the centers for disease control and prevention, 2009-2010. Infect Control Hosp Epidemiol 2013; 34(1): 1-14.

[6]   Ramage G, Rajendran R, Sherry L, Williams C. Fungal biofilm resistance. Int J Microbiol 2012; 2012: 1.

[7]   Chambers HF. Methicillin resistance in staphylococci: Molecular and biochemical basis and clinical implications. Clin Microbiol Rev 1997; 10(4): 781-91.

[8]   The bacterial challenge: Time to react. Stockholm: European Centre for Disease Prevention and Control/European Medicines Agency (ECDC/EMEA). 2009.

[9]   Orsi GB, Ciorba V. Vancomycin resistant enterococci healthcare associated infections. Ann Ig 2013; 25(6): 485-92.

[10]   Sievert DM, Rudrik JT, Patel JB, McDonald LC, Wilkins MJ, Hageman JC. Vancomycin-resistant staphylococcus aureus in the united states, 2002-2006. Clin Infect Dis 2008; 46(5): 668-74.

[11]   von Eiff C, Peters G, Heilmann C. Pathogenesis of infections due to coagulase-negative staphylococci. Lancet Infect Dis 2002; 2(11): 677-85.

[12]   Donlan RM, Costerton JW. Biofilms: Survival mechanisms of clinically relevant microorganisms. Clin Microbiol Rev 2002; 15(2): 167-93.

[13]   Lewis K. Riddle of biofilm resistance. Antimicrob Agents Chemother 2001; 45(4): 999-1007.

[14]   Moore NM, Flaws ML. Antimicrobial resistance mechanisms in pseudomonas aeruginosa. Clin Lab Sci 2011; 24(1): 47-51.

[15]   Strateva T, Yordanov D. Pseudomonas aeruginosa - a phenomenon of bacterial resistance. J Med Microbiol 2009; 58(9): 1133-48.

[16]   Magiorakos AP, Srinivasan A, Carey RB, et al. Multidrug-resistant, extensively drug-resistant and pandrug-resistant bacteria: An international expert proposal for interim standard definitions for acquired resistance. Clin Microbiol Infect 2012; 18(3): 268-81.

[17]   Canton R, Akova M, Carmeli Y, et al. Rapid evolution and spread of carbapenemases among enterobacteriaceae in europe. Clin Microbiol Infect 2012; 18(5): 413-31.

[18]   Pitout JDD, Sanders CC, Sanders WE. Antimicrobial resistance with focus on beta-lactam resistance in gram-negative bacilli. Am J Med 1997; 103(1): 51-9.

[19]   Wisplinghoff H, Seifert H, Wenzel RP, Edmond MB. Current trends in the epidemiology of nosocomial bloodstream infections in patients with hematological malignancies and solid neoplasms in hospitals in the united states. Clin Infect Dis 2003; 36(9): 1103-10.

[20]   Krcmery V, Barnes AJ. Non-albicans candida spp. Causing fungaemia: Pathogenicity and antifungal resistance. J Hosp Infect 2002; 50(4): 243-60.

[21]   Paramythiotou E, Frantzeskaki F, Flevari A, Armaganidis A, Dimopoulos G. Invasive fungal infections in the icu: How to approach, how to treat. Molecules 2014; 19(1): 1085-119.

[22]   Brondz I, Olsen I. Microbial chemotaxonomy - chromatography, electrophoresis and relevant profiling techniques. J Chromatogr 1986; 379: 367-411.

[23]   Miljković-Selimović B, Kocić B, Babić T, Ristić L. Bacterial typing methods. Acta Fac med Naiss 2009; 26(4): 225-33.

[24]   Patel RM. The guiding principles on antimicrobial susceptibility testing. Bull Pharm Res 2012; 2(3): 146-53.

[25]   Eucast [http://www.Eucast.Org/]. Växjö: Antimicrobial susceptibility testing [cited: 9th july 2015]. European Committee on Antimicrobial Susceptibility Testing (EUCAST). Available from: http://www.eucast.org/ast_of_bacteria/

[26]   Carter MW, Oakton KJ, Warner M, Livermore DM. Detection of extended-spectrum beta-lactamases in klebsiellae with the oxoid combination disk method. J Clin Microbiol 2000; 38(11): 4228-32.

[27]   French GL. Methods for screening for methicillin-resistant staphylococcus aureus carriage. Clin Microbiol Infect 2009; 15: 10-6.

[28]   Fluit AC, Visser MR, Schmitz FJ. Molecular detection of antimicrobial resistance. Clin Microbiol Rev 2001; 14(4): 836-71.

[29]   Danial J, Noel M, Templeton KE, et al. Real-time evaluation of an optimized real-time pcr assay versus brilliance chromogenic mrsa agar for the detection of meticillin-resistant staphylococcus aureus from clinical specimens. J Med Microbiol 2011; 60(3): 323-8.

[30]   Salplachta J, Kubesova A, Horka M. Latest improvements in cief: From proteins to microorganisms. Proteomics 2012; 12(19-20): 2927-36.

[31]   Schnabel U, Groiss F, Blaas D, Kenndler E. Determination of the pi of human rhinovirus serotype 2 by capillary isolectric focusing. Anal Chem 1996; 68(23): 4300-3.

[32]   Kenndler E, Blaas D. Capillary electrophoresis of macromolecular biological assemblies: Bacteria and viruses. TrAC, Trends Anal Chem 2001; 20(10): 543-51.

[33]   Kremser L, Blaas D, Kenndler E. Capillary electrophoresis of biological particles: Viruses, bacteria, and eukaryotic cells. Electrophoresis 2004; 25(14): 2282-91.

[34]   Poortinga AT, Bos R, Norde W, Busscher HJ. Electric double layer interactions in bacterial adhesion to surfaces. Surf Sci Rep 2002; 47(1): 3-32.

[35]   Dominguez-Vega E, Perez-Fernandez V, Luis Crego A, Angeles Garcia M, Luisa Marina M. Recent advances in ce analysis of antibiotics and its use as chiral selectors. Electrophoresis 2014; 35(1): 28-49.

[36]   Shimura K. Recent advances in capillary isoelectric focusing: 1997-2001. Electrophoresis 2002; 23(22-23): 3847-57.

[37]   Silvertand LHH, Torano JS, van Bennekom WP, de Jong GJ. Recent developments in capillary isoelectric focusing. J Chromatogr A 2008; 1204(2): 157-70.

[38]   Shimura K. Recent advances in ief in capillary tubes and microchips. Electrophoresis 2009; 30(1): 11-28.

[39]   Kilar F. Recent applications of capillary isoelectric focusing. Electrophoresis 2003; 24(22-23): 3908-16.

[40]   Hutterer K, Dolnik V. Capillary electrophoresis of proteins 2001-2003. Electrophoresis 2003; 24(22-23): 3998-4012.

[41]   Dolnik V. Capillary electrophoresis of proteins 2003-2005. Electrophoresis 2006; 27(1): 126-41.

[42]   Dolnik V. Capillary electrophoresis of proteins 2005-2007. Electrophoresis 2008; 29(1): 143-56.

[43]   Righetti PG, Candiano G. Recent advances in electrophoretic techniques for the characterization of protein biomolecules: A poker of aces. J Chromatogr A 2011; 1218(49): 8727-37.

[44]   Rodriguez MA, Armstrong DW. Separation and analysis of colloidal/nano-particles including microorganisms by capillary electrophoresis: A fundamental review. J Chromatogr B 2004; 800(1-2): 7-25.

[45]   Rijnaarts HHM, Norde W, Lyklema J, Zehnder AJB. The isoelectric point of bacteria as an indicator for the presence of cell surface polymers that inhibit adhesion. Colloids Surf, B 1995; 4(4): 191-7.

[46]   Jucker BA, Harms H, Zehnder AJB. Adhesion of the positively charged bacterium stenotrophomonas (xanthomonas) maltophilia 70401 to glass and teflon. J Bacteriol 1996; 178(18): 5472-9.

[47]   Busscher HJ, Bellonfontaine MN, Mozes N, et al. An interlaboratory comparison of physicochemical methods for studying the surface-properties of microorganisms - application to streptococcus-thermophilus and leuconostoc-mesenteroides. J Microbiol Methods 1990; 12(2): 101-15.

[48]   Ruzicka F, Horka M, Hola V. Extracellular polysaccharides in microbial biofilm and their influence on the electrophoretic properties of microbial cells. In: Volpi N, editor. Capillary electrophoresis of carbohydrates: From monosaccharides to complex polysaccharides. New York: Humana Press 2011; pp. 105-26.

[49]   Rijnaarts HHM, Norde W, Bouwer EJ, Lyklema J, Zehnder AJB. Reversibility and mechanism of bacterial adhesion. Colloids Surf, B 1995; 4(1): 5-22.

[50]   Rijnaarts HHM, Norde W, Bouwer EJ, Lyklema J, Zehnder AJB. Bacterial adhesion under static and dynamic conditions. Appl Environ Microbiol 1993; 59(10): 3255-65.

[51]   Vanloosdrecht MCM, Lyklema J, Norde W, Schraa G, Zehnder AJB. Electrophoretic mobility and hydrophobicity as a measure to predict the initial steps of bacterial adhesion. Appl Environ Microbiol 1987; 53(8): 1898-901.

[52]   Beveridge TJ, Graham LL. Surface layers of bacteria. Microbiol Rev 1991; 55(4): 684-705.

[53]   Armstrong DW, Schulte G, Schneiderheinze JM, Westenberg DJ. Separating microbes in the manner of molecules. 1. Capillary electrokinetic approaches. Anal Chem 1999; 71(24): 5465-9.

[54]   Bos R, van der Mei HC, Busscher HJ. Physico-chemistry of initial microbial adhesive interactions - its mechanisms and methods for study. FEMS Microbiol Rev 1999; 23(2): 179-230.

[55]   Shirtliff ME, Mader JT, Camper AK. Molecular interactions in biofilms. Chem Biol 2002; 9(8): 859-71.

[56]   Ruzicka F, Horka M, Hola V, Votava M. Capillary isoelectric focusing - useful tool for detection of the biofilm formation in staphylococcus epidermidis. J Microbiol Methods 2007; 68(3): 530-5.

[57]   Kostal V, Arriaga EA. Recent advances in the analysis of biological particles by capillary electrophoresis. Electrophoresis 2008; 29(12): 2578-86.

[58]   Horka M, Kubicek O, Ruzicka F, Hola V, Malinovska I, Slais K. Capillary isoelectric focusing of native and inactivated microorganisms. J Chromatogr A 2007; 1155(2): 164-71.

[59]   Gao P, Xu GW, Shi XZ, Yuan KL, Tian J. Rapid detection of staphylococcus aureus by a combination of monoclonal antibody-coated latex and capillary electrophoresis. Electrophoresis 2006; 27(9): 1784-9.

[60]   Klodzinska E, Dahm H, Rozycki H, Szeliga J, Jackowski M, Buszewski B. Rapid identification of escherichia coli and helicobacter pylori in biological samples by capillary zone electrophoresis. J Sep Sci 2006; 29(8): 1180-7.

[61]   Harden VP, Harris JO. The isoelectric poin of bacterial cells. J Bacteriol 1953; 65(2): 198-202.

[62]   Hjerten S, Zhu MD. Adaptation of the equipment for high-performance electrophoresis to isoelectric focusing. J Chromatogr 1985; 346(OCT): 265-70.

[63]   Shen YF, Berger SJ, Smith RD. Capillary isoelectric focusing of yeast cells. Anal Chem 2000; 72(19): 4603-7.

[64]   Horka M, Planeta J, Ruzicka F, Slais K. Sol-gel column technology for capillary isoelectric focusing of microorganisms and biopolymers with uv or fluorometric detection. Electrophoresis 2003; 24(9): 1383-90.

[65]   Horka M, Ruzicka F, Hola V, Slais K. Ce separation of proteins and yeasts dynamically modified by peg pyrenebutanoate with fluorescence detection. Electrophoresis 2007; 28(13): 2300-7.

[66]   Horka M, Ruzicka F, Horky J, Hola V, Slais K. Capillary isoelectric focusing of proteins and microorganisms in dynamically modified fused silica with uv detection. J Chromatogr B 2006; 841(1-2): 152-9.

[67]   Horka M, Ruzicka F, Hola V, Slais K. Capillary isoelectric focusing of microorganisms in the ph range 2-5 in a dynamically modified fs capillary with uv detection. Anal Bioanal Chem 2006; 385(5): 840-6.

[68]   Horka M, Ruzicka F, Horky J, Hola V, Slais K. Capillary isoelectric focusing and fluorometric detection of proteins and microorganisms dynamically modified by poly(ethylene glycol) pyrenebutanoate. Anal Chem 2006; 78(24): 8438-44.

[69]   Horka M, Ruzicka F, Hola V, Kahle V, Moravcova D, Slais K. Capillary electromigration separation of proteins and microorganisms dynamically modified by chromophoric nonionogenic surfactant. Anal Chem 2009; 81(16): 6897-904.

[70]   Horka M, Ruzicka F, Kubesova A, Slais K. Dynamic labeling of diagnostically significant microbial cells in cerebrospinal fluid by red chromophoric non-ionogenic surfactant for capillary electrophoresis separations. Anal Chim Acta 2012; 728: 86-92.

[71]   Slais K, Horka M, Novackova J, Friedl Z. Fluorescein-based pI markers for capillary isoelectric focusing with laser-induced fluorescence detection. Electrophoresis 2002; 23(11): 1682-8.

[72]   Horka M, Karasek P, Ruzicka F, Dvorackova M, Sittova M, Roth M. Separation of methicillin-resistant from methicillin-susceptible staphylococcus aureus by electrophoretic methods in fused silica capillaries etched with supercritical water. Anal Chem 2014; 86(19): 9701-8.

[73]   Horka M, Ruzicka F, Hola V, Slais K. Separation of similar yeast strains by ief techniques. Electrophoresis 2009; 30(12): 2134-41.

[74]   Ruzicka F, Horka M, Hola V, Kubesova A, Pavlik T, Votava M. The differences in the isoelectric points of biofilm-positive and biofilm-negative candida parapsilosis strains. J Microbiol Methods 2010; 80(3): 299-301.

[75]   Horka M, Ruzicka F, Kubesova A, Nemcova E, Slais K. Separation of phenotypically indistinguishable candida species, c. Orthopsilosis, c. Metapsilosis and c. Parapsilosis, by capillary electromigration techniques. J Chromatogr A 2011; 1218(25): 3900-7.

[76]   Horka M, Ruzicka F, Kubesova A, Hola V, Slais K. Capillary electrophoresis of conidia from cultivated microscopic filamentous fungi. Anal Chem 2009; 81(10): 3997-4004.

[77]   Hjerten S, Elenbring K, Kilar F, et al. Carrier-free zone electrophoresis, displacement electrophoresis and isoelectric-focusing in a high-performance electrophoresis apparatus. J Chromatogr 1987; 403: 47-61.

[78]   Ebersole RC, McCormick RM. Separation and isolation of viable bacteria by capillary zone electrophoresis. Bio-Technology 1993; 11(11): 1278-82.

[79]   Pfetsch A, Welsch T. Determination of the electrophoretic mobility of bacteria and their separation by capillary zone electrophoresis. Fresenius J Anal Chem 1997; 359(2): 198-201.

[80]   Sonohara R, Muramatsu N, Ohshima H, Kondo T. Difference in surface properties between escherichia coli and staphylococcus aureus as revealed by electrophoretic mobility measurements. Biophys Chem 1995; 55(3): 273-7.

[81]   Armstrong DW, Schneiderheinze JM. Rapid identification of the bacterial pathogens responsible for urinary tract infections using direct injection ce. Anal Chem 2000; 72(18): 4474-6.

[82]   Schneiderheinze JM, Armstrong DW, Schulte G, Westenberg DJ. High efficiency separation of microbial aggregates using capillary electrophoresis. FEMS Microbiol Lett 2000; 189(1): 39-44.

[83]   Moon YG, Lee YI, Kang SH, Kim Y. Capillary electrophoresis of microbes. Bull Korean Chem Soc 2003; 24(1): 81-5.

[84]   Buszewski B, Klodzinska E. Determination of pathogenic bacteria by cze with surface-modified capillaries. Electrophoresis 2008; 29(20): 4177-84.

[85]   Jackowski M, Szeliga J, Klodzinska E, Buszewski B. Application of capillary zone electrophoresis (cze) to the determination of pathogenic bacteria for medical diagnosis. Anal Bioanal Chem 2008; 391(6): 2153-60.

[86]   Song L, Li W, Li G, et al. Rapid detection of bacteria in urine samples by the "three-plug-injection" method using capillary electrophoresis. J Chromatogr B 2013; 935: 32-5.

[87]   Horka M, Tesarova M, Karasek P, et al. Determination of methicillin-resistant and methicillin-susceptible staphylococcus aureus bacteria in blood by capillary zone electrophoresis. Anal Chim Acta 2015; 868: 67-72.

[88]   Hrynkiewicz K, Klodzinska E, Dahm H, Szeliga J, Jackowski M, Buszewski B. Combination of capillary electrophoresis, pcr and physiological assays in differentiation of clinical strains of staphylococcus aureus. FEMS Microbiol Lett 2008; 286(1): 1-8.

[89]   Horka M, Ruzicka F, Hola V, Slais K. Dynamic modification of microorganisms by pyrenebutanoate for fluorometric detection in capillary zone electrophoresis. Electrophoresis 2005; 26(3): 548-55.

[90]   Tong M-Y, Jiang C, Armstrong DW. Fast detection of candida albicans and/or bacteria in blood plasma by "sample-self-focusing" using capillary electrophoresis-laser-induced fluorescence. J Pharm Biomed Anal 2010; 53(1): 75-80.

[91]   Lantz AW, Bisha B, Tong M-Y, Nelson RE, Brehm-Stecher BF, Armstrong DW. Rapid identification of candida albicans in blood by combined capillary electrophoresis and fluorescence in situ hybridization. Electrophoresis 2010; 31(16): 2849-53.

[92]   Torimura M, Ito S, Kano K, Ikeda T, Esaka Y, Ueda T. Surface characterization and on-line activity measurements of microorganisms by capillary zone electrophoresis. J Chromatogr B 1999; 721(1): 31-7.

[93]   Buszewski B, Szumski M, Klodzinska E, Dahm H. Separation of bacteria by capillary electrophoresis. J Sep Sci 2003; 26(11): 1045-9.

[94]   Lo AAL, Hu A, Ho Y-P. Identification of microbial mixtures by lc-selective proteotypic-peptide analysis(spa). J Mass Spectrom 2006; 41(8): 1049-60.

[95]   Zheng SP, Schneider KA, Barder TJ, Lubman DM. Two-dimensional liquid chromatography protein expression mapping for differential proteomic analysis of normal and o157 : H7 escherichia coli. BioTechniques 2003; 35(6): 1202-12.

[96]   Gatlin CL, Pieper R, Huang ST, et al. Proteomic profiling of cell envelope-associated proteins from staphylococcus aureus. Proteomics 2006; 6(5): 1530-49.

[97]   Hewelt-Belka W, Nakonieczna J, Belka M, Baczek T, Namiesnik J, Kot-Wasik A. Comprehensive methodology for staphylococcus aureus lipidomics by liquid chromatography and quadrupole time-of-flight mass spectrometry. J Chromatogr A 2014; 1362: 62-74.

[98]   Blonder J, Goshe MB, Xiao WZ, et al. Global analysis of the membrane subproteome of pseudomonas aeruginosa using liquid chromatography-tandem mass. J Proteome Res 2004; 3(3): 434-44.

[99]   Guina T, Wu MH, Miller SI, et al. Proteomic analysis of pseudomonas aeruginosa grown under magnesium limitation. J Am Soc Mass Spectrom 2003; 14(7): 742-51.

[100] Ravipaty S, Reilly JP. Comprehensive characterization of methicillin-resistant staphylococcus aureus subsp aureus col secretome by two-dimensional liquid chromatography and mass spectrometry. Mol Cell Proteomics 2010; 9(9): 1898-919.

[101] Vemula H, Bobba S, Putty S, Barbara JE, Gutheil WG. Ion-pairing liquid chromatography-tandem mass spectrometry-based quantification of uridine diphosphate-linked intermediates in the staphylococcus aureus cell wall biosynthesis pathway. Anal Biochem 2014; 465: 12-9.

[102] Schallenberger MA, Niessen S, Shao C, Fowler BJ, Romesberg FE. Type i signal peptidase and protein secretion in staphylococcus aureus. J Bacteriol 2012; 194(10): 2677-86.

[103] Chen X, Wu H, Cao Y, et al. Ion-pairing chromatography on a porous graphitic carbon column coupled with time-of-flight mass spectrometry for targeted and untargeted profiling of amino acid biomarkers involved in candida albicans biofilm formation. Mol Biosyst 2014; 10(1): 74-85.

[104] Wang T, Chen X, Li L, et al. Characterization of nucleotides and nucleotide sugars in candida albicans by high performance liquid chromatography-mass spectrometry with a porous graphite carbon column. Anal Lett 2014; 47(2): 234-49.

[105] Lee MY, Park HM, Son GH, Lee CH. Liquid chromatography-mass spectrometry-based chemotaxonomic classification of aspergillus spp. And evaluation of the biological activity of its unique metabolite, neosartorin. J Microbiol Biotechnol 2013; 23(7): 932-41.

[106] Bajad SU, Lu W, Kimball EH, Yuan J, Peterson C, Rabinowitz JD. Separation and quantitation of water soluble cellular metabolites by hydrophilic interaction chromatography-tandem mass spectrometry. J Chromatogr A2006. p. 76-88.

[107] Jury F, Al-Mahrous M, Apostolou M, et al. Rapid cost-effective subtyping of meticillin-resistant staphylococcus aureus by denaturing hplc. J Med Microbiol 2006; 55(8): 1053-60.

[108] Lay JO. Maldi-tof mass spectrometry of bacteria. Mass Spectrom Rev 2001; 20(4): 172-94.

[109] Giebel R, Worden C, Rust SM, Kleinheinz GT, Robbins M, Sandrin TR. Microbial fingerprinting using matrix-assisted laser desorption ionization time-of-flight mass spectrometry (maldi-tof ms): Applications and challenges. In: Laskin AI, Sariaslani S, Gadd GM, Eds. Advances in applied microbiology, vol 71. 1st ed. San Diego: Elsevier 2010; pp. 149-84.

[110] De Respinis S, Vogel G, Benagli C, Tonolla M, Petrini O, Samuels GJ. Maldi-tof ms of trichoderma: A model system for the identification of microfungi. Mycol Progress 2010; 9(1): 79-100.

[111] Lasch P, Nattermann H, Erhard M, et al. Maldi-tof mass spectrometry compatible inactivation method for highly pathogenic microbial cells and spores. Anal Chem 2008; 80(6): 2026-34.

[112] Anhalt JP, Fenselau C. Identification of bacteria using mass spectrometry. Anal Chem 1975; 47(2): 219-25.

[113] Krishnamurthy T, Ross PL. Rapid identification of bacteria by direct matrix-assisted laser desorption/ionization mass spectrometric analysis of whole cells. Rapid Commun Mass Spectrom 1996; 10(15): 1992-6.

[114] Claydon MA, Davey SN, EdwardsJones V, Gordon DB. The rapid identification of intact microorganisms using mass spectrometry. Nat Biotechnol 1996; 14(11): 1584-6.

[115] Demirev PA, Ho YP, Ryzhov V, Fenselau C. Microorganism identification by mass spectrometry and protein database searches. Anal Chem 1999; 71(14): 2732-8.

[116] Wilkins CL, Lay JO. Identification of microorganisms by mass spectrometry. Hoboken: John Wiley & Sons 2006; 376 p.

[117] Hathout Y, Demirev PA, Ho YP, et al. Identification of bacillus spores by matrix-assisted laser desorption ionization-mass spectrometry. Appl Environ Microbiol 1999; 65(10): 4313-9.

[118] Murray PR. Matrix-assisted laser desorption ionization time-of-flight mass spectrometry: Usefulness for taxonomy and epidemiology. Clin Microbiol Infect 2010; 16(11): 1626-30.

[119] Fenselau C, Demirev PA. Characterization of intact microorganisms by maldi mass spectrometry. Mass Spectrom Rev 2001; 20(4): 157-71.

[120] Wunschel SC, Jarman KH, Petersen CE, et al. Bacterial analysis by maldi-tof mass spectrometry: An inter-lab oratory comparison. J Am Soc Mass Spectrom 2005; 16(4): 456-62.

[121] Rezzonico F, Vogel G, Duffy B, Tonolla M. Application of whole-cell matrix-assisted laser desorption ionization-time of flight mass spectrometry for rapid identification and clustering analysis of pantoea species. Appl Environ Microbiol 2010; 76(13): 4497-509.

[122] Sedo O, Sedlacek I, Zdrahal Z. Sample preparation methods for maldi-ms profiling of bacteria. Mass Spectrom Rev 2011; 30(3): 417-34.

[123] Santos C, Paterson RRM, Venancio A, Lima N. Filamentous fungal characterizations by matrix-assisted laser desorption/ionization time-of-flight mass spectrometry. J Appl Microbiol 2010; 108(2): 375-85.

[124] Ryzhov V, Fenselau C. Characterization of the protein subset desorbed by maldi from whole bacterial cells. Anal Chem 2001; 73(4): 746-50.

[125] Keller BO, Suj J, Young AB, Whittal RM. Interferences and contaminants encountered in modern mass spectrometry. Anal Chim Acta 2008; 627(1): 71-81.

[126] Clark AE, Kaleta EJ, Arora A, Wolk DM. Matrix-assisted laser desorption ionization-time of flight mass spectrometry: A fundamental shift in the routine practice of clinical microbiology. Clin Microbiol Rev 2013; 26(3): 547-603.

[127] Havlicek V, Lemr K, Schug KA. Current trends in microbial diagnostics based on mass spectrometry. Anal Chem 2013; 85(2): 790-7.

[128] Dierig A, Frei R, Egli A. The fast route to microbe identification matrix assisted laser desorption/ionization-time of flight mass spectrometry (maldi-tof ms). Pediatr Infect Dis J 2015; 34(1): 97-9.

[129] Chen JHK, Ho P-L, Kwan GSW, et al. Direct bacterial identification in positive blood cultures by use of two commercial matrix-assisted laser desorption ionization-time of flight mass spectrometry systems. J Clin Microbiol 2013; 51(6): 1733-9.

[130] Croxatto A, Prod'hom G, Greub G. Applications of maldi-tof mass spectrometry in clinical diagnostic microbiology. FEMS Microbiol Rev 2012; 36(2): 380-407.

[131] Seng P, Drancourt M, Gouriet F, et al. Ongoing revolution in bacteriology: Routine identification of bacteria by matrix-assisted laser desorption ionization time-of-flight mass spectrometry. Clin Infect Dis 2009; 49(4): 543-51.

[132] Cherkaoui A, Hibbs J, Emonet S, et al. Comparison of two matrix-assisted laser desorption ionization-time of flight mass spectrometry methods with conventional phenotypic identification for routine identification of bacteria to the species level. J Clin Microbiol 2010; 48(4): 1169-75.

[133] Mellmann A, Bimet F, Bizet C, et al. High interlaboratory reproducibility of matrix-assisted laser desorption ionization-time of flight mass spectrometry-based species identification of nonfermenting bacteria. J Clin Microbiol 2009; 47(11): 3732-4.

[134] Blondiaux N, Gaillot O, Courcol RJ. Maldi-tof mass spectrometry to identify clinical bacterial isolates: Evaluation in a teaching hospital. Pathol Biol 2010; 58(1): 55-7.

[135] van Veen SQ, Claas ECJ, Kuijper EJ. High-throughput identification of bacteria and yeast by matrix-assisted laser desorption ionization-time of flight mass spectrometry in conventional medical microbiology laboratories. J Clin Microbiol 2010; 48(3): 900-7.

[136] Prod'hom G, Bizzini A, Durussel C, Bille J, Greub G. Matrix-assisted laser desorption ionization-time of flight mass spectrometry for direct bacterial identification from positive blood culture pellets. J Clin Microbiol 2010; 48(4): 1481-3.

[137] Bessede E, Angla-gre M, Delagarde Y, Hieng SS, Menard A, Megraud F. Matrix-assisted laser-desorption/ionization biotyper: Experience in the routine of a university hospital. Clin Microbiol Infect 2011; 17(4): 533-8.

[138] Martiny D, Busson L, Wybo I, El Haj RA, Dediste A, Vandenberg O. Comparison of the microflex lt and vitek ms systems for routine identification of bacteria by matrix-assisted laser desorption ionization-time of flight mass spectrometry. J Clin Microbiol 2012; 50(4): 1313-25.

[139] Buchan BW, Riebe KM, Ledeboer NA. Comparison of the maldi biotyper system using sepsityper specimen processing to routine microbiological methods for identification of bacteria from positive blood culture bottles. J Clin Microbiol 2012; 50(2): 346-52.

[140] Ferreira L, Sanchez-Juanes F, Porras-Guerra I, et al. Microorganisms direct identification from blood culture by matrix-assisted laser desorption/ionization time-of-flight mass spectrometry. Clin Microbiol Infect 2011; 17(4): 546-51.

[141] La Scola B. Intact cell maldi-tof mass spectrometry-based approaches for the diagnosis of bloodstream infections. Expert Rev Mol Diagn 2011; 11(3): 287-98.

[142] Stevenson LG, Drake SK, Murray PR. Rapid identification of bacteria in positive blood culture broths by matrix-assisted laser desorption ionization-time of flight mass spectrometry. J Clin Microbiol 2010; 48(2): 444-7.

[143] Hartmeyer GN, Jensen AK, Bocher S, et al. Mass spectrometry: Pneumococcal meningitis verified and brucella species identified in less than half an hour. Scand J Infect Dis 2010; 42(9): 716-8.

[144] Segawa S, Sawai S, Murata S, et al. Direct application of maldi-tof mass spectrometry to cerebrospinal fluid for rapid pathogen identification in a patient with bacterial meningitis. Clin Chim Acta 2014; 435: 59-61.

[145] Ferreira L, Sanchez-Juanes F, Gonzalez-Avila M, et al. Direct identification of urinary tract pathogens from urine samples by matrix-assisted laser desorption ionization-time of flight mass spectrometry. J Clin Microbiol 2010; 48(6): 2110-5.

[146] Koehling HL, Bittner A, Mueller K-D, et al. Direct identification of bacteria in urine samples by matrix-assisted laser desorption/ionization time-of-flight mass spectrometry and relevance of defensins as interfering factors. J Med Microbiol 2012; 61(3): 339-44.

[147] Ferreira L, Sanchez-Juanes F, Munoz-Bellido JL, Gonzalez-Buitrago JM. Rapid method for direct identification of bacteria in urine and blood culture samples by matrix-assisted laser desorption ionization time-of-flight mass spectrometry: Intact cell vs. Extraction method. Clin Microbiol Infect 2011; 17(7): 1007-12.

[148] March Rossello GA, Gutierrez Rodriguez MP, de Lejarazu Leonardo RO, Orduna Domingo A, Bratos Perez MA. Procedure for microbial identification based on matrix-assisted laser desorption/ionization-time of flight mass spectrometry from screening-positive urine samples. APMIS 2014; 122(9): 790-5.

[149] March Rossello GA, Gutierrez Rodriguez MP, de Lejarazu Leonardo RO, Orduna Domingo A, Bratos Perez MA. New procedure for rapid identification of microorganisms causing urinary tract infection from urine samples by mass spectrometry (maldi-tof). Enferm Infecc Microbiol Clin 2015; 33(2): 89-94.

[150] Wang XH, Zhang G, Fan YY, Yang X, Sui WJ, Lu XX. Direct identification of bacteria causing urinary tract infections by combining matrix-assisted laser desorption ionization-time of flight mass spectrometry with uf-1000i urine flow cytometry. J Microbiol Methods 2013; 92(3): 231-5.

[151] Burillo A, Rodriguez-Sanchez B, Ramiro A, Cercenado E, Rodriguez-Creixems M, Bouza E. Gram-stain plus maldi-tof ms (matrix-assisted laser desorption ionization-time of flight mass spectrometry) for a rapid diagnosis of urinary tract infection. PLoS One 2014; 9(1).

[152] Drancourt M. Detection of microorganisms in blood specimens using matrix-assisted laser desorption ionization time-of-flight mass spectrometry: A review. Clin Microbiol Infect 2010; 16(11): 1620-5.

[153] La Scola B, Raoult D. Direct identification of bacteria in positive blood culture bottles by matrix-assisted laser desorption ionisation time-of-flight mass spectrometry. PLoS One 2009; 4(11).

[154] Schieffer KM, Tan KE, Stamper PD, et al. Multicenter evaluation of the sepsityper (tm) extraction kit and maldi-tof ms for direct identification of positive blood culture isolates using the bd bactec (tm) fx and versatrek((r)) diagnostic blood culture systems. J Appl Microbiol 2014; 116(4): 934-41.

[155] Ferroni A, Suarez S, Beretti J-L, et al. Real-time identification of bacteria and candida species in positive blood culture broths by matrix-assisted laser desorption ionization-time of flight mass spectrometry. J Clin Microbiol 2010; 48(5): 1542-8.

[156] Christner M, Rohde H, Wolters M, Sobottka I, Wegscheider K, Aepfelbacher M. Rapid identification of bacteria from positive blood culture bottles by use of matrix-assisted laser desorption-ionization time of flight mass spectrometry fingerprinting. J Clin Microbiol 2010; 48(5): 1584-91.

[157] Lagace-Wiens PRS, Adam HJ, Karlowsky JA, et al. Identification of blood culture isolates directly from positive blood cultures by use of matrix-assisted laser desorption ionization-time of flight mass spectrometry and a commercial extraction system: Analysis of performance, cost, and turnaround time. J Clin Microbiol 2012; 50(10): 3324-8.

[158] Kok J, Thomas LC, Olma T, Chen SCA, Iredell JR. Identification of bacteria in blood culture broths using matrix-assisted laser desorption-ionization sepsityper (tm) and time of flight mass spectrometry. PLoS One 2011; 6(8).

[159] Loonen AJM, Jansz AR, Stalpers J, Wolffs PFG, van den Brule AJC. An evaluation of three processing methods and the effect of reduced culture times for faster direct identification of pathogens from bact/alert blood cultures by maldi-tof ms. Eur J Clin Microbiol Infect Dis 2012; 31(7): 1575-83.

[160] Martiny D, Dediste A, Vandenberg O. Comparison of an in-house method and the commercial sepsityper (tm) kit for bacterial identification directly from positive blood culture broths by matrix-assisted laser desorption-ionisation time-of-flight mass spectrometry. Eur J Clin Microbiol Infect Dis 2012; 31(9): 2269-81.

[161] Saffert RT, Cunningham SA, Ihde SM, Jobe KEM, Mandrekar J, Patel R. Comparison of bruker biotyper matrix-assisted laser desorption ionization-time of flight mass spectrometer to bd phoenix automated microbiology system for identification of gram-negative bacilli. J Clin Microbiol 2011; 49(3): 887-92.

[162] Szabados F, Michels M, Kaase M, Gatermann S. The sensitivity of direct identification from positive bact/alert (tm) (biomerieux) blood culture bottles by matrix-assisted laser desorption ionization time-of-flight mass spectrometry is low. Clin Microbiol Infect 2011; 17(2): 192-5.

[163] Spanu T, Posteraro B, Fiori B, et al. Direct maldi-tof mass spectrometry assay of blood culture broths for rapid identification of candida species causing bloodstream infections: An observational study in two large microbiology laboratories. J Clin Microbiol 2012; 50(1): 176-9.

[164] Kostrzewa M, Sparbier K, Maier T, Schubert S. Maldi-tof ms: An upcoming tool for rapid detection of antibiotic resistance in microorganisms. Proteomics Clin Appl 2013; 7(11-12): 767-78.

[165] Hrabak J, Chudackova E, Walkova R. Matrix-assisted laser desorption ionization-time of flight (maldi-tof) mass spectrometry for detection of antibiotic resistance mechanisms: From research to routine diagnosis. Clin Microbiol Rev 2013; 26(1): 103-14.

[166] Sparbier K, Schubert S, Weller U, Boogen C, Kostrzewa M. Matrix-assisted laser desorption ionization-time of flight mass spectrometry-based functional assay for rapid detection of resistance against beta-lactam antibiotics. J Clin Microbiol 2012; 50(3): 927-37.

[167] Hrabak J, Walkova R, Studentova V, Chudackova E, Bergerova T. Carbapenemase activity detection by matrix-assisted laser desorption ionization-time of flight mass spectrometry. J Clin Microbiol 2011; 49(9): 3222-7.

[168] Burckhardt I, Zimmermann S. Using matrix-assisted laser desorption ionization-time of flight mass spectrometry to detect carbapenem resistance within 1 to 2.5 hours. J Clin Microbiol 2011; 49(9): 3321-4.

[169] Kempf M, Bakour S, Flaudrops C, et al. Rapid detection of carbapenem resistance in acinetobacter baumannii using matrix-assisted laser desorption ionization-time of flight mass spectrometry. PLoS One 2012; 7(2).

[170] Alvarez-Buylla A, Picazo JJ, Culebras E. Optimized method for acinetobacter species carbapenemase detection and identification by matrix-assisted laser desorption ionization-time of flight mass spectrometry. J Clin Microbiol 2013; 51(5): 1589-92.

[171] Demirev PA, Hagan NS, Antoine MD, Lin JS, Feldman AB. Establishing drug resistance in microorganisms by mass spectrometry. J Am Soc Mass Spectrom 2013; 24(8): 1194-201.

[172] Adaway JE, Keevil BG. Therapeutic drug monitoring and lc-ms/ms. J Chromatogr B 2012; 883-884: 33-49.

[173] Pickering MK, Brown SD. Assays for determination of ertapenem for applications in therapeutic drug monitoring, pharmacokinetics and sample stability. Biomed Chromatogr 2014; 28(11): 1525-31.

[174] Lara FJ, del Olmo-Iruela M, Cruces-Blanco C, Quesada-Molina C, Garcia-Campana AM. Advances in the determination of beta-lactam antibiotics by liquid chromatography. TrAC, Trends Anal Chem 2012; 38: 52-66.

[175] Samanidou VF, Evaggelopoulou EN, Papadoyannis IN. Chromatographic analysis of penicillins in pharmaceutical formulations and biological fluids. J Sep Sci 2006; 29(12): 1879-908.

[176] Sharma PC, Jain A, Jain S, Pahwa R, Yar MS. Ciprofloxacin: Review on developments in synthetic, analytical, and medicinal aspects. J Enzyme Inhib Med Chem 2010; 25(4): 577-89.

[177] Sime FB, Roberts MS, Roberts JA, Robertson TA. Simultaneous determination of seven beta-lactam antibiotics in human plasma for therapeutic drug monitoring and pharmacokinetic studies. J Chromatogr B 2014; 960: 134-44.

[178] Colin P, De Bock L, T'Jollyn H, Boussery K, Van Bocxlaer J. Development and validation of a fast and uniform approach to quantify beta-lactam antibiotics in human plasma by solid phase extraction-liquid chromatography-electrospray-tandem mass spectrometry. Talanta 2013; 103: 285-93.

[179] Briscoe SE, McWhinney BC, Lipman J, Roberts JA, Ungerer JP. A method for determining the free (unbound) concentration of ten beta-lactam antibiotics in human plasma using high performance liquid chromatography with ultraviolet detection. J Chromatogr B Analyt Technol Biomed Life Sci 2012; 907: 178-84.

[180] Ohmori T, Suzuki A, Niwa T, et al. Simultaneous determination of eight beta-lactam antibiotics in human serum by liquid chromatography-tandem mass spectrometry. J Chromatogr B 2011; 879(15-16): 1038-42.

[181] Dailly E, Bouquie R, Deslandes G, Jolliet P, Le Floch R. A liquid chromatography assay for a quantification of doripenem, ertapenem, imipenem, meropenem concentrations in human plasma: Application to a clinical pharmacokinetic study. J Chromatogr B 2011; 879(15-16): 1137-42.

[182] Rigo-Bonnin R, Juvany-Roig R, Leiva-Badosa E, et al. Measurement of meropenem concentration in different human biological fluids by ultra-performance liquid chromatography-tandem mass spectrometry. Anal Bioanal Chem 2014; 406(20): 4997-5007.

[183] Casals G, Hernandez C, Hidalgo S, et al. Development and validation of a uhplc diode array detector method for meropenem quantification in human plasma. Clin Biochem 2014; 47(16-17): 223-7.

[184] Kameda K, Ikawa K, Ikeda K, et al. Hplc method for measuring meropenem and biapenem concentrations in human peritoneal fluid and bile: Application to comparative pharmacokinetic investigations. J Chromatogr Sci 2010; 48(5): 406-11.

[185] la Marca G, Giocaliere E, Villanelli F, et al. Development of an uplc-ms/ms method for the determination of antibiotic ertapenem on dried blood spots. J Pharm Biomed Anal 2012; 61: 108-13.

[186] Mundkowski RG, Majcher-Peszynska J, Burkhardt O, Welte T, Drewelow B. A new simple hplc assay for the quantification of ertapenem in human plasma, lung tissue, and broncho-alveolar lavage fluid. J Chromatogr B Analyt Technol Biomed Life Sci 2006; 832(2): 231-5.

[187] Baietto L, D'Avolio A, De Rosa FG, et al. Development and validation of a simultaneous extraction procedure for hplc-ms quantification of daptomycin, amikacin, gentamicin, and rifampicin in human plasma. Anal Bioanal Chem 2010; 396(2): 791-8.

[188] Oertel R, Neumeister V, Kirch W. Hydrophilic interaction chromatography combined with tandem-mass spectrometry to determine six aminoglycosides in serum. J Chromatogr A 2004; 1058(1-2): 197-201.

[189] Zawilla NH, Li B, Hoogmartens J, Adams E. Improved reversed-phase liquid chromatographic method combined with pulsed electrochemical detection for the analysis of amikacin. J Pharm Biomed Anal 2007; 43(1): 168-73.

[190] Brajanoski G, Hoogmartens J, Allegaert K, Adams E. Determination of amikacin in cerebrospinal fluid by high-performance liquid chromatography with pulsed electrochemical detection. J Chromatogr B 2008; 867(1): 149-52.

[191] Serrano JM, Silva M. Determination of amikacin in body fluid by high-performance liquid-chromatography with chemiluminescence detection. J Chromatogr B 2006; 843(1): 20-4.

[192] Shou D, Dong Y, Shen L, et al. Rapid quantification of tobramycin and vancomycin by uplc-tqd and application to osteomyelitis patient samples. J Chromatogr Sci 2014; 52(6): 501-7.

[193] Isoherranen N, Soback S. Determination of gentamicins c-i, c-ia, and c-2 in plasma and urine by hplc. Clin Chem 2000; 46(6): 837-42.

[194] Nemutlu E, Kir S, Katlan D, Beksac MS. Simultaneous multiresponse optimization of an hplc method to separate seven cephalosporins in plasma and amniotic fluid: Application to validation and quantification of cefepime, cefixime and cefoperazone. Talanta 2009; 80(1): 117-26.

[195] Samanidou VF, Hapeshi EA, Papadoyannis IN. Rapid and sensitive high-performance liquid chromatographic determination of four cephalosporin antibiotics in pharmaceuticals and body fluids. J Chromatogr B 2003; 788(1): 147-58.

[196] Sousa J, Alves G, Fortuna A, Pena A, Lino C, Falcao A. Development and validation of a fast isocratic liquid chromatography method for the simultaneous determination of norfloxacin, lomefloxacin and ciprofloxacin in human plasma. Biomed Chromatogr 2011; 25(5): 535-41.

[197] Watabe S, Yokoyama Y, Nakazawa K, et al. Simultaneous measurement of pazufloxacin, ciprofloxacin, and levofloxacin in human serum by high-performance liquid chromatography with fluorescence detection. J Chromatogr B 2010; 878(19): 1555-61.

[198] Samanidou VF, Demetriou CE, Papadoyannis IN. Direct determination of four fluoroquinolones, enoxacin, norfloxacin, ofloxacin, and ciprofloxacin, in pharmaceuticals and blood serum by hplc. Anal Bioanal Chem 2003; 375(5): 623-9.

[199] Canada-Canada F, Espinosa-Mansilla A, Munoz de la Pena A. Separation of fifteen quinolones by high performance liquid chromatography: Application to pharmaceuticals and ofloxacin determination in urine. J Sep Sci 2007; 30(9): 1242-9.

[200] Muchohi SN, Thuo N, Karisa J, Muturi A, Kokwaro GO, Maitland K. Determination of ciprofloxacin in human plasma using high-performance liquid chromatography coupled with fluorescence detection: Application to a population pharmacokinetics study in children with severe malnutrition. J Chromatogr B 2011; 879(2): 146-52.

[201] Grondin C, Zhao W, Fakhoury M, Jacqz-Aigrain E. Determination of ciprofloxacin in plasma by micro-liquid chromatography-mass spectrometry: An adapted method for neonates. Biomed Chromatogr 2011; 25(7): 827-32.

[202] Wu S-S, Chein C-Y, Wen Y-H. Analysis of ciprofloxacin by a simple high-performance liquid chromatography method. J Chromatogr Sci 2008; 46(6): 490-5.

[203] Wang Y, Zhang P, Jiang N, et al. Simultaneous quantification of metronidazole, tinidazole, ornidazole and morinidazole in human saliva. J Chromatogr B Analyt Technol Biomed Life Sci 2012; 899: 27-30.

[204] Suyagh MF, Iheagwaram G, Kole PL, et al. Development and validation of a dried blood spot-hplc assay for the determination of metronidazole in neonatal whole blood samples. Anal Bioanal Chem 2010; 397(2): 687-93.

[205] Silva M, Schramm S, Kano E, Koono E, Porta V, Serra C. Development and validation of a hplc-ms-ms method for quantification of metronidazole in human plasma. J Chromatogr Sci 2009; 47(9): 781-4.

[206] Chepyala D, Tsai IL, Sun HY, Lin SW, Kuo CH. Development and validation of a high-performance liquid chromatography-fluorescence detection method for the accurate quantification of colistin in human plasma. J Chromatogr B 2015; 980: 48-54.

[207] Gobin P, Lemaitre F, Marchand S, Couet W, Olivier JC. Assay of colistin and colistin methanesulfonate in plasma and urine by liquid chromatography-tandem mass spectrometry. Antimicrob Agents Chemother 2010; 54(5): 1941-8.

[208] Hagihara M, Sutherland C, Nicolau DP. Development of hplc methods for the determination of vancomycin in human plasma, mouse serum and bronchoalveolar lavage fluid. J Chromatogr Sci 2013; 51(3): 201-7.

[209] Abu-Shandi KH. Determination of vancomycin in human plasma using high-performance liquid chromatography with fluorescence detection. Anal Bioanal Chem 2009; 395(2): 527-32.

[210] Zhang T, Watson DG, Azike C, et al. Determination of vancomycin in serum by liquid chromatography-high resolution full scan mass spectrometry. J Chromatogr B 2007; 857(2): 352-6.

[211] Catena E, Perez G, Sadaba B, Azanza JR, Campanero MA. A fast reverse-phase high performance liquid chromatographic tandem mass spectrometry assay for the quantification of clindamycin in plasma and saliva using a rapid resolution package. J Pharm Biomed Anal 2009; 50(4): 649-54.

[212] Cho SH, Im HT, Park WS, Ha YH, Choi YW, Lee KT. Simple method for the assay of clindamycin in human plasma by reversed-phase high-performance liquid chromatography with uv detector. Biomed Chromatogr 2005; 19(10): 783-7.

[213] Henry H, Sobhi HR, Scheibner O, Bromirski M, Nimkar SB, Rochat B. Comparison between a high-resolution single-stage orbitrap and a triple quadrupole mass spectrometer for quantitative analyses of drugs. Rapid Commun Mass Spectrom 2012; 26(5): 499-509.

[214] Farowski F, Cornely OA, Vehreschild JJ, et al. Quantitation of azoles and echinocandins in compartments of peripheral blood by liquid chromatography-tandem mass spectrometry. Antimicrob Agents Chemother 2010; 54(5): 1815-9.

[215] Decosterd LA, Rochat B, Pesse B, et al. Multiplex ultra-performance liquid chromatography-tandem mass spectrometry method for simultaneous quantification in human plasma of fluconazole, itraconazole, hydroxyitraconazole, posaconazole, voriconazole, voriconazole-n-oxide, anidulafungin, and caspofungin. Antimicrob Agents Chemother 2010; 54(12): 5303-15.

[216] Couchman L, Buckner SL, Morgan PE, Ceesay MM, Pagliuca A, Flanagan RJ. An automated method for the simultaneous measurement of azole antifungal drugs in human plasma or serum using turbulent flow liquid chromatography-tandem mass spectrometry. Anal Bioanal Chem 2012; 404(2): 513-23.

[217] Beste KY, Burkhardt O, Kaever V. Rapid hplc-ms/ms method for simultaneous quantitation of four routinely administered triazole antifungals in human plasma. Clin Chim Acta 2012; 413(1-2): 240-5.

[218] Chhun S, Rey E, Tran A, Lortholary O, Pons G, Jullien V. Simultaneous quantification of voriconazole and posaconazole in human plasma by high-performance liquid chromatography with ultra-violet detection. J Chromatogr B 2007; 852(1-2): 223-8.

[219] Alffenaar JWC, Wessels AMA, van Hateren K, Greijdanus B, Kosterink JGW, Uges DRA. Method for therapeutic drug monitoring of azole antifungal drugs in human serum using lc/ms/ms. J Chromatogr B 2010; 878(1): 39-44.

[220] Khoschsorur G, Fruehwirth F, Zelzer S. Isocratic high-performance liquid chromatographic method with ultraviolet detection for simultaneous determination of levels of voriconazole and itraconazole and its hydroxy metabolite in human serum. Antimicrob Agents Chemother 2005; 49(8): 3569-71.

[221] Jeans AR, Howard SJ, Al-Nakeeb Z, et al. Combination of voriconazole and anidulafungin for treatment of triazole-resistant aspergillus fumigatus in an in vitro model of invasive pulmonary aspergillosis. Antimicrob Agents Chemother 2012; 56(10): 5180-5.

[222] Eldem T, Arican-Cellat N. Determination of amphotericin b in human plasma using solid-phase extraction and high-performance liquid chromatography. J Pharm Biomed Anal 2001; 25(1): 53-64.

[223] Deshpande NM, Gangrade MG, Kekare MB, Vaidya VV. Determination of free and liposomal amphotericin b in human plasma by liquid chromatography-mass spectroscopy with solid phase extraction and protein precipitation techniques. J Chromatogr B 2010; 878(3-4): 315-26.

[224] Alebic-Kolbah T, Modesitt MS. Anidulafungin-challenges in development and validation of an lc-ms/ms bioanalytical method validated for regulated clinical studies. Anal Bioanal Chem 2012; 404(6-7): 2043-55.

[225] Burhenne H, Kielstein JT, Burkhardt O, Kaever V. Quantitative analysis of the antifungal drug anidulafungin by lc-online spe-ms/ms in human plasma. Biomed Chromatogr 2012; 26(6): 681-3.

[226] Hermawan D, Ali NAM, Ibrahim WAW, Sanagi MM. Analysis of fluconazole in human urine sample by high performance liquid chromatography method. J Phys Conf Ser 2013; 423.

[227] Gao S, Tao X, Sun L, et al. An liquid chromatography-tandem mass spectrometry assay for determination of trace amount of new antifungal drug iodiconazole in human plasma. J Chromatogr B 2009; 877(4): 382-6.

[228] Cendejas-Bueno E, Cuenca-Estrella M, Gomez-Lopez A. A simple, sensitive hplc-pda method for the quantification of itraconazole and hydroxy itraconazole in human serum: A reference laboratory experience. Diagn Microbiol Infect Dis 2013; 76(3): 314-20.

[229] Srivatsan V, Dasgupta AK, Kale P, et al. Simultaneous determination of itraconazole and hydroxyitraconazole in human plasma by high-performance liquid chromatography. J Chromatogr A 2004; 1031(1-2): 307-13.

[230] Nakagawa S, Kuwabara N, Kobayashi H, Shimoeda S, Ohta S, Yamato S. Simple column-switching hplc method for determining levels of the antifungal agent micafungin in human plasma and application to patient samples. Biomed Chromatogr 2013; 27(5): 551-5.

[231] Neubauer W, Koenig A, Bolek R, et al. Determination of the antifungal agent posaconazole in human serum by hplc with parallel column-switching technique. J Chromatogr B 2009; 877(24): 2493-8.

[232] Cendejas-Bueno E, Forastiero A, Rodriguez-Tudela JL, Cuenca-Estrella M, Gomez-Lopez A. Hplc/uv or bioassay: Two valid methods for posaconazole quantification in human serum samples. Clin Microbiol Infect 2012; 18(12): 1229-35.

[233] Cunliffe JM, Noren CF, Hayes RN, Clement RP, Shen JX. A high-throughput lc-ms/ms method for the quantitation of posaconazole in human plasma: Implementing fused core silica liquid chromatography. J Pharm Biomed Anal 2009; 50(1): 46-52.

[234] Pennick GJ, Clark M, Sutton DA, Rinaldi MG. Development and validation of a high-performance liquid chromatography assay for voriconazole. Antimicrob Agents Chemother 2003; 47(7): 2348-50.

[235] Racil Z, Winterova J, Kouba M, et al. Monitoring trough voriconazole plasma concentrations in haematological patients: Real life multicentre experience. Mycoses 2012; 55(6): 483-92.

[236] Pauwels S, Vermeersch P, Van Eldere J, Desmet K. Fast and simple lc-ms/ms method for quantifying plasma voriconazole. Clin Chim Acta 2012; 413(7-8): 740-3.

[237] Langman LJ, Boakye-Agyeman F. Measurement of voriconazole in serum and plasma. Clin Biochem 2007; 40(18): 1378-85.

[238] Mak J, Sujishi KK, French D. Development and validation of a liquid chromatography-tandem mass spectrometry (lc-ms/ms) assay to quantify serum voriconazole. J Chromatogr B 2015; 986-987: 94-9.

[239] Sun H, Wei L, Zuo Y, Wu Y. Effective separation and simultaneous detection of gatifloxacin, aminomethylbenzoic acid, cefazolin and cefminox in human urine by capillary zone electrophoresis. J Iran Chem Soc 2011; 8(4): 1043-51.

[240] Sun H, Zuo Y. Effective separation and simultaneous detection of ceftriaxone sodium and levofloxacin in human urine by capillary zone electrophoresis. Curr Anal Chem 2013; 9(1): 157-62.

[241] Hernandez M, Borrull F, Calull M. Analysis of antibiotics in biological samples by capillary electrophoresis. TrAC, Trends Anal Chem 2003; 22(7): 416-27.

[242] Garcia-Ruiz C, Marina ML. Recent advances in the analysis of antibiotics by capillary electrophoresis. Electrophoresis 2006; 27(1): 266-82.

[243] Perez-Fernandez V, Dominguez-Vega E, Crego AL, Angeles Garcia M, Luisa Marina M. Recent advances in the analysis of antibiotics by ce and cec. Electrophoresis 2012; 33(1): 127-46.

[244] Castro-Puyana M, Crego AL, Marina ML. Recent advances in the analysis of antibiotics by ce and cec. Electrophoresis 2008; 29(1): 274-93.

[245] Castro-Puyana M, Crego AL, Luisa Marina M. Recent advances in the analysis of antibiotics by ce and cec. Electrophoresis 2010; 31(1): 229-50.

[246] Pinero M-Y, Garrido-Delgado R, Bauza R, Arce L, Valcarcel M. Easy sample treatment for the determination of enrofloxacin and ciprofloxacin residues in raw bovine milk by capillary electrophoresis. Electrophoresis 2012; 33(19-20): 2978-86.

[247] Hernandez-Mesa M, Cruces-Blanco C, Garcia-Campana AM. Determination of 5-nitroimidazoles and metabolites in environmental samples by micellar electrokinetic chromatography. Anal Bioanal Chem 2012; 404(2): 297-305.

[248] Huang H-Y, Liu W-L, Singco B, Hsieh S-H, Shih Y-H. On-line concentration sample stacking coupled with water-in-oil microemulsion electrokinetic chromatography. J Chromatogr A 2011; 1218(42): 7663-9.

[249] Ding Y, Bai L, Suo X, Meng X. Post separation adjustment of ph to enable the analysis of aminoglycoside antibiotics by microchip electrophoresis with amperometric detection. Electrophoresis 2012; 33(21): 3245-53.

[250]   Cheng Y-J, Huang S-H, Singco B, Huang H-Y. Analyses of sulfonamide antibiotics in meat samples by on-line concentration capillary electrochromatography-mass spectrometry. J Chromatogr A 2011; 1218(42): 7640-7.

[251]   Liu W-L, Wu C-Y, Li Y-T, Huang H-Y. Penicillin analyses by capillary electrochromatography-mass spectrometry with different charged poly(stearyl methacrylate divinylbenzene) monoliths as stationary phases. Talanta 2012; 101: 71-7.

[252]   Ma T-Y, Vickroy TW, Shien J-H, Chou C-C. Improved nonaqueous capillary electrophoresis for tetracyclines at subparts per billion level. Electrophoresis 2012; 33(11): 1679-82.

[253]   da Silva IS, Rajh Vidal DT, do Lago CL, Angnes L. Fast simultaneous determination of trimethoprim and sulfamethoxazole by capillary electrophoresis with capacitively coupled contactless conductivity detection. J Sep Sci 2013; 36(8): 1405-9.

[254]   Ho J-aA, Fan N-c, Jou AF-j, Wu L-c, Sun T-p. Monitoring the subcellular localization of doxorubicin in cho-k1 using mekc-lif: Liposomal carrier for enhanced drug delivery. Talanta 2012; 99: 683-8.

[255]   Wang L, Wu J, Wang Q, et al. Rapid and sensitive determination of sulfonamide residues in milk and chicken muscle by microfluidic chip electrophoresis. J Agric Food Chem 2012; 60(7): 1613-8.

[256]   Sun H, Zuo Y, Qi H, Lv Y. Accelerated solvent extraction combined with capillary electrophoresis as an improved methodology for simultaneous determination of residual fluoroquinolones and sulfonamides in aquatic products. Anal Methods 2012; 4(3): 670-5.

[257]   Mu G, Liu H, Xu L, Tian L, Luan F. Matrix solid-phase dispersion extraction and capillary electrophoresis determination of tetracycline residues in milk. Food Anal Methods 2012; 5(1): 148-53.

[258]   Ibarra IS, Rodriguez JA, Elena Paez-Hernandez M, Santos EM, Miranda JM. Determination of quinolones in milk samples using a combination of magnetic solid-phase extraction and capillary electrophoresis. Electrophoresis 2012; 33(13): 2041-8.

[259]   Wen Y, Li J, Zhang W, Chen L. Dispersive liquid-liquid microextraction coupled with capillary electrophoresis for simultaneous determination of sulfonamides with the aid of experimental design. Electrophoresis 2011; 32(16): 2131-8.

[260]   Gao W, Chen G, Chen Y, Zhang X, Yin Y, Hu Z. Application of single drop liquid-liquid-liquid microextraction for the determination of fluoroquinolones in human urine by capillary electrophoresis. J Chromatogr B 2011; 879(3-4): 291-5.

[261]   Herrera-Herrera AV, Ravelo-Perez LM, Hernandez-Borges J, Afonso MM, Antonio Palenzuela J, Angel Rodriguez-Delgado M. Oxidized multi-walled carbon nanotubes for the dispersive solid-phase extraction of quinolone antibiotics from water samples using capillary electrophoresis and large volume sample stacking with polarity switching. J Chromatogr A 2011; 1218(31): 5352-61.

[262]   Horka M, Vykydalova M, Ruzicka F, et al. Cief separation, uv detection, and quantification of ampholytic antibiotics and bacteria from different matrices. Anal Bioanal Chem 2014; 406(25): 6285-96.

[263]   Wang Y, Baeyens WRG, Huang C, Fei G, He L, Ouyang J. Enhanced separation of seven quinolones by capillary electrophoresis with silica nanoparticles as additive. Talanta 2009; 77(5): 1667-74.

[264]   Cheng C-L, Fu C-H, Chou C-H. Determination of norfloxacin in rat liver perfusate using capillary electrophoresis with laser-induced fluorescence detection. J Chromatogr B 2007; 856(1-2): 381-5.

[265]   Zhou S, Ouyang J, Baeyens WRG, Zhao H, Yang Y. Chiral separation of four fluoroquinolone compounds using capillary electrophoresis with hydroxypropyl-beta-cyclodextrin as chiral selector. J Chromatogr A 2006; 1130(2): 296-301.

[266]   Sun H, Li L, Wu Y. Capillary electrophoresis with electrochemiluminescence detection for simultaneous determination of proline and fleroxacin in human urine. Drug Testing and Analysis 2009; 1(1-2): 87-92.

[267]   Liu Y-M, Cao J-T, Tian W, Zheng Y-L. Determination of levofloxacin and norfloxacin by capillary electrophoresis with electrochemiluminescence detection and applications in human urine. Electrophoresis 2008; 29(15): 3207-12.

[268]   Sun H, Li L, Su M. Simultaneous determination of proline and pipemidic acid in human urine by capillary electrophoresis with electrochemiluminescence detection. J Clin Lab Anal 2010; 24(5): 327-33.

[269]   Sun H, Su M, Li L. Simultaneous determination of tetracaine, proline, and enoxacin in human urine by ce with ecl detection. J Chromatogr Sci 2010; 48(1): 49-54.

[270]   Fu Z, Wang L, Li C, Liu Y, Zhou X, Wei W. Ce-ecl detection of gatifloxacin in biological fluid after clean-up using spe. J Sep Sci 2009; 32(22): 3925-9.

[271]   Liu Y-M, Shi Y-M, Liu Z-L. Determination of enoxacin and ofloxacin by capillary electrophoresis with electrochemiluminescence detection in biofluids and drugs and its application to pharmacokinetics. Biomed Chromatogr 2010; 24(9): 941-7.

[272]   Deng B, Su C, Kang Y. Determination of norfloxacin in human urine by capillary electrophoresis with electrochemiluminescence detection. Anal Bioanal Chem 2006; 385(7): 1336-41.

[273]   Morales-Cid G, Fekete A, Simonet BM, et al. In situ synthesis of magnetic multiwalled carbon nanotube composites for the clean-up of (fluoro)quinolones from human plasma prior to ultrahigh pressure liquid chromatography analysis. Anal Chem 2010; 82(7): 2743-52.

[274]   Liu Y-M, Mei L, Yue H-Y, Shi Y-M, Liu L-J. Highly sensitive chemiluminescence detection of norfloxacin and ciprofloxacin in ce and its applications. Chromatographia 2010; 72(3-4): 337-41.

[275]   Thomas A, Upoma OK, Inman JA, Kaul AK, Beeson JH, Roberts KP. Quantification of penicillin g during labor and delivery by capillary electrophoresis. J Biochem Bioph Methods 2008; 70(6): 992-8.

[276]   Solangi AR, Memon SQ, Bhanger MI, Khuhawar MY. Quantitative analysis of eight cephalosporin antibiotics in pharmaceutical products and urine by capillary zone electrophoresis. Acta Chromatogr 2007; 19: 81-96.

[277]   Petsch M, Mayer-Helm BX, Sauermann R, Joukhadar C, Kenndler E. Capillary electrophoresis analysis of fosfomycin in biological fluids for clinical pharmacokinetic studies. Electrophoresis 2004; 25(14): 2292-8.

[278]   Solangi AR, Memon SQ, Mallah A, Memon N, Khuhawar MY, Bhanger MI. Development and implication of a capillary electrophoresis methodology for ciprofloxacin, paracetamol and diclofenac sodium in pharmaceutical formulations and simultaneously in human urine samples. Pak J Pharm Sci 2011; 24(4): 539-44.

[279]   Berzas Nevado JJ, Castaneda Penalvo G, Guzman Bernardo FJ. Micellar electrokinetic chromatography method for the determination of sulfamethoxazole, trimethoprim and their main metabolites in human serum. J Sep Sci 2005; 28(6): 543-8.

[280]   Andrasi M, Gaspar A, Klekner A. Analysis of cephalosporins in bronchial secretions by capillary electrophoresis after simple pretreatment. J Chromatogr B 2007; 846(1-2): 355-8.

[281]   Injac R, Kac J, Kreft S, Strukelj B. Determination of doxycycline in pharmaceuticals and human urine by micellar electrokinetic capillary chromatography. Anal Bioanal Chem 2007; 387(2): 695-701.

[282]   Eder AR, Chen JS, Arriaga EA. Separation of doxorubicin and doxorubicinol by cyclodextrin-modified micellar electrokinetic capillary chromatography. Electrophoresis 2006; 27(16): 3263-70.

[283]   Petsch M, Mayer-Helm BX, Sauermann R, Joukhadar C, Kenndler E. Determination of fosfomycin in pus by capillary zone electrophoresis. J Chromatogr A 2005; 1081(1): 55-9.

[284]   Klekner A, Ga'spa'r A, Kardos S, Szabo J, Cse'csei G. Cefazolin prophylaxis in neurosurgery monitored by capillary electrophoresis. J Neurosurg Anesthesiol 2003; 15(3): 249-54.

[285]   Lin Y-F, Wang Y-C, Chang SY. Capillary electrophoresis of aminoglycosides with argon-ion laser-induced fluorescence detection. J Chromatogr A 2008; 1188(2): 331-3.

[286]   Law WS, Kuban P, Yuan LL, Zhao JH, Li SFY, Hauser PC. Determination of tobramycin in human serum by capillary electrophoresis with contactless conductivity detection. Electrophoresis 2006; 27(10): 1932-8.

[287]   Kaale E, Long YH, Fonge HA, et al. Gentamicin assay in human serum by solid-phase extraction and capillary electrophoresis. Electrophoresis 2005; 26(3): 640-7.

[288]   Peng X, Wang Z, Li J, Le G, Shi Y. Electrochemiluminescence detection of clarithromycin in biological fluids after capillary electrophoresis separation. Anal Lett 2008; 41(7): 1184-99.

[289]   Liu Y-M, Shi Y-M, Liu Z-L, Tian W. A sensitive method for simultaneous determination of four macrolides by ce with electrochemiluminescence detection and its applications in human urine and tablets. Electrophoresis 2010; 31(2): 364-70.

[290]   McGlinchey TA, Rafter PA, Regan F, McMahon GP. A review of analytical methods for the determination of aminoglycoside and macrolide residues in food matrices. Anal Chim Acta 2008; 624(1): 1-15.

[291]   Wang Z, Yang Z, Ye J, Tan G, Xu H, Liu Y. Capillary electrophoresis-electrochemiluminescence method for simultaneous detection of azithromycin, roxithromycin and erythromycin ethylsuccinate. Chem Anal (Warsaw) 2009; 54(5): 883-94.

[292]   Cunha BA, Ristuccia AM. Clinical usefulness of vancomycin. Clin Pharm 1983; 2(5): 417-24.

[293]   Somerville AL, Wright DH, Rotschafer JC. Implications of vancomycin degradation products on therapeutic drug monitoring in patients with end-stage renal disease. Pharmacotherapy 1999; 19(6): 702-7.

[294]   Kitahashi T, Furuta R. Determination of vancomycin in human serum by micellar electrokinetic capillary chromatography with direct sample injection. Clin Chim Acta 2001; 312(1-2): 221-5.

[295]   Higgins DL, Chang R, Debabov DV, et al. Telavancin, a multifunctional lipoglycopeptide, disrupts both cell wall synthesis and cell membrane integrity in methicillin-resistant staphylococcus aureus. Antimicrob Agents Chemother 2005; 49(3): 1127-34.

[296]   Liao H-W, Lin S-W, Wu U-I, Kuo C-H. Rapid and sensitive determination of posaconazole in patient plasma by capillary electrophoresis with field-amplified sample stacking. J Chromatogr A 2012; 1226: 48-54.

[297]   Crego AL, Gomez J, Marina ML, Lavandera JL. Application of capillary zone electrophoresis with off-line solid-phase extraction to in vitro metabolism studies of antifungals. Electrophoresis 2001; 22(12): 2503-11.

[298]   Lin S-C, Lin S-W, Chen J-M, Kuo C-H. Using sweeping-micellar electrokinetic chromatography to determine voriconazole in patient plasma. Talanta 2010; 82(2): 653-9.

[299]   Theurillat R, Zimmerli S, Thormann W. Determination of voriconazole in human serum and plasma by micellar electrokinetic chromatography. J Pharm Biomed Anal 2010; 53(5): 1313-8.

[300]   Lin S-C, Liu H-Y, Lin S-W, et al. Simultaneous determination of triazole antifungal drugs in human plasma by sweeping-micellar electrokinetic chromatography. Anal Bioanal Chem 2012; 404(1): 217-28.

[301]   vonHeeren F, Tanner R, Theurillat R, Thormann W. Determination of fluconazole in human plasma by micellar electrokinetic capillary chromatography with detection at 190 nm. J Chromatogr A 1996; 745(1-2): 165-72.

[302]   Wan Ibrahim WA, Abd Wahib SM, Hermawan D, Sanagi MM, Aboul-Enein HY. Separation of selected imidazole enantiomers using dual cyclodextrin system in micellar electrokinetic chromatography. Chirality 2013; 25(6): 328-35.

[303]   Schmutz A, Thormann W. Rapid-determination of the antimycotic drug flucytosine in human serum by micellar electrokinetic capillary chromatography with direct sample injection. Ther Drug Monit 1994; 16(5): 483-90.

[304]   Crego AL, Marina ML, Lavandera JL. Optimization of the separation of a group of antifungals by capillary zone electrophoresis. J Chromatogr A 2001; 917(1-2): 337-45.

[305]   Kitahashi T, Furuta I. Analysis of micafungin in serum by capillary zone electrophoresis. J Chromatogr Sci 2007; 45(1): 28-32.

CHAPTER 6

Antimalarial Herbal Medicine: From Natural Products to Drug Molecules

Norma Rivera Fernández[1,*] and Perla Y. López Camacho[2]

[1]*Laboratory of Malariology, Department of Microbiology and Parasitology, Faculty of Medicine, National Autonomous University of Mexico. Mexico City, 04510, Mexico and* [2]*Department of Natural Sciences, Metropolitan Autonomous University, Cuajimalpa, Mexico City, 11850, Mexico*

Abstract: Malaria is still the most important parasitic disease in the world. Traditional medicines have been used to treat malaria for thousands of years and are the source of artemisinin and quinine derivatives. With the increasing levels of drug resistance, the high cost of artemisinin-based combination therapies and fake antimalarial drugs, traditional medicine has become an important and sustainable source of malaria treatment in endemic areas. The use of herbal medicines believed to have therapeutic properties is becoming increasingly widespread. These remedies are usually taken by patients on their own initiative without prescription from a physician. The discovery and use of natural compounds require a thorough investigation of their safety and efficacy before their release into the market because herbal medicines present the greatest risk of adverse effects relative to all complementary therapies. Nevertheless, natural products have been a major source of new drugs due to the high diversity of their natural compounds that often provide specific biological activities. In this chapter, we review the results achieved in the use of extracts, fractions and compounds obtained from natural sources that have antimalarial efficacy. We also provide a panoramic view of the updated literature on the challenges and strategies associated with contemporary antimalarial natural drug research.

Keywords: Antimalarial, antimalarial natural drug research, drug design, extracts, herbal medicine, malaria, malaria complementary therapies, malaria treatment, natural medicine, *Plasmodium falciparum*.

INTRODUCTION

Malaria is the most important parasitic disease globally and is attributed to four Plasmodium species: *Plasmodium falciparum, Plasmodium vivax, Plasmodium ovale* and *Plasmodium malariae*. *P. falciparum* is distributed worldwide throughout all malaric areas, predominantly in sub-Saharan Africa. *P. malariae*

***Corresponding author Norma Rivera Fernández:** Laboratory of Malariology, Department of Microbiology and Parasitology, Faculty of Medicine, National Autonomous University of Mexico. Mexico City, 04510, Mexico; Tel: 562-32465; E-mail: normariv@unam.mx

Atta-ur-Rahman (Ed)
All rights reserved-© 2016 Bentham Science Publishers

has a similar distribution as *P. falciparum* but occurs less frequently. *P. vivax* predominates in Central America and India, and *P. ovale* is rarely found outside Africa [1]. *Plasmodium knowlesi* is emerging as a relevant zoonotic pathogen that is exported by travelers from endemic areas around the world; the infection could be potentially propagated through blood transfusions, bone marrow transplants and congenital infections [2]. In accordance with the World and Health Organization (WHO) report published in 2011, there are 106 known countries with malaria transmission distributed in the tropical and sub-tropical areas, with millions of clinical cases and thousands of deaths registered annually [3]. The most alarming situation occurs in the African countries that are south of the Sahara, with children under 5 years old particularly exposed [4]. Worldwide surveillance systems do not capture all malaria cases and deaths occurring in a country; therefore, estimates are obtained by adjusting the number of reported cases to take into account the estimated proportion of cases that are not reported. The estimated number of malaria cases fell from 227 million in 2000 to 198 million in 2013, with 128 million people infected with *P. falciparum* in sub-Saharan Africa, with an estimated 584 000 deaths; the average infection prevalence in children aged 2 to 10 years has declined by 46% between 2000 and 2013; 82% of these cases were reported in the African Region, 12% were reported in South-East Asia, and the remaining cases were reported in the Mediterranean Region. Approximately 47% of the reported cases outside of Africa were due to *P. vivax*, with the major percentage of cases occurring in the Americas (62%) [4].

For the first time, two countries with malaria transmission reported zero indigenous cases in 2013. Argentina, Armenia, Iraq, Georgia, Kyrgyzstan, Morocco, Oman, Paraguay, Turkmenistan and Uzbekistan maintained zero cases. Algeria, Cabo Verde, Costa Rica and El Salvador reported fewer than 10 local cases. Argentina and Kyrgyzstan have asked the WHO how to start the process for certifying their achievement of malaria elimination [5].

Malaria Biology

Parasitic diseases have been one of the most significant public health problems for centuries with noteworthy mortality and devastating social and economic consequences. Parasites belonging to the protozoa subkingdom are important pathogens that cause several human infections with globally massive impacts [6]. The protozoan phylum Apicomplexa includes species such as *Plasmodium*, *Toxoplasma gondii* and *Cryptosporidium,* among others, that are threatening the life and health of humans and domestic animals [7]. Apicomplexa are unicellular eukaryotic organisms and are tricky invaders with complex and beautiful structures that allow them to hide from the host immune response [8].

During the life cycle of the Apicomplexan, the interaction between the host and the parasite is mediated by three apical secretory organelles: micronemes, rhoptries and dense granules [9]; these 'apical organelles' store proteins that are secreted sequentially during invasion and intracellular proliferation [10]. Micronemes proteins (MIC), stored in the micronemes are secreted during gliding motility and adhesion to the host cell membrane [11]. Rhoptries proteins (ROP), stored in the rhoptries are secreted after the apical end of the parasite is pushed down over the host cell membrane during the early stages of invasion, and dense granules proteins (GRA) stored in dense granules are exclusively secreted during proliferation and within the intravascular space of the parasitophorous vacuole [9].

The malaria parasite develops both in humans and in the female *Anopheles* mosquitoes and undergoes different parasite stages during its life cycle. The parasites initially multiply inside liver cells and then in successive intraerythrocytic cycles, causing the symptoms of the disease [12]. When a female *Anopheles* mosquito bites a person infected with malaria, the parasite journey in the mosquito begins [13]. In the mosquito midgut lumen, *Plasmodium* female and male gametocytes mature into gametes, undergo fusion and develop a motile ookinete, which will become an oocyst at the midgut epithelium. The oocysts mature and release sporozoites into the mosquito hemolymph; these sporozoites will migrate into the salivary glands of the insect; then, an infected female *Anopheles* mosquito bites a person, injecting *Plasmodium* sporozoites into the bloodstream, and within 30-60 minutes [14], the parasites invade hepatocytes and mature to schizonts, which rupture and release merozoites that continue the intraerythrocytic cycle. The *P. vivax* and *P. ovale* dormant stage, called hypnozoites, can persist in the liver of the host and cause recurrences [15]. Malaria life cycle is depicted in Fig. (**1**).

Merozoites represent the parasite stage responsible for malaria symptoms. Once released from the liver, merozoites actively invade red blood cells (RBCs) by forming a junction between its apical end and the erythrocyte membrane and developing an incipient parasitophorous vacuole in the junction area; then, the junction between the parasite and host cell becomes ring-shaped. The ring-shaped parasite grows and develops into a trophozoite. The trophozoite starts feeding, the schizont stage begins, and new merozoites are finally released. Some of these released parasites differentiate into gametocytes, which do not cause pathology in humans and disappear from circulation if not taken up by a mosquito [16].

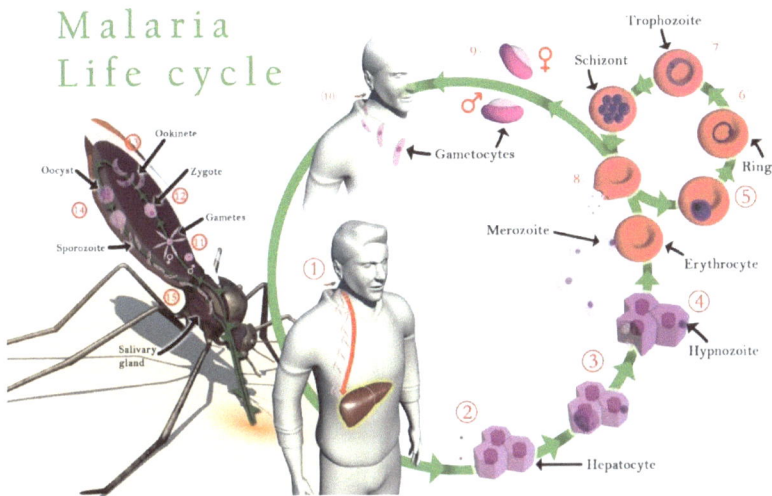

Fig. (1). Malaria life cycle. When feeding, female Anopheles mosquito infected with malaria, injects sporozoites into the blood stream of the human host (1). Sporozoites migrate to the liver and invade hepatocytes (2) and in about two weeks, a replicative process called schizogony is carried out (3), resulting in the liberation of thousands of parasitic haploid forms called merozoites. In the case of *Plasmoidum vivax* and *Plasmodium ovale*, parasites remain as a dormant stage called "hipnozoites" (4) that may cause relapses weeks or even years later. When liberated from the hepatocytes, the merozoites invade red blood cells (5) and an intraerythrocytic schizogony begins with the development of different parasites stages: ring (6), trophozoite (7), schizont and the release of new merozoites (8). Some merozoites continue with the asexual intraerythrocytic replication by invading new red blood cells, and others differentiate into sexual erythrocytic stages called gametocytes (9) that are ingested by the Anopheles female mosquito during blood feeding (10). In the mosquito lumen, female and male gametes (11) fuse to produce diploid zygotes (12) that will develop into motile ookinetes (13). The ookinetes cross the mosquito midgut epithelium and basal lamina and form occysts (14). Mature oocysts release thousands of sporozoites that migrate and invade the lobes of the salivary glands of the mosquito (15) and the cycle re-starts when the Anopheles female mosquito bites a new human host (1).

Malaria Pathogenesis

The pathological expression of malaria infection in the host depends largely on the immunopathologic response induced by the parasite [17]. Inappropriate immuno-responses to some malarial antigens can generate major complications as a result of malaria infection [18]. The damage made by the mosquito in the dermis of the host during infection induces the release of pro-inflammatory cytokines and the influx of leukocytes [19]. The pathogenesis of all malaria species is related to the shizonts rupture and the release of new merozoites, toxins and pro-inflammatory cytokines from the infected red blood cell (iRBC). The discharge of these molecules triggers a systemic inflammatory process that initially controls parasite multiplication but later favors the damage to the host cells and tissues, and starts the febrile paroxysm [20, 21]. The released components during the lysis of the iRBC stimulate the macrophages and the discharge of TNF (Tumor Necrosis Factor), IL-1 (Interleukin) and IL-6. TNF induces the release of prostaglandin E2 (PE2), which attaches to the surface of the neurons of the thermoregulatory nucleus and modifies the baseline body temperature. When the baseline temperature rises to 40 °C, the neurons still record a temperature of 37°C, and then the neurons of the supraoptic nucleus need to be activated to increase the temperature. The mechanisms to increase energy costs include thermoregulatory behavior to reduce heat loss (adinamia), cutaneous vasoconstriction to conserve heat in the body core (pale teguments), piloerection (chills), hypoventilation (abnormal breathing) and shivering thermogenesis in the skeletal muscle (teeth chattering). In this phase of the malaric paroxysm, the patient feels an intense cold and cephalea. Then, the temperature increases and reaches the febrile state, even though the patient continues to feel cold. The sensation of cold disappears when the corporal temperature equals the reference temperature of the thermoregulatory neurons. This febrile temperature remains as long as the stimulation of the macrophages by the parasites persists, and sometimes this stimulation could last up to 10 hours. When the production of TNF-prostaglandins returns to a normal level, the reference temperature automatically returns to a normal value of 37 ± 0.5 °C. Nevertheless, in this moment, the body temperature recorded by the neurons is 40 °C; the neurons of the paraventricular nucleus are then activated and send a message to stop producing heat and dissipate the existing heat. In response, metabolism is reduced, the skeletal muscles relax, the peripheral blood vessels dilate, the skin turns hot and red because of the heat loss by radiation, and there is hyperventilation (panting) and diaphoresis (sweating); finally, the patient is exhausted and falls asleep. When awake and still weak, the patient is able to continue with their regular activities until the next paroxysm repeats every 36, 48 or 72 hours, depending on the strain of the plasmodium that has infected him. If the infection is left to develop freely without treatment, and if the patient is not re-infected, the paroxysms return less intensely and for shorter periods and finally disappear in approximately 6 months. Although the symptoms disappear, the parasites may continue circulating in the blood for a variable time period, and in a small number of infections; in the case of *P. malariae*, the parasites persist for between 30 and 40 years, during which symptoms may return. The natural evolution of infections with *P. vivax* and *P. ovale* brings the parasite to a latent stage in the liver called hypnozoite, and relapses occur weeks or months later after the infection [21].

Severe or complicated malaria is defined by clinical or laboratory evidence of vital organ dysfunction [22]. Nearly all deaths from severe malaria result from infections with *P. falciparum*. Although death in *P. vivax* infections has been recognized for over a century, the last decade has seen a remarkable increase in case reports, series and studies describing severe and fatal *P. vivax* malaria [23]. TNF levels are raised in patients with severe malaria, even more so than in CM (cerebral malaria) and placental malaria, and are associated with low birth weight [24, 25]. NO (nitric oxide) synthesis requires extracellular arginine, and recent studies found an association between hypoargininemia and severe malaria and death in children. In recent studies in the *P. berghei* ANKA model, levels of indoleamine 2, 3-deaminase (IDO) in patients were increased 40-fold compared to those in controls, at the point of cerebral symptom development [24]. Recent studies reported the role of perforin in the pathogenesis of severe murine malaria through disruption of the blood-brain barrier (BBB) [25]. Rivera *et al.* (2015) described disruption of the cerebrospinal fluid brain barrier (CSFBB) in a murine malaria model [22]. The sequestration of falciparum in non-infected and infected red blood cells (iRBC) in endothelial cells leads to profound endothelial alterations that trigger immunopathological changes, varying degrees of brain edema and blood flow alterations [18].

Clinical Manifestations of Malaria

The clinical manifestations of malaria vary with geography, epidemiology, immunity and age. In hyper endemic areas, children up to 36 months and pregnant women are at highest risk for severe disease [26]. In areas where malaria is transmitted throughout the year, older children and adults develop partial immunity after repeated infections and are at relatively low risk for severe disease. Travelers from non-endemic areas are consider a high risk group as well because they have no previous exposure to parasites [27]. Thus, it is important to consider malaria in all febrile patients returning from malaria endemic areas. The incubation period of malaria in most cases varies from 7 to 30 days. The shorter periods are observed most frequently with *P. falciparum*, and the longer periods are observed with *P. malariae* (CDC). In relapsing species such as *P. vivax* and *P. ovale,* clinical manifestations can occur months or even years after the initial infection due to activation of hypnozoites in the liver. *P. falciparum* and *P. malariae* have no hypnozoites and therefore do not relapse [28].

Uncomplicated malaria can occur with any *Plasmodium* species. The typical but rarely observed clinical manifestation of uncomplicated malaria consists of shivering, fever, cephalea, nausea, vomiting, diaphoresis, asthenia, malaise, cough, anorexia, diarrhea, arthralgias, myalgias, and in young children, seizures. Malaria paroxysms occur every second day with *P. falciparum*, *P. vivax*, and

P. ovale and every third day with *P. malariae*. Unlike endemic areas where people usually recognize the initial symptoms of malaria and seek treatment, in non-endemic areas, these clinical manifestations could be due to other infectious diseases. Physical findings may include hepatomegaly, splenomegaly, tachypnea and tachycardia, and laboratory findings may include mild anemia, thrombocytopenia, jaundice, high levels of aminotransferases, elevated BUN and creatinine and blood smears with <0.1% parasitemia [29].

Patients with complicated or severe malaria have parasitemia levels of ≥5 to 10%. Clinical features of severe malaria include impaired consciousness (including unrousable coma); prostration and generalized weakness; multiple convulsions: more than two episodes within 24 h; deep breathing and respiratory distress; acute pulmonary edema and acute respiratory distress syndrome; circulatory collapse or shock, systolic blood pressure < 80 mm Hg in adults and < 50 mm Hg in children; acute kidney injury; clinical jaundice plus evidence of other vital organ dysfunction; and abnormal bleeding. The manifestations of severe malaria can occur singly or, more commonly, in combination in the same patient. In hyperendemic areas, the risk for severe falciparum malaria is greatest among young children and visitors (of any age) from non-endemic areas. Risk is increased in the second and third trimesters of pregnancy, in patients with HIV/AIDS and in people who have undergone splenectomy [30]. Anemia is a common complication of malarial infection, although the consequences are more pronounced with *P. falciparum* malaria [31]. In patients with falciparum malaria (FM), hyperbilirubinemia and jaundice may be considered as a warning sign associated with liver and kidney dysfunction, and sometimes with severe illness with a higher incidence of complications and poor prognosis. Acute renal failure is an important complication of severe malaria, particularly in adults and older children, and has a poor prognosis. Renal injury in malaria is caused by acute tubular necrosis that is reversible in survivors. The exact mechanism of acute renal failure in FM is not known. Some studies indicated that acute renal failure in FM is due to the exaggerated induction of proinflammatory cytokines, primarily TNF, leading to vasoconstriction and increased vascular permeability [32]. Hypoglycemia is another important complication of severe FM, and the mechanisms seem to be multifactorial including the depletion of glucose stores due to starvation, parasite utilization of glucose, and cytokine-induced impairment of gluconeogenesis [33]. Malaria hemoglobinuria, commonly known as black water fever (BWF), is the term used to designate the occurrence of hemoglobin pigments in the urine of patients infected with malaria parasites. BWF is more often associated with *Plasmodium falciparum* infection in man. The pathogenesis of BWF has not been satisfactorily explained [34]. BWF is essentially a syndrome of acute intravascular hemolysis, occurring typically in individuals who have experienced repeated and severe attacks of falciparum malaria. The symptomatology appears abruptly with discharge of port wine-colored urine, icterus, pallor, nausea, fever, and acute renal failure [35]. In some clinically important syndromes of human malaria such as malaria-associated acute renal failure in adults and BWF, very little data are available on the clinical or pathological correlates in animal models [36]. Repeated attacks of malaria and the consequent destruction of red blood cells induce the formation of autoimmune actors, which in turn produce hemolysis [31]. Since the introduction of primaquine for the radical cure of *vivax* malaria and the consequent discovery of glucose-6-phosphate-dehydrogenase (G6PD) deficiency as a cause of hemolysis in patients receiving primaquine or other oxidant drugs, G6PD deficiency has been added to the differential diagnosis of BWF [37].

Cerebral malaria (CM) is the most severe neurological complication of infection with *Pf*, and children in sub-Saharan Africa are the most affected [38]. CM is usually secondary to *Pf* infection; however, there are infrequent reports of cerebral malaria associated with *P. vivax* infection [39]. In malaria falciparum, the sequestration of the non-infected and infected, red blood cells (iRBC) leads to profound endothelial alterations that trigger immunopathological changes, varying degrees of brain edema and blood flow alterations [18]. Hypotheses that imply that only the parasitized red cells are altered do not explain why CM does not occur in all individuals with massive infections. In the mouse model, the sequestration of parasitized red cells is absent or marginal, while hemorrhagic necrosis is fully developed, which indicates that the sequestration of red cells may not be necessary for the development of CM [40]. Malaria parasites can damage the BBB and CSFBB, which causes these nervous system structure barriers to increase their permeability and allow access to an increased amount of proinflammatory cytokines that result in damage to the brain tissues and CM [41]. Rivera *et al.* (2015) confirmed that CD1 male mice infected with the *Plasmodium yoelii* lethal strain exhibit damage to the CSFBB and ependymal cells. The severity of the damage to the epithelium was observed to be dependent on the extent of parasitemia [22].

Malaria Prophylaxis

Malaria remains one of the most devastating diseases threatening the human race, affecting populations in the tropical and subtropical regions of the world. Despite the effort made to control malaria for over a century, it remains a leading cause of morbidity and mortality in the world's least-developed regions [42]. The global distribution of malaria shows a remarkable correlation between malaria and poverty and lower rates of economic growth [43]. The battle against malaria started with its discovery by Ross and Grassi in 1898, who demonstrated that the transmission of malaria parasites occurs through the bite of an infected mosquito [44, 45].

Malaria control requires an integrated approach, including prevention (primarily vector control) and prompt treatment with effective antimalarial agents. The last 10 years have seen increased economic resources to prevent malaria from institutions such as the Global Fund to fight AIDS, Tuberculosis and Malaria, the World Bank, the US President's Malaria Initiative (PMI), and the Bill and Melinda Gates Foundation [46]. Most countries with high malaria burdens have changed their treatment algorithms by adopting more efficacious but expensive artemisinin-based drug combinations [47] and increasing coverage of malaria chemoprophylatic treatments for pregnant women and children [48], universal testing to diagnose malaria by microscopy or rapid improved diagnostic test [47] and the free distribution of insecticide treated nets, particularly in sub-Saharan African countries [49].

The CDC recommends drugs for travelers to each country to prevent malaria. No antimalarial drug is 100% protective and must be combined with the use of personal protective measures, such as insect repellent, long sleeves, long pants, sleeping in a mosquito-free setting or using an insecticide-treated bednet [50]. Atovaquone/Proguanil are effective for last-minute travelers because the drug is started 1-2 days before traveling to an area where malaria transmission occurs, and pediatric tablets are available but cannot be used by pregnant or breastfeeding women, children under 5 kg and patients with severe renal impairment. Cloroquine (CQ) has to be started 1 to 2 weeks before travel and could be taken once a week and in all three trimesters of pregnancy. However, CQ cannot be used in CQ or mefloquine (MQ) resistance areas [50]. Doxycycline is given every 24 h and seems to be the less expensive antimalarial. Mefloquine is taken weekly, can be used during pregnancy but cannot be used in areas with mefloquine resistance. Mefloquine seems to have more neuropsychiatric adverse events than atovaquone/proguanil and doxycycline. Risk factors for the occurrence of neuropsychiatric adverse events in response to mefloquine have been established and include being female and having a personal or family history of seizures or affective disorder [50]. Ringqvist *et al.* (2015) have reported anxiety, phobic anxiety, depression, time-limited psychotic symptoms, illusions/hallucinations more frequently observed among women, hypomania/mania and significant long-term mental health in mefloquine-treated people [51].

Malaria Treatment

Progress toward developing malaria vaccines has accelerated in the recent years. Three candidate vaccines are in Phase 2B clinical trials, and one has completed Phase 3, with a total of 25 projects in the pipeline [52]. Venegas *et al.* (2014) described a novel symmetric double dimer and condensed linear constructs for presenting selected peptide multi-copies from the apical sushi protein expressed in *Plasmodium falciparum*; these molecules have shown strong protective efficacy in rodents challenged with two *Plasmodium* species; nevertheless, efforts to develop an effective malaria vaccine are yet to be successful, and thus, chemotherapy remains the primary malaria control strategy [53].

Malaria treatment should not be initiated until the diagnosis has been confirmed; presumptive treatment can be used in exceptional circumstances as in the case of severe malaria, which is almost always fatal without treatment. The WHO recommends that artemisinin-based combination therapies (ACTs) be used for the treatment of malaria. ACT is the simultaneous use of two or more blood schizontocidal medicines with independent modes of action that could prevent or delay the emergence of resistance. Non-artemisinin-based combination treatments include sulfadoxine-pyrimethamine plus chloroquine or amodiaquine [54]. Most common antimalarial drugs are shown in Table **1**.

Artemisinin-Based Combination Therapies (ACT)

In the recent years, parasites have developed resistance to conventional antimalarial drugs such as chloroquine, sulfadoxine and pyrimethamine. Recommendations, combination therapy that include artemisinin derivatives are now advised, widely known as ACT. It is known that when administered in adherence with treatment guidelines, combination therapies are more effective than monotherapies and besides administration of two drugs reduces the chance of resistance to emerge. It has been demonstrated that ACT results in remission of symptoms, clearance of parasites and gametocyte carriage reduction [54]. Artemisinin-based combination treatments (ACTs) are now generally accepted as the best treatments for uncomplicated falciparum malaria.

WHO currently recommends five different ACT: Artesunate- mefloquine, artesunate-sulfadoxine-pyrimethamine, artesunate-amodiaquine, artemether-lumefantrine and dihydroartemisinin-piperaquine. In general, ACT is a combination of an artemisinin derivative and another structurally unrelated and more slowly eliminated antimalarial drug. Efficacy is determined by the drug partnering the artemisinin derivative [54].

Table 1. Antimalarial drugs recommended by the World and Health Organization; (2010).

Uncomplicated *Plasmodium falciparum* Malaria	Complicated *Plasmodium falciparum* Malaria	*Plasmodium vivax* Malaria
For adults*: Arthemether plus*: lumefantrine, artesunate amodiaquine, mefloquine. *Artesunate plus*: Sulfadoxine-pyrimethamine. *Artesunate plus*: Tetracycline or doxycycline or clindamycin. *Quinine plus*: Tetracycline or doxycycline or clindamycin (could be used during pregnancy). During lactation dapsone, primaquine and tetracyclines should be avoid. **For Children**: *ACTs* for first-line treatment. **For Travelers returning to non-endemic areas:** Atovaquone-proguanil; artemether-lumefantrine; quinine plus doxycycline or clindamycin.	Artesunate plus clindamycin, artemether, quinine, quinine plus clindamycin, doxycycline.	Cloroquine plus primaquine; ACTs are recommended.

Despite efforts to control malaria, a dramatic revival of the disease is ongoing due to the increasing resistance of vectors to insecticides, the disproportional access to bed nets, especially among poor households, and to the progressive resistance of the parasite to antimalarial drugs [49, 55]. This situation is aggravated by reports from Southeast Asia of the parasite becoming resistant to artemisinin, the last line of defense in malaria chemotherapy [56, 57]. Petersen *et al.* (2011) discussed that the emergence of *Plasmodium* resistance depends on multiple factors such as the mutation rate of the parasites, the overall parasite load, the strength of drug selection, and the treatment compliance [45].

Malaria parasites rapidly evolve mechanisms to escape drug pressure to survive [58]. The genes responsible for resistance to the most important antimalarial drugs are the CQ resistance transporter gene (*pf*crt), *P. falciparum* multidrug resistance transporter 1 (*pf*mdr1), multidrug resistance-associated protein *Pf*mrp, *P. falciparum* Na+/H+ exchanger (*pf*nhe), cytochrome b gene (cytb, mal_mito_3) that leads to atovaquone resistance and *pf*dhfr and *pf*dhps genes that are implicated in resistance to sulfadoxine-pyrimethamine. These genes have been implemented as molecular markers in screening for the emergence of resistance and to assess its spread, as a means to inform rational drug policy decisions. Artemisinins are potent inhibitors of *Plasmodium falciparum* phosphatidylinositol-3-kinase (PfPI3K). In resistant clinical strains, increased PfPI3K was associated with the C580Y mutation in *P. falciparum* Kelch13 (PfKelch13), a primary marker of artemisinin resistance [59].

The emergence and spread of multidrug-resistant malaria are the key factors contributing to the complexity of malaria control [60]. Resistance to antimalarials has been documented for *P. falciparum*, *P. malariae* and *P. vivax*. In *P. falciparum*, resistance has been observed to all currently used antimalarials (amodiaquine, chloroquine, mefloquine, quinine, and sulfadoxine-pyrimethamine) and, more recently, in artemisinin derivatives [56, 61]. The increasing spread of malaria together with the emergence of resistance against conventional antimalarial drugs has put enormous pressure on public health systems to introduce new therapeutics. Research efforts on the discovery of new antimalarial drugs have generated only a few successful compounds suitable for the treatment and prevention of acute malaria [62].

The Discovery of Antimalarials from Medicinal Plants

Medicinal plants have been used since the origin of manhood to treat illnesses. In the Ebers Papyrus, more than 800 remedies (including a variety of plants) for diverse diseases are listed. In the document: "*De Materia Medica*", more than 600 plants used as medicinal herbs are described in Helenic, and it could be considered to be the first compendium of pharmacy. Galen (129 - 199 AD) prescribed "galenics" (mixtures of natural medicines). During the 15th century, different printed herbal documents were developed and the use of herbal medicines became more common; in 1498, the "*Nuovo Receptario*" was compiled and printed in Florence as the first official pharmacopoeia [63, 64].

Actually, in developing countries, herbal medicines are important because they are affordable to the general population. The WHO has encouraged studies of old remedies used in traditional medicine because their secular use could confirm their medicinal efficacy; in 1999, they published a WHO monograph on selected medicinal plants, containing 28 monographs; in 2003, volume two included 30 additional monographs; in 2007, the third volume presented 31 additional monographs; and in 2009, the fourth volume contained an additional 28 monographs describing the quality control and use of selected medicinal plants [65-68]. Plants with antimalarial activity compiled by the WHO are depicted in Table **2**.

Table 2. Plants with antimalarial activity compiled by the World and Health Organization Monographs on selected medicinal plants.

Scientific name	Family	Material of Interest	Geographical Distribution	Studied Chemical Composition	Antimalarial Activity
Brucea javanica. (L.) Merr.	Simaroubaceae	Dried ripe fruit or seed	China, India, Indonesia, and Viet Nam	Quassinoid, triterpenes	Efficacy against Pf *in vitro* and *in vivo, in vitro* against chloroquine-resistant *Pf, in vivo* against *P. berghei* [117,118]
Bupleurum falcatum L. or *B. falcatum* L. var. *scorzonerifolium*	Apiaceae	Dried roots	Indigenous to northern Asia, northern China, and Europe	Triterpene, saponins,	Antipyretic activity in patients with fever [119]
Coptis chinensis Franch, *Coptis deltoides* C.Y. Cheng et Hsiao, *Coptis japonica* Makino	Ranunculaceae	Dried rhizome	China	Berberine and related protoberberine alkaloids	Antimalarial use not supported by experimental data
Andrographis paniculata (Burm. f.) Nees	Acanthaceae	Dried aerial parts	South-East Asia and India	Diterpene, lactones	Ethanol extract efficient against *Plasmodium berghei in vitro* and *in vivo* [120,121]
Eucalyptus globulus Labill	Myrtaceae	Essential oil Dried leaves	Australia, Africa, South America Asia southern Europe and the United States of America	1,8-cineole, terpenol, tannins, ellagitannins, triterpenes	Uses described in folk medicine, not supported by experimental or clinical data [122, 123]
Ocimum sanctum L.	Lamiaceae	Fresh or dried leaves	India, north and eastern Africa, Island, Taiwan, China	Tannins (4.6%) and essential oil	Antimalarial use, not supported by experimental data

Table 2: contd…

Azadirachta indica A. Juss.	Meliaceae	Dried leaves Fixed oil	India, South and South-East Asia, Australia, Florida and California, United States, South and Central America	Oxidized tetranortriterpenes	Extracts inhibited *Pf in vitro* growth, no effect against against *P. berghei* [124, 125]
Psidium guajava L.	Myrtaceae	Dried or young leaves	America, but now pantropical	Tannins, essential oils, flavonoids, and terpenes	Extracts have activity against *Pf in vitro* [126]
Phellodendron amurense Rupr. or *Phellodendron chinense* Schneid.	Rutaceae	Dried bark	China, Japan, Korea	Isoquinoline alkaloids	Antimalarial use not supported by experimental data
Picrorhiza kurrooa Royle; *Neopicrorhiza scrophulariiflora* Hong	Scrophulariaceae	Dried rhizome with root	North-western Himalayas	Iridoid glycosides, cucurbitacin, triterpenes and simple phenols	Antimalarial use not supported by experimental data
Bidens tripartita L.	Asteraceae	Dried aerial parts	Asia, Africa, Australia, Europe, North America and New Zealand	Flavonoids, chalcones, coumarins, tannins, essential oil	Ethanol extract active against *Pf in vitro* [127]
Hypericum perforatum L.	Clusiaceae	Dried flowering tops or aerial part	Africa, South Africa, South America, Asia, Australia, Europe and New Zealand, United States of America	Naphthodianthrones, flavonoids, tannins	Antimalarial use not supported by experimental data
Peganum harmala L.	Zygophyllaceae	Dried aerial parts	North Africa and southern Europe, Australia, Central Asia	Indole alkaloids	Extracts have *in vitro* activity against *Pf* [128-130]

Historically, compounds containing novel structures of natural origin represent a major source of the discovery and development of new drugs for several diseases [69]. The vast number of components found in medicinal plants provides an ideal source for drug discovery and drug design and are the primary compounds used for the development of new anti-infectives [70]. Traditional medicines have been used to treat malaria for thousands of years and are the source of artemisinin and quinine derivatives, two of the most used drugs for the treatment of malaria. Malaric patients, especially in rural areas, have no access to novel antimalarials such as artemisinin, for which the average cost per dose ranges from 5 to 8€. Consequently, affected people have to turn to traditional medicine to control the disease [71]. The discovery of the curative properties of cinchona bark (which contains the alkaloid quinine) is unclear. It is believed that Peruvian Indians drank hot infusions of stembark to treat shivering and fever. The active components of cinchona bark were isolated by Pelletier and Caventou in 1820 [72]. For almost three centuries, quinine was the only active principle effective against *Plasmodium falciparum*, and it has been considered to be responsible for the development of synthetic antimalarial drugs belonging to the 4- and 8-aminoquinoline classes after the Second World War [73]. Quinine became limited during the First World War. During this time, Bayer Company developed a synthetic antimalarial compound named plasmoquine, which was not approved for human use, and in 1932, they described the antimalarial properties of atebrine, which led to the discovery of cloroquine and sontochin. In the US, amodiaquine was synthetized but had lethal side effects. Primquine was then found to be the most active compound of the 8-aminoquinolines. The 8-aminoquinolines emerged during the 20th century and are considered the only antimalarial compounds effective against the different life-cycle stages of the human malaria. Mefloquine and halofantrine were then generated in the US [74]. The drugs that are used in the ACTs share their origins in nature, as most of them are variants of the natural product quinine. They are separated into two chemical classes: the amino-alcohols (sharing the closest similarity to quinine) such as mefloquine and lumefantrine, and the 4-aminoquinolines such as chloroquine, amodiaquine, piperaquine and pyronaridine [75]. In 1979, the Chinese reported the antimalarial activity of *Artemesia annua*, which has been used in traditional Chinese medicine for more than 2000 years. Later extensive clinical trials describe its active molecule, artemisinin; its derivatives artesunate, artemether and arteether, are now accepted as potent and fast-acting antimalarial agents [54].

It is clear enough that there is an urgent need for the development of new drugs to treat and control malaria. Around the world and even more so in the tropics, many countries have a vast collection of plants that are used as medicinal products to heal malaise and fever caused by malaria. It must be take into consideration that natural medicinal products have specific characteristics that differentiate them from commercial drugs; their composition may vary as a function of geographical origin and mode of preparation, so the complete composition of an extract is difficult to unravel and they will probably always contain toxic components. The search "antimalarial plant extracts" retrieved 1397 citations in PubMed. The term "antimalarial plant extracts toxicity" retrieved 221 citations, and "antimalarial plant extracts genotoxicity" retrieved only eight citations. For the benefit of those who consume medicinal plants as infusions, extracts, micronized stem bark, and through other modalities, scientific information concerning their efficacy and toxicity must be provided in detail to prevent toxic side effects when consumed.

Malaria control is recognized as one of the priorities of the WHO. Modern antimalarial drugs have been developed from only two plants: *Cinchona* spp. and *Artemisia annua.* According to the Research Initiative on Traditional Antimalarial Methods (RITAM), founded in 1999, there are 1200 plant species that are used to treat malaria and fever, most of them found on the three tropical continents and belonging to the following families: Annonaceae, Anacardiaceae, Crassulaceae, Cucurbitaceae, Euphorbiaceae, Fabaceae, Malvaceae, Menispermaceae and Zingiberaceae [76].

The modern pharmaceutical industry was born from botanical medicine, which is a prolific source for drugs because nature tends to form oxides by the hydrolysis of organic compounds; in contrast, medicinal chemistry centers on nitrogen and frequently includes additional atoms such as sulfur or halogens that are quite rare in nature [77]. In many cases, the crude extract has more pharmacological efficacy than its purified compounds because natural products have a mixture of diverse ingredients of varying potency and have an innate affinity for biological receptors; thus, their biological action is often highly selective [78]. Some emerging antimalarials from plants and their sources are described in a recent and very complete review [77].

New Synthetic Antimalarials

There are many challenges in the treatment of malaria. One challenge is the attempt to have a simple treatment regimen in the form of a single dose cure [79]. Another challenge is that most of the patients are under 5 years old. Furthermore, malaria is particularly prevalent in pregnant women, so understanding the safety profiles is of great importance [80]. Additionally, we believe that it necessary to develop drugs capable of breaking the cycle of infection, which could block transmission. Even more, it is known that the hypnozoites of *P. vivax* and *P. ovale* have the capacity to relapse over a period of time, causing a disease outbreak [79]. Finally, it is necessary and urgent to have new medicines because of the appearance of resistance to the treatment of malaria, particularly to artemisinin [79].

Some methods have been developed to find molecules capable of treating malaria. Some approaches have evolved from rationally designed molecules, using information from validated targets [81]. Other approaches are a result of high-throughput screens, testing millions of compounds on the whole parasite [82].

In recent years, there have been many reports of antimalarial drugs resistance, especially to artemisinin. Combining drugs has been an effective strategy to limit resistance, but even with combined treatments, resistance has risen. It is thus necessary to develop new drugs [83].

New drugs have to meet a series of criteria. They have to be fast acting, safe for children and pregnant women and easily administrable in a single dose.

Artemisinin Derivatives

One way to obtain artemisinin involves extraction from sweet wormwood [84]; an alternative production method uses a yeast fermentation process to obtain the precursor, followed by a photochemical oxidation process [85]. Synthetic routes have also been reported. In the search for new drugs, artemisinin has worked as a natural product model [86].

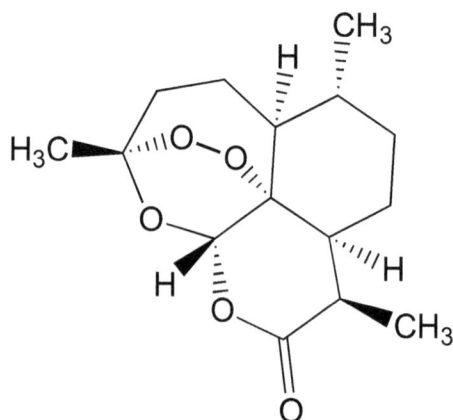

Artemisinin

Artemisinin and its first derivatives are metabolically instable due to their susceptibility to hydrolysis or oxidative-dealkylation to dihydroartemisinin [87].

Dihydroartemisinin has demonstrated more antimalarial efficacy than artemisinin [88], but it has also been demonstrated to be neurotoxic [89].

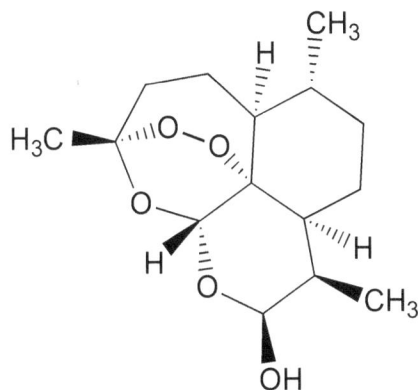

Dihydroartemisinin

To prevent metabolic instability and the toxicity of artemisinin derivatives, semi-synthetic derivatives have been developed with a backbone of C10 deoxyartemisinin functionalized at C9 or at C14 and C5 [90]. These derivatives include new groups at C10, or artemisinin-derived dimers that have been described [91, 92]. Specifically, artemisone has demonstrated remarkable antimalarial activity and has been evaluated in clinical Phase II trials [93, 94].

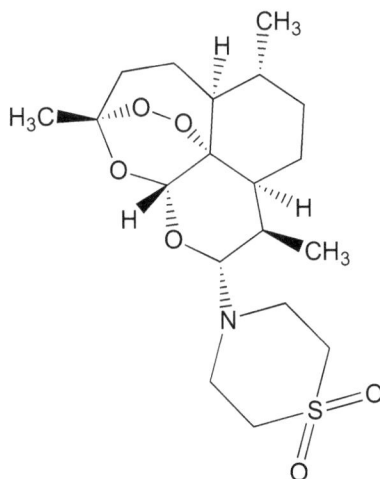

Artemisone

Artesunate is recommended by WHO in preference to quinidine for the treatment of severe malaria and has been used worldwide for many years. On June 21, 2007, the Food and Drug Administration (FDA) approved Intravenous Artesunate for Treatment of Severe Malaria in the United States, and according to CDC, High quality-intravenous artesunate is available only to malaria patients hospitalized in the United States who need intravenous treatment because of: severe malaria disease, high levels of malaria parasites in the blood, inability to take oral medications, lack of timely access to intravenous quinidine, quinidine intolerance or contraindications, quinidine failure.

It has been demonstrated that the peroxide functional group present in the artemisinin structure is directly related to antimalarial activity: if the peroxide bond is reduced, antimalarial activity is lost [95]. Thus, a series of semisynthetic derivatives, containing 1,2,4-trioxanes, 1,2,4-trioxolanes and mixed 1,2,4,5-tetraoxanes 1,2,4-trioxane heterocycle moieties, were prepared [96]. Another series of peroxides and the corresponding antimalarial activities have been reported, of which tetraoxane WR 148999 is the most active [97, 98].

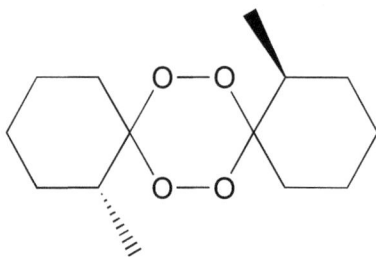

WR 148999

Preparing 1,2,4-trioxolanes (ozonides, OZs) is relatively simple [99]. Specifically, OZ277 (arterolane) has been proven to be a highly active antimalarial in preclinical studies [100] and has shown superior pharmacokinetic results, although it has significantly lower bioavailability. OZ277 has been advanced to Phase III clinical trials [101].

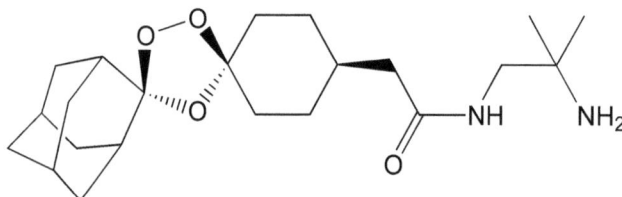

OZ277

OZ439, another ozonide, has been designed to overcome the low bioavailability of OZ277, and it has demonstrated enhanced stability in the treatment of infected blood malaria. Additionally, it can function as a single dose oral cure [102].

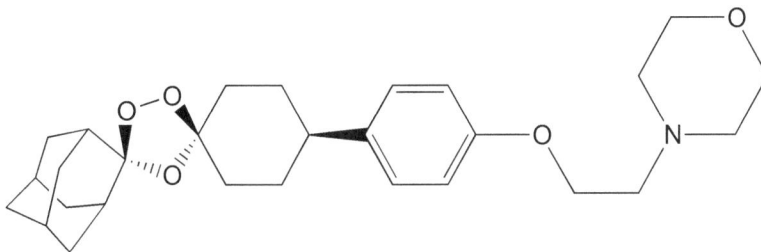

OZ439

Chloroquine Derivatives

Quinine is one of the traditional antimalarial agents and is extracted from cinchona tree bark. From this compound, it was possible to design and synthesize analogues such as 4-aminoquinoline chloroquine. However, in recent years, as a result of the development of parasite resistance, it is not an actual alternative for malaria treatment [103].

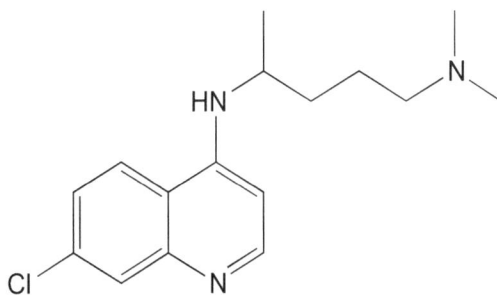

Cloroquine

Short-chain analogues, organometallic compounds and trioxaquine derivatives have been developed using the chloroquine structure template, [103-106].

AQ-13 is a short-chain compound with a better pharmacokinetic profile than chloroquine. It has low toxicity, increased clearance and high efficacy. It is in Phase II clinical trials [104].

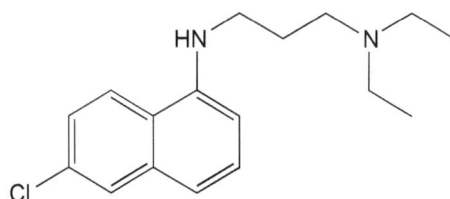

AQ-13

Organometallic compounds have particular physicochemical properties; thus, new compounds incorporating metal fragments into chloroquine have resulted in molecules with a higher efficacy and no acute toxicity. Specifically, some complex chloroquine-transition metals have been synthesized and have high *in vitro* antimalarial activity. Ferroquine was the first organometallic candidate to begin clinical trials [105, 106].

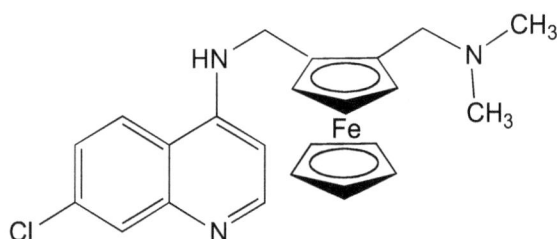

Ferroquine

Hybrid molecules covalently connect two distinct drug entities in one molecule. For the treatment of malaria, hybrid molecules with compounds bearing a biologically active natural product such as chloroquine have been developed [107, 108]. The hybrid is designed to target the parasite by two distinct mechanisms. Several trioxaquines have been developed and tested. SAR116242 has been shown to be potent against chloroquine and pyrimethamine-resistant strains and has improved antimalarial activity compared with its individual components. SAR 116242 is undergoing pre-clinical trials by Sanofi-Aventis.

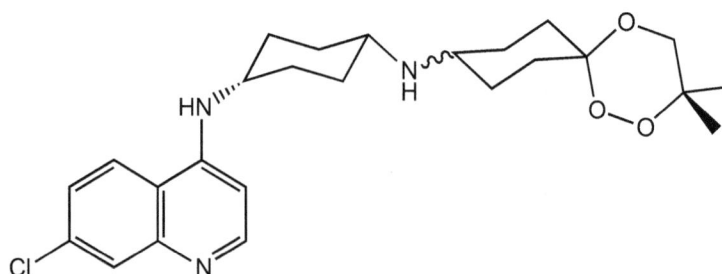

SAR116242

Novel Antimalarial Drug Delivery System

Mefloquine is a synthetic analogue of quinine, which is of limited use currently because of its pharmacokinetic profile, slow clearance, poor solubility, variation in oral absorption, and its mild to severe adverse reactions [109]. The neurological effects of mefloquine have been established by numerous case studies and by neurotoxicity investigations [110, 111]. Mefloquine is highly lipophilic and has low solubility [112]. As an alternative to the use of this drug, lipid-based submicron emulsions have been formulated. Lipid-based drug delivery systems are designed to improve bioavailability and to reduce side effects [113], thereby enhancing drug solubility. The novel antimalarial drug delivery system, named Pheroid technology, is a patented colloidal system of lipid bilayers constructed of natural essential fatty acids necessary for normal cell function. The vesicles are submicron-sized structures that are formed when the oil phase is dispersed in a nitrous oxide saturated water solution [114].

Pheroid vesicles integrate both hydrophilic and hydrophobic drugs and have been demonstrated to increase the bioavailability of poorly soluble drugs such as artemisone and mefloquine [115, 116].

Artemisinin Derivatives

Artesuante

According to WHO, Artemether is a lipid-soluble methyl ether of dihydroartemisinin which has very rapid schizontocidal activity against blood forms of *P. falciparum* and *P. vivax*. Mostly, treatment of slide-confirmed severe falciparum malaria in areas where there is evidence that quinine is ineffective, is with a full dose of an effective oral antimalarial such as mefloquine. After intramuscular administration, peak plasma concentrations are attained within about 6 hours. Artemether has been reported to clear fever in severe falciparum malaria within 30-84 hours.

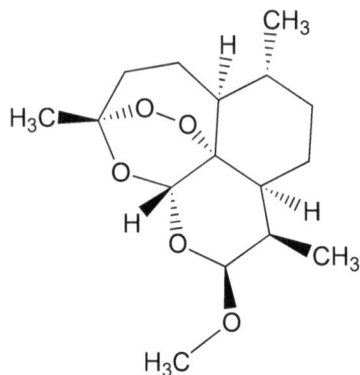

Artemether

Arteether is an ethyl ether derivative of artemisinin. It has efficacy in laboratory malaria models, being active against *P. falciparum* strains that were resistant to chloroquine, mefloquine, halofantrine, quinine, pyrimethamine, cycloquanil and amodiaquine. The two available formulations are: Artemotil (previously known as beta arteether) and alpha/beta arteether. Alpha/beta arteether is recommended for both children and adults with severe malaria. High doses of arteether may cause heart and nervous system damage.

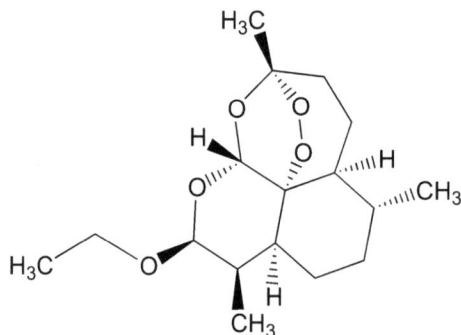

Arteether

CONCLUDING REMARKS

Although herbal medicine is used to treat malaria in endemic countries because it is more available and affordable than antimalarial drugs, most of the plants used in this way have not been scientifically researched and are consumed without a physician's prescription. Ethno-medical research has discovered many natural products with *in vitro* activity against *Pf*; nevertheless, no effective molecules have been identified apart from quinine and artemisinin derivatives. The active components of a plant extract that exhibit efficacy *in vitro* seem to have reduced or no activity when tested *in vivo*, besides having toxic side effects. Tests conducted *in vitro* are not able to mimic *in vivo* conditions due to different absorption and pharmacokinetic factors, and much time is wasted studying herbal compounds that will be useless in the experimental host or in the patient. More clinical trials on herbal antimalarial remedies are desirable before these remedies can be recommended to affected patients. An urgent call to the scientific guild working in this and other areas of malaria research is needed to give serious consideration to the potential of antimalarial herbal medicine.

CONFLICT OF INTEREST

The authors confirm that this chapter content has no conflict of interest.

ACKNOWLEDGEMENTS

The authors are grateful to the projects: PAPIIT-DGAPA UNAM IA203015 and CONACyT 182003. Malaria life cycle illustrations made by DCV Brenda Esquivel Flores, Department of Visualization and Virtual Reality, DGTIC-UNAM.

REFERENCES

[1]   Baird JK. Malaria zoonoses. Trav Med Inf Dis 2009; 7(5):267-69.
[2]   Carrasco RE, Malagón GF. La malaria como una zoonosis. Pacal Med Lab 2013; 5(2): 4-10.
[3]   The world medicine situation 2011. World Health Organization [homepage on the internet]. Geneva, Switzerland   [cited   4th   April   2015].   Available   from: http://www.who.int/medicines/areas/policy/world_medicines_situation/WMS_ch6_wPricing_v6.pdf
[4]   Charlette SL, Nongkynrih B. Can intermittent preventive treatment for malaria reduce child mortality? Nat Med J India 2013; 26(1):37.
[5]   World Health Organization. World Malaria Report 2014 [homepage on the internet] [cited 6th April 2015].   Available   from: http://www.who.int/malaria/publications/world_malaria_report_2014/report/en/
[6]   Martins M, Marreo-Ponce Y, Meneses M, *et al*. Antiprotozoan lead discovery by aligning dry and wet screening. Bioorg Med Chem 2014; 22:1568-85.
[7]   Gubbels MJ, Striepen B. Studying the cell biology of apicomplexan parasites using fluorescent proteins. Microsc Microanal 2004; 10, 568-579.
[8]   Striepen B, Jordan NC, Reiff S, van Dooren GG. Building the perfect parasite: Cell division in apicomplexa. Plos Pathog 2007; 3(6): 691-698.
[9]   Counihan NA, Kalanon Ming, Coppel RL, *et al*. Plasmodium proteins: why order is important. Trends Parasitol 2013; 29 (5): 228-36.
[10]   Ravindran S, Boothroyd JC. Secretion of proteins into host cells by Apicomplexan parasites. Traffic 2008; 9:647-656.
[11]   Soldati D, Dubremetz JF, Lebrun M. Microneme proteins: structural and functional requirements to promote adhesion and invasion by the Apicomplexan parasite *Toxoplasma gondii*. Int J Parasitol 2001; 31:1293-1302.
[12]   Mac-Daniel L, Ménard R. Plasmodium and mononuclear phagocytes. Microb Pathog 2015; 78:43-5.

[13] Vlachou D, Schlegelmilch T, Runn E, Mendes A, Kafatos FC. The developmental migration of Plasmodium in mosquitoes. Curr Opin Genet Dev 2006; 16(4):384-91.

[14] Kappe SH, Kaiser K, Matuschewski K. The Plasmodium sporozoite journey: a rite of passage. Trends Parasitol 2003; 19(3):135-43.

[15] Malaria biology [homepage on the internet]. Atlanta, GA: Centers for Disease Control and Prevention [updated 23th September 2015; 2015cited 14th April 2015]. Available from: http://www.cdc.gov/malaria/about/biology/

[16] Baker DA. Malaria gametocytogenesis. Mol Biochem Parasitol 2010; 172(2):57-65.

[17] Hayder AG, Mustafa IE, Ishraga EA, Thoraya ME, Gadir EL. Biomodal transmission of cerebral malaria and severe malaria anemia and reciprocal co-existence of sexual and asexual parasitemia in an area of seasonal malaria transmission. Parasitol 2008; 103(1):81-5.

[18] Grau GE, El-Assad F, Combes V. Experimental models of microvascular immunopathology: The example of cerebral malaria. J Neuroinfect Dis 2013; 5:134.

[19] Demeure C, Brahimi K, Hacini F, et al. Anopheles mosquito bites activate cutaneous mast cells leading to a local inflammatory response and lymph node hyperplasia. J Immunol 2005; 174: 3932-40.

[20] Chua CLL, G. Brown G, Hamilton JA, Rogerson P. Monocytes and macrophages in malaria: protection or pathology? Trends Parasitol 2013; 29: 26-34.

[21] Malagón F. El origen del paroxismo malárico. Rev Med IMSS 2005; 43 (1): 83-88.

[22] Rivera N, Colín B, Romero S, et al. Ependymal damage in a *Plasmodium yoelii yoleii* lethal murine malaria model. Histol Histopathol 2015; 30:245-53.

[23] Rahimi BA, Thakkinstian A, White NJ, et al. Severe vivax malaria: a systematic review and meta-analysis of clinical studies since 1900. Malar J 2015; 8(13):481.

[24] Mackintosh CL, Beeson JG, Marsh K. Clinical features and pathogenesis of severe malaria. Trends Parasitol 2004; 20(12):597-603.

[25] Engwerda CR, Mynott TL, Sawhney S, et al. Locally up-regulated lymphotoxin alpha, not systemic tumor necrosis factor alpha, is the principle mediator of murine cerebral malaria. J Exp Med 2002; 195, 1371-1377.

[26] Breman JG. Clinical Manifestations of malaria. UpToDate 2015. Available from: http://www.uptodate.com/contents/clinical-manifestations-of-malaria [cited: 15th April 2015].

[27] Wilson ME, Weld LH, Boggild A, et al. Fever in returned travelers: results from the GeoSentinel Surveillance Network. Clin Infect Dis 2007; 44(12):1560.

[28] Lover AA, Zhao X, Gao Z, et al. The distribution of incubation and relapse times in experimental human infections with the malaria parasite Plasmodium vivax. BMC Infect Dis 2014; 4:14:539.

[29] Centers for Disease Control and Prevention. Malaria Disease [homepage on the internet]. Atlanta, GA [cited 14th April 2015]. Available from: http://www.cdc.gov/malaria/about/disease.html#incubation

[30] World Health Organization. Management of severe malaria, 3rd edition 2012 [homepage on the internet] [cited 8th April 2015]. Available from: http://apps.who.int/iris/bitstream/10665/79317/1/9789241548526_eng.pdf

[31] Ghosh K, Ghosh K. Pathogenesis of anemia in malaria: a concise review. Parasitol Res 2007; 101:1463-69.

[32] Das BS. Renal failure in malaria. J Vector Borne Dis 2008; 45:83-97.

[33] Jiménez BC, Cuadros-Tito P, Ruiz-Giardin JM, Rojo-Marcos G, Cuadros-González J, Canalejo E, et al. Imported malaria in pregnancy in Madrid. Malar J 2012; 11:112.

[34] Rivera N, Ponce YM, Arán VJ, Martínez C, Malagón F. Biological assay of a novel quinoxalinone with antimalarial efficacy on *Plasmodium yoelii yoelii*. Parasitol Res 2013; 112(4):1523-7.

[35] Bruneel F, Gachot B, Wolff M, et al. Blackwater fever. Presse Med 2002; 31(28):1329-34.

[36] Craig GA, Grau EG, Janse C, et al. The role of animal models for research on severe malaria. PLoS Pathog 2012; 8:1-9.

[37] Ganesan S, Tekwani BL, Sahu R, Tripathi LM, Walker LA. Cytochrome P (450)-dependent toxic effects of primaquine on human erythrocytes. Toxicol Appl Pharmacol 2009; 241(1):14-22.

[38] Idro R, Marsh K, John CC, Newton CR. Cerebral malaria: mechanisms of brain injury and strategies for improved neurocognitive outcome. Pediatr Res 2011; 68: 267-74.

[39] Ozen M., Gungor S., Atambay M. and Daldal N. Cerebral malaria owing to *Plasmodium vivax*: case report. Ann J Pediatr 2006; 26: 141-4.

[40]   Grau GE, Piguet PF, Lambert PH. Immunopathology of malaria: role of cytokine production and adhesion molecules. Mem Inst Oswaldo Cruz 1992; 87: 95-100.

[41]   Angulo I, Fresno M. Cytokines in the pathogenesis of and protection against malaria. Clin. Diagn. Lab Immunol 2002; 9:1145-52.

[42]   Peterson A, Calamandrei E (eds). Malaria, etiology, pathogenesis and treatment, 1st Edn. Nova Science 2012; New York, p 1.

[43]   Elsheikha MH, Sheashaa AH. Epidemiology, pathophysiology, management and outcome of renal dysfunction associated with plasmodia infection. Parasitol Res 2007; 101:1183-90.

[44]   Hay S, Guerra, Tatem C, Noor A, Snow R. The global distribution and population at risk of malaria: past, present, and future. Lancet Infect Dis 2004; 4: 327-36.

[45]   Petersen I, Eastman R, Lanzer M. Drug-resistant malaria: Molecular mechanisms and implications for public health. FEBS Letters 2011; 585: 1551-62.

[46]   Njau1 JD, Stephenson R, Menon M, Kachur SP, McFarland DA. Exploring the impact of targeted distribution of free bed nets on household's bed net ownership, socio-economic disparities and childhood malaria infection rates: analysis of national malaria survey data from three sub-Saharan Africa countries. Malar J 2013; 12: 245.

[47]   Bosman A, Mendis KN. A major transition in malaria treatment: the adoption and deployment of artemisinin-based combination therapies. Am J Trop Med Hyg 2007; 77:193-7.

[48]   Carneiro I, Smith L, Ross A, *et al.* Intermittent preventive treatment for malaria infants: a decision-support tool for sub-Saharan Africa. Bull World Health Organ 2010; 88:807-14.

[49]   Sexton A. Best practices for an insecticide-treated bed net distribution programme in sub-Saharan eastern Africa. Malar J 2011; 10: 157.

[50]   Centers for Disease Control and Prevention. Choosing a drug to prevent malaria [homepage on the internet].   Atlanta,   GA   [cited   02   April   2015].   Available   from: http://www.cdc.gov/malaria/travelers/drugs.html

[51]   Ringqvist A, Bech P, Glenthøj B, Petersen E. Acute and long-term psychiatric side effects of mefloquine: A follow-up on Danish adverse event reports. Trav Med Infect Dis 2015; 13: 80-8.

[52]   WHO. Tables of malaria vaccine projects globally [homepage on the internet] [update 28th September 2015;   cited: 9th   April   2015].   Available   from: http://www.who.int/immunization/research/development/Rainbow_tables/en/

[53]   Vanegas M, Bermúdez A, Guerrero YA, *et al.* Protecting capacity against malaria of chemically defined tetramer forms based on the Plasmodium falciparum apical sushi protein as potential vaccine components. Biochem Biophys Res Commun 2014; 15; 451(1):15-23.

[54]   WHO. Guidelines for the Treatment of Malaria, 3rd Edn 2010 [homepage on the internet]. Geneva, Switzerland   [cited   8th   April   2015].   Available   from: http://apps.who.int/iris/bitstream/10665/162441/1/9789241549127_eng.pdf?ua=1&ua=1

[55]   Chea PY, White NJ. Antimalarial mass drug administration: ethical considerations. Int Health 2016; 8(4): 235-8.

[56]   Traore MS, Baldé MA, Diallo MST, Baldé ES, Diané S, Camara A, *et al.* Ethnobotanical survey on medicinal plants used by Guinean traditional healers in the treatment of malaria. J Ethnopharmacol 2013; 150(3):1145-53.

[57]   Giha H. Artemisinin derivatves for treatment of uncomplicated Plasmodium falciparum malaria in Sudan: too early for too much hope. Parasitol Res 2010; 106:549-552.

[58]   Muregi FW, Kirira PG, Ishih A. Novel rational drug design strategies with potential to revolutionize malaria chemotherapy. Curr Med Chem 2011; 18(1):113-143.

[59]   Winzeler EA, Manary MJ. Drug resistance genomics of the antimalarial drug artemisinin. Genome Biol 2014; 15(11):544.

[60]   Mbengue A, Bhattacharjee S, Pandharkar T, Liu H, Estiu G, Stanhelin R, Rizk SS *et al.* A molecular mechanism of artemisinin resistance in *Plasmodium falciparum* malaria. Nature 2015; doi: 10.1038/nature14412. [Epub ahead of print].

[61]   Kesara N, Phunuch M, Ronnatari R, Wanna C, Juntra K. Identification of resistance of Plasmodium falciparum to artesunate-mefloquine combination in an area along the Thai-Myanmar border. Malar J 2013; 12:1-14.

[62]   Jensen M, Mehlhorn H. Seventy-five years of Resochin in the fight against malaria. Parasitol Res 2009; 105:609-627.

[63] Schlitzer M. Antimalarial drugs what is in use and what is in the pipeline. Arch Pharm 2008; 341:149-163.

[64] Hata Y, Ebrahimi SN, De Mieri M, *et al.* Antitrypanosomal isoflavan quinones from Abrus precatorius. Fitoterapia 2014; 93:81-7.

[65] Potterat, O, Hamburger M. Drug discovery and development with plant-derived compounds, Prog Drug Res 2008; 65 (45): 7-118.

[66] WHO monographs on selected medicinal plants Vol. 1 [homepage on the internet]. Geneva 1999 [cited: 23rd April 2015]. Available from: http://apps.who.int/medicinedocs/pdf/s2200e/s2200e.pdf

[67] WHO monographs on selected medicinal plants Vol. 2 [homepage on the internet]. Geneva 2003 [cited: 23rd April 2015]. Available from: http://apps.who.int/medicinedocs/es/d/Js4927e/

[68] WHO monographs on selected medicinal plants Vol. 3 [homepage on the internet]. Geneva 2007 [cited: 23rd April 2015]. Available from: http://apps.who.int/medicinedocs/es/m/abstract/Js14213e/

[69] WHO monographs on selected medicinal plants Vol. 4 [homepage on the internet]. Geneva 2009 [cited: 23rd April 2015]. Available from: http://apps.who.int/medicinedocs/es/m/abstract/Js16713e/

[70] Kaur K, Jain M, Kaur T, Jain R. Antimalarials from nature. Bioorg Med Chem 2009; 17:3229-3256.

[71] Nicolaou KC, Chen JS, Dalby SM. From nature to the laboratory and into the clinic. Bioorg Med Chem 2009; 17: 2290-2303.

[72] Silva GN, Rezende LC, Emery FS, Gosmann G, Gnoatto SC. Natural and Semisynthetic Antimalarial Compounds: Emphasis on the Terpene Class. Mini Rev Med Chem 2015; [Epub ahead of print].

[73] Guerra F. The introduction of cinchona in the treatment of malaria. J Trop Med Hyg 1977; 80: 112-118.

[74] Batista R, de Jesus Silva A, Braga de Oliveira A. Plant-Derived Antimalarial Agents: New Leads and Efficient Phytomedicines. Part II. Non-Alkaloidal Natural Products. Mol 2009; 14: 3037-3072.

[75] Greenwood D. Conflicts of interest: the genesis of synthetic antimalarial agents in peace and war. J Antimicrob Chemother 1995; 36: 857-872.

[76] Burrows JN, Burlot E, Campo B, *et al.* Antimalarial drug discovery the path towards eradication. Parasitol 2014; 141(1):128-39.

[77] RITAM Research Initiative on Traditional Antimalarial Methods [homepage on the internet] [cited: 23rd April 2015]. Available from: http://giftsofhealth.org/ritam/

[78] Negi AS, Gupta A, Hamid AA (2014). Combating malaria with plant molecules: a brief update. Curr Med Chem. 2014; 21(4):458-500.

[79] Feher M, Schmidt JM. Property Distributions: Differences between Drugs, Natural Products, and Molecules from Combinatorial Chemistry. J Chem Inf Comput Sci 2003; 43(1):218-227.

[80] Biamonte MA, Wanner J, Le Roch KG. Recent advances in malaria drug discovery. Bioorg Med Chem Lett 2013; 23: 2829-2843

[81] Staines HM, Krishna S, eds. Treatment and Prevention of Malaria: Antimalarial Drug Chemistry, Action and Use. Springer Science & Business Media, 2012.

[82] Ludin P, Woodcroft B, Ralph SA, Mäser P. *In silico* prediction of antimalarial drug target candidates. Int J Parasitol Drugs Drug Resist 2012; 191-199.

[83] Wells TN, Burrows JN, Baird JK. Targeting the hypnozoite reservoir of Plasmodium vivax: the hidden obstacle to malaria elimination. Trends Parasitol 2010; 26(3): 145-151.

[84] Lin JT, Juliano JJ, Wongsrichanalai C. Drug-resistant malaria: the era of ACT. Curr Infect Dis Rep 2010; 12: 165-173.

[85] Milhous WK, Weina PJ. The Botanical Solution for Malaria. Science 2010; 327 (5963): 279-280.

[86] Levesque F, Seeberger PH. Continuous-Flow Synthesis of the Anti-Malaria Drug Artemisinin. Angew. Chem. Int. Ed. 2012; 51: 1706 -1709.

[87] Zhu C, Cook SP. A concise synthesis of (+)-artemisinin. J Am Chem Soc. 2012; 134(33):13577-13579.

[88] Lin AJ, Miller RE. Antimalarial Activity of New Dihydroartemisinin Derivatives. 6. -Alkylbenzylic Ethers. J Med Chem 1995; 38 (5): 764-770.

[89] Lin AJ, Lee M, Klayman DL. Antimalarial activity of new water-soluble dihydroartemisinin derivatives. 2. Stereospecificity of the ether side chain. J Med Chem 1989; 32:1249-1252.

[90] Fishwick J, McLean WG, Edwards G, Ward SA. The toxicity of artemisinin and related compounds on neuronal and glial cells in culture. Chem Biol Interact 1995; 96:263-271.

[91]   Avery MA, Alvim-Gaston M, Vroman JA, Wu B, Ager A, Peters W, Robinson BL, Charman W. Structure-activity relationships of the antimalarial agent artemisinin. 7. Direct modification of (+)-artemisinin and *in vivo* antimalarial screening of new potential preclinical antimalarial candidates. J Med Chem 2002; 45:4321-4335.

[92]   Chadwick J, Mercer AE, Park BK, Cosstick R, O'Neill PM. Synthesis and biological evaluation of extraordinarily potent C-10 carba artemisinin dimers against *P. falciparum* malaria parasites and HL-60 cancer cells. Bioorg Med Chem 2009; 17:1325-1338.

[93]   Posner GH, Ploypradith P, Parker MH, O'Dowd H, Woo SH, Northrop J, Krasavin M, Dolan P, Kensler TW, Xie S *et al*. Antimalarial, antiproliferative, and antitumor activities of artemisinin-derived, chemically robust, trioxane dimers. J Med Chem 1999; 42:4275-4280.

[94]   Vivas L, Rattray L, Stewart LB, Robinson BL, Fugmann B, Haynes RK, Peters W, Croft SL. Antimalarial efficacy and drug interactions of the novel semi-synthetic endoperoxide artemisone *in vitro* and *in vivo*. J Antimicrob Chemother 2007; 59:658-665.

[95]   Schrader FC, Barho M, Steiner I, Ortmann R, Schlitzer M. The antimalarial pipeline - An update. Int J Med Microbiol 2012; 302 (4-5): 165-171.

[96]   Meshnick SR, Taylor TE, Kamchonwongpaisan S. Artemisinin and the Antimalarial Endoperoxides: from Herbal Remedy to Targeted Chemotherapy. Microbiol Rev 1996; 60 (2): 301-315.

[97]   Jefford CW. New developments in synthetic peroxidic drugs as artemisinin mimics. Drug Discov Today 2007; 12 (11-12): 487-495.

[98]   Vennerstrom JL, Ager AL, Andersen SL, Grace JM, Wongpanich V, Angerhofer CK, Hu JK, Wesche DL. Assessment of the antimalarial potential of tetraoxane WR 148999. Am J Trop Med Hyg 2000; 62(5): 573-578.

[99]   Dong Y, Matile H, Chollet J, Kaminsky R, Wood JK,| Vennerstrom JL. Synthesis and Antimalarial Activity of 11 Dispiro-1, 2, 4, 5-tetraoxane Analogues of WR 148999. 7, 8, 15, 16-Tetraoxadispiro [5.2.5.2] hexadecanes Substituted at the 1 and 10 Positions with Unsaturated and Polar Functional Groups. J Med Chem 1999; 42 (8): 1477-1480.

[100]   Tang Y, Dong Y, Karle JM, DiTusa CA, Vennerstrom JL. Synthesis of tetrasubstituted ozonides by the Griesbaum coozonolysis reaction: diastereoselectivity and functional group transformations by post-ozonolysis reactions. J Org Chem 2004; 69:6470-6473.

[101]   Olliaro P, Wells TNC. The global portfolio of new antimalarial medicines under development. Clin Pharmacol Ther 2009; 85:584-595.

[102]   Valecha N, Martensson, Looareesuwan S, *et al*. Arterolane, a new synthetic trioxolane for treatment of uncomplicated Plasmodium falciparum malaria: a phase II, multicenter, randomized, dose-finding clinical trial. Clin Infect Dis 2010; 51: 684-691.

[103]   Charman SA, Arbe-Barnes S, Bathurst IC, Brun R, Campbell M, Charman WN, *et al*. Synthetic ozonide drug candidate OZ439 offers new hope for a single-dose cure of uncomplicated malaria. PNAS 2011; 108: 4400-4405.

[104]   U.S. National Institute of Health. Studies of a Candidate Aminoquinoline Antimalarial (AQ-13); http://clinicaltrials.gov/show/ NCT01614964 (last accessed: 2015, may 5th).

[105]   Teixeira C, Vale N, Pérez B, Gomes A, Gomes JR, Gomes P. "Recycling" Classical Drugs for Malaria. Chem Rev 2014; 114(22): 11164-11220.

[106]   Sánchez-Delgado RA, Navarro M, Pérez H, Urbina JA. Toward a novel metal-based chemotherapy against tropical diseases. 2. Synthesis and antimalarial activity *in vitro* and *in vivo* of new ruthenium- and rhodium-chloroquine complexes. J Med Chem 1996; 39:1095-1099.

[107]   Dubar F, Khalife J, Brocard J, Dive D, Biot C. Ferroquine, an ingenious antimalarial drug - thoughts on the mechanism of action. Molecules 2008; 13:2900-2907.

[108]   Meunier, B. Hybrid Molecules with a Dual Mode of Action: Dream or Reality? Acc Chem Res 2007; 41(1): 69-77.

[109]   Oliveira R, Miranda D, Magalhães J, Capela R, Perry MJ, O'Neill PM, *et al*. From hybrid compounds to targeted drug delivery in antimalarial therapy. Bioorg Med Chem 2015; doi: 10.1016/j.bmc.2015.04.017. [Epub ahead of print].

[110]   Rosenthal P. Antiprotozoal drugs. In: Katzung BG, ed. Basic & Clinical Phar- macology. Boston: McGrawHill, 2004: 845-877.

[111]   Meier CR etal. The risk of severe depression, psychosis or panic attacks with prophylactic antimalarials. Drug Saf 2004; 27: 203-213.

[112] Dow G *et al*. Mefloquine induces dose-related neurological effects in a rat model. Antimicrob Agents Chemother 2006; 50: 1045-1053.

[113] Basco LK. Field Application of *in Vitro* Assays for the Sensitivity of Human Malaria Parasites to Antimalarial Drugs 2007 [home page on the internet]. Geneva, Switzerland: World Health Organization [cited 8th April 2015]. Available from: http://whqlibdoc.who.int/publications/2007/9789241595155_eng.pdf

[114] Gardner CR. Drug delivery - Where now? In: Johnson P, Lloyd-Jones JG, eds. Drug Delivery Systems: Funda- mentals and Techniques. England: Ellis Horwood LTD, 1987: 11-31.

[115] Speiser PP. Poorly soluble drugs, a challenge in drug delivery. In: Müller RH *et al.*, ed. Emulsions and Nanosuspensions for the Formulation of Poorly Soluble Drugs. Stuttgart: Medpharm, 1998: 15-28.

[116] Steyn JD *et al*. Absorption of the novel artemisinin derivatives artemisone and artemiside: potential application of PheroidTM technology. Int J Pharm 2011; 414: 260-266.

[117] Plessis LH, Helena C, Huysteen E, Wiesner L, Kotzé AF. (2014). Formulation and evaluation of Pheroid vesicles containing mefloquine for the treatment of malaria. J Pharm Pharmacol 2014; 66(1): 14-22.

[118] O'Neill MJ, Bray DH, Boardman P, *et al*. Plants as sources of antimalarial drugs: *in vitro* antimalarial activities of some quassinoids. Antimicrob Agents Chemother1986; 30:101-104.

[119] Pavanand K, Nutakul W, Dechatiwongse T, *et al*. *In vitro* antimalarial activity of *Brucea javanica* against multi-drug resistant *Plasmodium falciparum*. Planta Med 1986; 2:108-111.

[120] Chang HM, But PPH, eds. Pharmacology and applications of Chinese Materia Medica, Vol.2. Singapore, World Scientific Publishing 1987.

[121] Misra P, Guru PY, Katiyar JC, Tandon JS. Antimalarial activity of traditional plants against erythrocytic stagesof *Plasmodium berghei*. Int J Pharmacog 1991; 29 (1):19-23.

[122] Misra P, Pal NL, Guru PY, Katiyar JC, Srivastava V, Tandon JS. Antimalarial activity of Andrographis paniculata (kalmegh) against *Plasmodium berghei* NK 65 in Mastomys natalensis. Int J Pharmacog 1992; 30:263-274.

[123] Brandao M. Antimalarial experimental chemotherapy using natural products. Ciência e Cultura Sociedad Brasileira para o Progresso da Ciência 1985; 37:1152-1163.

[124] Spencer CF, Koniuszy FR. Survey of plants for antimalarial activity. Lloydia, 1947, 10:145-174.

[125] Abatan MO, Makinde MJ. Screening *Azadirachta indica* and *Pisum sativum* for possible antimalarial activities. J Ethnopharm 1986; 17:85-93.

[126] Bray DH, Warhurst DC, Connolly JD, O'Neill MJ, Phillipson JD. Plants as sources of antimalarial drugs. Part 7. Activity of some species of Meliaceae plants and their constituents limonoids. Phytother Res 1990; 4:29-35.

[127] Gessler MC, Nkunya MH, Mwasumbi LB, Heinrich M, Tanner M. Screening Tanzanian medicinal plants for antimalarial activity. Acta Trop 1994; 56(1):65-77.

[128] Brandão MG, Krettli AU, Soares LS, Nery CG, Marinuzzi HC. Antimalarial activity of extracts and fractions from Bidens pilosa and other Bidens species (Asteraceae) correlated with the presence of acetylene and flavonoid compounds. J Ethnopharmacol 1997; 57(2):131-8.

[129] Sathiyamoorthy P, Lugasi-Evgi H, Schlesinger P, Kedar I, Gopas J, Pollack Y. Screening for cytotoxic and antimalarial activities in desert plants of the Negev and Bedouin market plant products. Pharm Biol 1999; 37 (3):188-195.

[130] WHO Monographs on Medicinal Plants Commonly Used in the Newly Independent States (NIS) [homepage on the internet]. Geneva 2010 [cited: 23rd April 2015]. Available from: http://apps.who.int/medicinedocs/es/m/abstract/Js17534en/

CHAPTER 7

Drug Delivery Systems for Vaginal Infections

Sandra Borges, Joana Barbosa and Paula Teixeira[*]

CBQF-Centro de Biotecnologia e Química Fina – Laboratório Associado, Escola Superior de Biotecnologia, Universidade Católica Portuguesa/Porto, Rua Arquiteto Lobão Vital, Apartado 2511, 4202-401 Porto, Portugal

Abstract: Vaginal infections are one of the most common gynecological problems. The lower female genital tract can be infected by various pathogens such as virus (*human immunodeficiency virus,* HIV), bacteria (*Gardnerella vaginalis*), fungi (*Candida* spp.) or parasites (*Trichomonas vaginalis*).

The vagina is the local site for the delivery of therapeutic agents. Depending on the antimicrobial agents, different dosage forms have been developed, comprising of douches, creams, ointments, gels, foams, tablets, ovules, rings, tampons and, more recently, vaginal films. Innovative approaches, like encapsulation technologies, have emerged in an attempt to overcome several limitations of the existing systems for vaginal administration of therapeutic agents.

This review explores the antimicrobial agents that can be used for vaginal infections therapy, the various vaginal dosage forms to deliver these therapeutic agents, their advantages and limitations and the novel advances in the area of vaginal drug delivery.

Keywords: Antimicrobials, encapsulation, mucoadhesion, therapeutic systems, vaginal delivery, vaginal dosage forms, vaginal infection, vaginal tract.

INTRODUCTION

The vaginal microbiota is constituted by a variety of aerobic and anaerobic microorganisms, being lactobacilli the more prevalent with 10^7 and 10^8 cfu/g of vaginal fluid [1, 2]. The normal vaginal microbiota plays an important function in the vaginal health, preventing the colonization and/or infection by pathogens [2]. This population can be disturbed, occuring a loss of beneficial bacteria due to antibiotic treatment, sexual intercourse, hormone deficiency and contraceptives [3, 4]. Thus, vaginal tract can be infected by diverse pathogens resulting in

*Corresponding author Paula Teixeira: CBQF-Centro de Biotecnologia e Química Fina – Laboratório Associado, Escola Superior de Biotecnologia, Universidade Católica Portuguesa/Porto, Rua Arquiteto Lobão Vital, Apartado 2511, 4202-401 Porto, Portugal; Tel: 351225580095; Fax: 35122 509 0351;
E-mail: pcteixeira@porto.ucp.pt

Atta-ur-Rahman (Ed)
All rights reserved-© 2016 Bentham Science Publishers

diseases such as syndrome of bacterial vaginosis (BV), vulvovaginal candidiasis (VVC), trichomoniasis, urinary tract infections, aerobic vaginitis and sexually transmitted diseases as those caused by *Chlamydia trachomatis, Neisseria gonorrhoeae, Treponema pallidum,* human immunodeficiency virus (HIV), human simplex virus, and human papillomavirus [5, 6]. Various antimicrobial compounds have been studied to treat these gynaecological problems by vaginal administration, including antibacterial [7], antifungal [8], antiparasital [9] and antiviral agents [10].

The vaginal drug delivery is known since ancient Egyptian times, being a route used for contraceptives. Several pharmaceutical ingredients have been used intravaginally as antimicrobial, spermicides, hormone therapy and labor induction, among other [11]. Thus, vaginal formulations can be used to produce a local or systemic effect [12]. This route presents numerous advantages such as: accessibility of delivery, it is simple since it allows self-insertion/removal and it is non-invasive (did not cause pain, tissue damage and associated infections) [11]. Vaginal drug delivery presents advantages when compared with oral administration, since this route avoids hepatic first-pass metabolism, prevents the presystemic elimination within gastrointestinal tract, possesses a well-developed blood supply and a large surface, allowing an excellent route for systemic and local drug delivery [6].

Several products have been developed for vaginal application, such as: douches, gels, tablets, suppositories, rings and films. The selection of dosage form depends on the desired effect, for example, semi-solid or solid system with fast dissolution for local effect; or intravaginal ring for a systemic effect. The development of an ideal dosage form is a pharmaceutical challenge, because vagina has unique characteristics relatively to microbiota, hormonal cyclic and pH [13]. The design of the vaginal products should consider the vehicles used for the active drug delivery, in order to protect, support and increase the stability and bioavailability of the pharmaceutical ingredient as well as be safe and acceptable for the user [14].

The vaginal drug delivery system must respect a number of requirements: i) it should be dissolved at vaginal environment, ii) it should not be toxic and irritating, iii) it should not have any meta-stable form, iv) it should have properties of wetting, emulsifying and viscosity, and v) it should have an appropriate contact time [15]. Simultaneously, the delivery system must necessarily be designed in order to be acceptable for the patient, such as it should not have adverse effect on sexual intercourse, not have odor nor color, should not lead to leakage, messiness, irritation, itching and burning [16].

The development of vaginal products shows diverse problems caused by the histology and physiology of the vagina, which contributes to an easily removal of drug. This leads to a decrease of contact time, which requires a multiple daily doses to achieve the therapeutic effect. To solve this issue, encapsulation has been explored for vaginal administration [17]. The technology of encapsulation allows the development of novel formulations, besides the conventional dosage forms, in order to improve the vaginal drug delivery through the increase of retention time and permeation of vaginal epithelium [18]. The design of these controlled delivery systems permits a long-term of drug concentration with a unique dose [19]. As a drug delivery system, the encapsulated drugs can be co-formulated with traditional dosage forms as their carrier to enhance the distribution of the pharmaceutical ingredient [18].

Another way to prolong the contact time is the use of mucoadhesives that allow the interaction between the polymer (natural or synthetic) and the mucus [19]. It can be possible to combine the mucoadhesive polymers with the encapsulation technology in order to obtain multiple-unit mucoadhesive carriers such as microparticles or nanoparticles, achieving a delivery drug system with multiple advantageous features. These novel delivery systems enable a high uniform dispersion in vaginal cavity, a greater drug adsorption and a reduced local irritation [20].

This review highlights diverse vaginal infections and the use of therapeutic agents, considering the various drug delivery systems for vaginal administration.

Anatomy, Histology and Physiology of Vagina

Vagina has an S-shaped fibromuscular collapsible tubes between 6 and 10 cm lengthening from the cervix of the uterus. The vaginal wall is composed of different layers: the epithelial layer, the muscular coat and the *tunica* [12, 21]. The surface of the vagina is constituted for several folds, designated for *rugae*. These folds afford distensibility, support and enhance the surface area of the vaginal wall. The vagina presents a great elasticity due to the presence of smooth elastic fibers in the muscular coat. The loose connective tissue of the *tunica* is also an important element for the elasticity of vagina.

The vaginal fluid contains cervical secretion and transudation from the blood vessels with desquamated vaginal cells and leucocytes. Secretions from the endometrium and fallopian tubes also contribute to the production of vaginal fluid [12]. Thus, vaginal fluid may comprise of contributions from different routes:

vaginal transudate, Bartholin's and Skenes's glands, exfoliated epithelial cells, residual urine, and fluids from the upper reproductive tract. Vaginal secretions possess a complex mixture of components, such as diverse salts, proteins, carbohydrates and low molecular weight organic compounds [22]. Zegels and coworkers [23] collected cervical-vaginal fluid during colposcopy and identified 339 proteins, which included antimicrobial peptides such as human β-defensin 2 and cathelicidin. The enzymatic activity of the vaginal tract is lower than the gastrointestinal tract but several enzymes are present such as nucleases, lysozymes and esterases [21].

Previous studies propose that the daily production of vaginal fluid is about 6 g/day, with approximately 0.5-0.75 g present in the vagina at any one time. The volume of vaginal fluid has been shown to increase significantly during periods of sexual stimulation [22]. The qualitative and quantitative analysis of human vaginal fluid has been performed by many researchers for a variety of reasons. These include the diagnosis of pathologies such as BV, urinary tract infection, cancer, premature rupture of membranes during pregnancy, assessment of the presence of semen for forensic analysis, estimation of the time of ovulation, and the study of organic acids that may act as sexual attractants.

The vaginal pH is acidic because *Lactobacillus* spp. present in vagina can produce lactic acid from glycogen [24]. This pH is also preserved through organic acids secretion by cells of vaginal epithelium [25]. The normal vaginal pH ranges from 3.5 to 4.5 in pre-menopausal women [26-28]. An increase of pH values can be associated with various factors such as reduction of vaginal lactobacilli [27, 29], menstruation and unprotected sexual activity [30]. This disorder can be related with colonization by various pathogenic microorganisms [31, 32].

Vaginal Infections

Gynaecological infections can be located at the level of vulva or internally in the vagina, cervix, uterus and fallopian tubes. The most common of infectious vaginitis are bacterial vaginosis (22-50%) [33], vulvovaginal candidiasis (17-39%) [34] and trichomoniasis (4-35%) [35]. These infections are a risk factor for the transmission and acquisition of HIV. Vaginal infections are not obligatory reportable, so the exact number of cases is not known. Additionally, these infections are often asymptomatic and thence underestimated [36]. When the infections are symptomatic the diagnosis is established taking into account the patient history or the discharge visualization, failing the screen of infections.

Health professionals commonly diagnose a yeast infection using this empirical diagnosis, although the most prevalent infection is BV [37].

Infections of the genital tract can cause discomfort and pain and may affect the sexual function and reproductive capability. Therefore, medical care should have the ability to carry out a differential diagnosis and treat correctly the vaginal infections [35].

Bacterial Vaginosis

Bacterial vaginosis is the main cause of abnormal vaginal discharge in women of reproductive age. Generally, patients report an abnormal excessive white vaginal discharge with an aggressive fishy-smelling, while 50% of women are asymptomatic when this disorder is diagnosed. Beyond the symptoms, this syndrome should be confirmed by microscopy with other additional tests [38]. The key for the development of epidemiology of BV has been the validation of a standardized, reliable and reproducible method to diagnose BV [33]. Nugent and coworkers [39] proposed that BV should be diagnosed by vaginal smears analyzed following Gram's stain, which consists in a cell population score. The clinical evaluation of Amsel criteria considers parameters as odor, pH, presence of clue cells and vaginal fluid appearance. This clinical evaluation and the microscopic examination based on the Nugent score are the methods currently used for BV diagnosis [3].

There appears to be a linkage between absence (or low numbers) of *Lactobacillus* populations and the development of this disorder. In women with BV, the vaginal microbiota is constituted more frequently and in higher numbers by *Gardnerella vaginalis*, *Mycoplasma hominis*, *Prevotella* spp., *Peptostreptococcus* spp., *Mobiluncus* spp., *Bacteroides* spp., *Atopium vaginae* and *Megasphera* spp. [40, 41]. *Gardnerella vaginalis* is an important microorganism of pathogenesis of BV due to its ability to produce biofilms, corresponding to 90% of the bacteria present in the biofilm [42].

Bacterial vaginosis is associated with an increase of pH values, a reduction in antimicrobial activity of the vaginal secretions and local injury of the innate immune pathways [43]. A classic characteristic of BV is the absence of inflammation. A small increase in interleukin I and a low production of interleukin 8, blocking the attraction of inflammatory cells such as macrophages and neutrophils has been observed [24].

Vulvovaginal Candidiasis

Vulvovaginal candidiasis is the most known vaginal infection in the general population, being notorious by the vast number of antifungal medication available [37]. This disorder is the second most frequent vaginal infection after BV. It is estimated that 75% of women in reproductive age have at least one episode of VVC, with 40 to 45% having at least two episodes [44].

Candida albicans is the yeast most frequently isolated from the vagina (90% of the cases), but other species of *Candida* can induce vaginitis such as *Candida tropicalis*, *Candida krusei* and *Candida glabrata* [44]. *Candida albicans* can form a biofilm that turns its more resistant to antifungal compounds as compared to their planktonic cells [45].

Risk factors for episode of VVC which have been documented are oral contraception, intra-uterine device, antibiotics, diabetes, sugar and alcohol consumption [46].

Candidiasis may have a variety of symptoms: vulvar pruritus; the vaginal discharge varies from watery to homogeneously being designated as "cottage cheese-like"; vaginal pain, irritation and burning and can be observed an erythema and swelling of the labia and vulva [47]. However, candidiasis can also be asymptomatic, yeasts have been isolated from vagina of 20% of asymptomatic women in reproductive age [44].

Trichomoniasis

Trichomoniasis is a sexually transmitted infection caused by *Trichomonas vaginalis* which possesses five flagella that are responsible for its motility and their shape is typically pyriform but occasionally amoeboid [48, 49]. Worldwide, this infection is the most frequent non-viral sexually transmitted disease. The World Health Organization (WHO) has assessed that the incidence of trichomoniasis in 2008 was 276 million cases per year [50]. Besides sexual transmission,
T. vaginalis may also be transmitted perinatally from infected mothers [51]. This infection is gender-related predominately affecting women, in men the infection is quickly cleared, suggesting the genital environment is an important element in *T. vaginalis* pathobiology [52]. The factors associated to sexual transmission are non-use of condoms, smoking and low socioeconomic class [53]. The prevalence is also related with a high number of sexual partners and an early initiation of sexual activity [35].

The symptoms of trichomonisis are: vaginal discharge with abnormal color (yellowish-green) and odor, irritation and erythema of vagina and vulva. This infection presents a clinical condition with colpitis macularis (an erythematous cervix with pinpoint areas of exudation) and an increased vaginal pH [54]. Half of the infections can also be asymptomatic [48], these cases are often detected by routine Papanicolaou smear that is 57% sensitive and 97% specific [55].

Human Immunodeficiency Virus

Vaginal infections increase the susceptibility to acquire HIV, which is a lentivirus (slowly replicating retrovirus) that causes the acquired immunodeficiency syndrome (AIDS), where the immune system fails, allowing the development of opportunistic infections [56]. Therefore, immune cells ($CD4^+T$ cells, monocytes, macrophages and dendritic cells) are the target of HIV, being the decline of $CD4^+T$ cells the principal accountable for the immune suppression of the advanced stage of AIDS [57]. Two types of viruses (HIV-1 and HIV-2) are able to infect and generate disease in humans, however, HIV-2 is less efficiently transmitted and is related with a more slow progression of immunodeficiency [58, 59].

Approximately, 17 millions women live with HIV, most of them living in Sub-Saharan Africa and aging between 15-49 years [60]. This virus is transmitted through blood, semen, vaginal fluids and breastmilk. In adults, it is generally acquired by unprotected sexual intercourse and in children is acquired before or during labor or by breastfeeding [61].

Antimicrobial Compounds as Therapeutic Agents

Women should avoid the use of local irritants (shower gels and perfumed soaps) and should be careful on the use of feminine hygiene products (wipes and sprays) that can disturb the normal vaginal microbiota or induce allergic reactions [62]. When women have vaginal infections some recommended treatments should be applied.

To treat BV, metronidazole and clindamycin are the antibiotics used. The standard treatment is 400-500 mg of metronidazole administered twice daily during 5-7 days or 2 g as a single oral dose [62]. The oral administration of metronidazole has some drawbacks, such as nausea, metallic taste, alcohol intolerance and allergic rashes. Oral clindamycin can also cause rashes. Intravaginal treatments can also be used such as 2% clindamycin cream once daily for seven days or 0.75% metronidazole gel once daily for five days [38]. The BV often recurs and an acidic vaginal gel can be used to reduce the recurrence [63] because that gel restores the acidic vaginal environment, being propitious to the growth of autochthonous microbiota. Approximately, 10% of women develop candidiasis after BV treatment [38].

For the treatment of VVC, itraconazole is orally administered 200 mg/day for three days or 400 mg for one day; or 150 mg single daily dose of fluconazole [44]. Diverse vaginal imidazole preparations can be administered such as clotrimazole, econazole and miconazole [62]. The azole derivatives have a mycological cure rate of 85-90%. Nystatin is also used and has a cure rate of 75-80% [44].

Trichomonas vaginalis infection is treated using 2 g of orally metronidazole in a single dose or 400-500 mg of metronidazole twice daily for five to seven days [53]. Metronidazole is a 5-nitroimidazole drug, other compounds of its family can also be used, like tinidazole and secnidazole, all these agents have been demonstrated a cure rate of 95% for trichomoniasis [64].

Topical microbicides have been investigated to avoid the HIV transmission through the formation of a barrier (chemical, biological or physical) to infection or by blocking and inactivating the HIV at the mucosal surface [65]. However, some microbicides showed to be ineffective in clinical trials, for example the repetitive use of nonoxynol-9, a recognized contraceptive spermicide, demonstrated to cause irritation and inflammation of genital tract and increased the acquisition of HIV [66]. There are also evidences that cellulose sulfate is another agent that enhances the risk of infection [67].

Several examples of antimicrobial compounds have been studied for vaginal administration in various dosage forms to treat different vaginal infections (Table **1**).

Table 1. Some examples of the most common therapeutic agents incorporated in different vaginal dosage forms.

Infection type	Therapeutic agent	Dosage form	Composition	Reference
Bacterial Vaginosis	Clindamycin	Cream	2% clindamycin phosphate	[68]
	Lactic acid	Hydrogel	Poly(ethylene glycol) Lactic acid	[69]
	Metronidazole	Gel	Metronidazole, sorbitan monostearate, sesame oil organogel and carbopol 934 hydrogel	[7]
		Tablet	Metronidazole, pregelatinised starch, polyacrylic acid and sodium stearylfumarate	[70]

Table 1: contd…

	Metronidazole plus miconazole	Pessary	750 mg of metronidazole and 200 mg of miconazole nitrate	[71]
	Metronidazole plus nystatin	Ovule	500 mg metronidazole 100,000 U nystatin	[72]
Vulvovaginal candidiasis	Butoconazole	Pessary	100 mg butoconazole nitrate	[73]
	Clotrimazole	Tablet	200 mg clotrimazole	[8]
		Pessary	500 mg clotrimazole	[74]
	Econazole	Tablet	150 mg econazole	[75]
		Suppository	150 mg econazole	[76]
	Itraconazole	Film	100 mg itraconazole, hydroxypropyl cellulose, polyethylene glycol 400	[77]
	Miconazole	Pessary	400 mg miconazole nitrate	[78]
	Nystatin	Cream	25,000 IU/g nystatin	[79]
	Terconazole	Pessary	80 mg terconazole	[80]
Trichomoniasis	Fenticonazole	Ovule	600 mg or 1000 mg fenticonazole	[81]
	Tinidazole	Tablet	500 mg tinidazole	[9]
HIV	Dapivirine	Ring	25 mg dapivirine Excipients similar to Estring® Silicone curing: platinum-catalyzed hydrosilylation reaction	[82]
	Tenofovir	Gel	40 mg of 9- [(R)-2-phosphonomethoxy)propyl]adenine monohydrate (PMPA) in a solution of purified water with edetate disodium, citric acid, glycerin, methylparaben, propylparaben, and hydroxyethycellulose (HEC)	[83]
	UAMC01398 (a novel non-nucleoside reverse transcriptase inhibitor)	Film	Hydroxypropylmethylcellulose (HPMC), polyethylene glycol 400 (PEG400) and UAMC01398	[10]

Alternative Treatments

The use of antibiotics to treat vaginal infections possesses negative effects such as the reduction of the amount of lactobacilli belonging to normal vaginal microbiota, it is not always effective due to microorganism resistance and sometimes there is a recurrence of infections [40]. Thereby, the use of probiotics to complement the conventional treatment of vaginal infection has been investigated. Various clinical studies were performed to evaluate the oral [84] or intravaginal [85, 86] administration of lactobacilli. Probiotic strain can be administered orally because the microorganism has the ability to ascend from the rectum to the vagina, but the time to obtain beneficial effects is obviously longer than direct vaginal administration [40, 87]. Probiotics are capable to colonize the vaginal tract of women with BV restoring the vaginal microbiota and reduce the colonization or even inhibit vaginal pathogens by secreting hydrogen peroxide, bacteriocins and lactic acid [88].

Dosage Forms for Vaginal Administration

In order to administer drugs intravaginally, it is required to incorporate them in adequate vehicles. The anatomical and physiological characteristics of vagina should be taken into account to the design of vaginal products [21]. The pharmaceutical companies are focused on various approaches to allow the vaginal administration and may lead to an extended product shelf life. Many vaginal drug delivery systems are already used for contraception, treatment of vaginal infections, sexually transmitted diseases and other gynecological conditions [89]. Several aspects should be addressed for their development such as the retention time in the vagina, the stabilization of an appropriate vaginal pH, a uniform distribution of the drug, the compatibility with co-administered drugs, simple to apply [15], non-toxic and non-irritating to the mucus membrane [6]. The vaginal drug delivery systems include a large variety of pharmaceutical forms such as liquid systems, semi-solid systems (gels, creams, ointments) and solid systems (tablets, vaginal suppositories, rings, films, tampons) (Fig. **1**). The selection of the appropriate dosage form depends on the physicochemical features of the delivered drug, the target for the drug and women acceptance [93].

Liquid Systems

Liquid systems comprise vaginal douches which allow to rinse and clean by forcing a certain solution into the vagina. The use of vaginal douches dating back to 1500 B.C., when women used preparations with garlic and wine for the treatment of menstrual disorders [94]. Nowadays, these preparations include compounds that can be pH-regulators (acetic acid, citric acid or sodium bicarbonate), antimicrobial agents (povidone-iodine, octoxynol-9) and fragrances [95]. The Food and Drug Administration (FDA) regulates these commercial products faintly, which can be pre-filled into bottles or hanged into refillable and expandable bags [96]. A douche bottle can be disposable (the solution can be directly inserted to the vagina without a douche nozzle or bulb) or reusable (being necessary a connection with tubing and a nozzle). Bag douches allow distributing a significantly higher volume of the preparation compared with douche bottles [96].

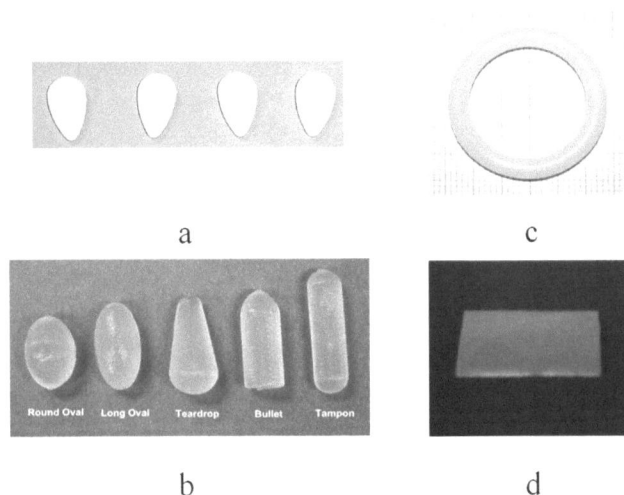

Fig. (1). Examples of solid systems of dosage forms: (**a**) vaginal tablets [90], (**b**) vaginal suppositories [91], (**c**) silicon elastomer vaginal ring [92] and (**d**) vaginal film [90].

Karnaky [97] investigated vaginal douches chemically and found that the pH of a vaginal douche solution alone is not sufficient to decrease the vaginal pH, being necessary the addition of a buffering agent, which maintains the pH of the solution, a surface-acting agent, which helps the penetration of the vaginal solution in the mucosa, and also vaginal adhesives.

Liquid systems are not often used since they are unsuitable for controlled drug release due to the very short residence time in the vagina [21].

Semi-Solid Systems

Semi-solids systems, such as gels and creams, are usually used for topical delivery of antimicrobial compounds and contraceptives.

Although possessing more solid-like character, gels belong to semi-solid systems as they have small quantities of solid dispersed in large quantities of liquid [98]. They can be sub-classified as hydrogels, which are chemically similar but physically different than gels [99]. Hydrogels are hydrophilic polymers, naturally elastic since they are capable to maintain their three-dimensional structure even after absorb, swell and retain large amounts of water [100]. Gels are three-dimensional polymeric networks with a high degree of physical or chemical reticulation, which are previously swollen to equilibrium. When in contact with a fluid, gels are merely diluted [99, 101]. Hydrogels, produced from natural, synthetic or semi-synthetic polymers, are used as drug delivery systems because they release the drug slowly and in a controlled way [6]. They have been developed for vaginal administration with devices of different shapes from cylindrical to torpedo-shaped [102, 103].

These vaginal dosage forms show diverse advantages as bioavailability, low cost and acceptance [12]. Moreover, in pathological situations wherein the vaginal mucosa is dry, lubrication and hydration are achieved by the rheological properties and water content of gels [13]. On the other hand, these dosage forms possess disadvantages as discomfort, leakage and a non-uniform distribution since they do not supply a precise dose [12]. However, the leakage and other negative features as activity loss and short residence time can be overtaken by the addition of mucoadhesive polymers (mentioned below).

Several clinical trials have been done with these dosage forms in order to test the effectiveness of some compounds in BV. A therapy with 0.75% metronidazole vaginal gel proved to be very effective and allowed a significant reduction in the recurrence rate of BV, after a treatment at a bedtime for 10 days [104]. Also in 1994, Livengood and collaborators [105] proposed intravaginal metronidazole gel as an effective, safe and well-tolerated treatment for BV. Another study was performed with 2% vaginal clindamycin cream to test whether it was capable to treat BV in pregnancy. During 3 days, 404 women with BV were treated randomly with 2% vaginal clindamycin cream or placebo. The authors concluded that the cream was tolerated by the mother and showed to be effective [106].

Solid Systems

The solid systems contain a high variety of vaginal formulations such as tablets, vaginal suppositories, rings, films and tampons.

Vaginal Tablets

Vaginal tablets are simple to produce and allow drug release over several hours [21]. After a short time following the administration, their presence is not noticed by women. The tablet adheres to vaginal mucosa and it is retained until dissolution and release is complete [6]. Binders, disintegrant and other excipients used in the manufacture of vaginal tablets are the same that are used for oral tablets. Polymers with mucoadhesive properties can be used in vaginal formulations in order to improve their residence time. Also the presence of surfactants can be added to increase the absorption, operating as penetration enhancers [12]. Itraconazole, clotrimazole and metronidazole are some of the drugs administered in vaginal tablets.

Voorspoels and collaborators [70] proposed the use of a vaginal bioadhesive tablet with metronidazole as an alternative to oral administration for the treatment of BV. In this study, 116 patients were randomly divided into different groups, according to the quantity of metronidazole per bioadhesive tablet: 100 mg; 250 mg and 500 mg metronidazole. No adverse reactions were observed and the cure rates obtained were of 64% (100 mg dose); 61.5% (250 mg dose) and 68% (500 mg dose). This alternative treatment of BV with a single application of only 100 mg metronidazole demonstrated to be a good choice, particularly among women that have gastric intolerance to this drug.

Another study compared the action of a commercial vaginal tablet (Canesten®) combined with Chinese herbal medicine for the treatment of VVC. There were 100 patients randomly selected (between 20 and 41 years old) and two groups were formed: one control group in which 50 patients were treated with only one tablet of Canesten® (500 mg of clotrimazole per tablet) and one treatment group in which 50 patients were treated previously with Chinese herbal medicine – Kushen powder that was submerged in water and boiled (patients' vulva was fumigated with the vapor and then washed with the solution) and then with one tablet of Canesten®. Both treatments (applied just once) were effective, being the previous treatment with Chinese herbal medicine able to improve the therapeutic effect from 96% to 100% [107]. It can be said that besides the usual treatment, the sinergism with other compounds could improve the treatment of vaginal infections.

Vaginal Suppositories

Vaginal suppositories (or ovules) are used for local infections, vaginal atrophy and contraception. These formulations are similar to rectal suppositories and their composition is based on water soluble bases (glycerol-gelatin base) or water miscible bases (polyethylene glycols) [13]. Instead of melting, vaginal suppositories dissolve after insertion due to their hygroscopicity. Some excipients can be added to improve their action such as surface active agents and preservatives [13].

Some clinical trials have been conducted with ovules to treat different types of vaginal infections. For intravaginal treatment of VVC, Upmalis and collaborators [108] compared miconazole nitrate vaginal ovule with miconazole nitrate cream.

Five hundred and fifty-eight women were treated with a single-dose of miconazole nitrate (1200 mg) ovule or seven consecutive doses of miconazole nitrate 100 mg cream. Symptom relief was faster with the treatment with ovule and was the dosage form preferred by women. The authors also concluded that miconazole nitrate vaginal ovule is a safe and effective way to treat VVC. In the treatment of vaginal trichomoniasis, Gorlero and coworkers [81] studied the effectiveness and tolerability of ovules containing different doses of fenticonazole. For two consecutive days, 21 patients were treated with 600 mg and 17 patients with 1000 mg of fenticonazole. After treatment, a negative result for *T. vaginalis* was observed in 65.0% and 58.8% of patients in the group of 600 mg and 1000 mg, respectively. Although there have been side effects of mild or moderate intensity in 3 patients treated with 1000 mg, as they were symptoms of the underlying disease, it can be said that fenticonazole in ovules is effective in the eradication of *T. vaginalis*.

Vaginal Rings

The use of vaginal pessary ring-shaped as sustained/controlled drug delivery system was firstly described in 70's [109]. There are several advantages of this system: it does not interfere with sexual intercourse, does not require daily administration of pills, and enables a continuous delivery of the drug [12].

Vaginal rings are circular, flexible and elastomeric drug delivery devices designed to provide a long-term, sustained or controlled release of drug in vagina [110]. Their diameter is approximately 5.5 cm with a circular cross section diameter of 4-9 mm [12]. The composition of vaginal rings comprises of elastomeric polymers like polydimethylsiloxane or silicone, although others polymers have been tested such as ethylene vinyl acetate and styrene butadiene block copolymer. Ethylene vinyl acetate improved optical features, increased flexibility and adhesion [111]. There are two types of rings: simple or sandwich vaginal rings. Simple vaginal devices contain the drug homogeneous within the ring, which means that the drug at the surface is released faster than the drug that is inside the ring. On the other hand, sandwich vaginal devices allow a constant release of the drug since a drug-containing layer is inserted below the surface of the ring and positioned between a non-medicated central core and a non-medicated outer band [12].

Commercial vaginal rings are already available for hormone therapy containing estradiol (Estring®, Pharmacia & Upjohn) and for contraception containing etonogestrel and ethinyl estradiol (NuvaRing®, Organon).

Vaginal Films

Vaginal films are solid dry dosage forms that dissolve when in contact with vaginal fluids, avoiding the leakage and messiness. This fact makes this product more acceptable by women when compared with vaginal gels. Other positive features associated with vaginal films are their low cost, the easy storage, the easy application and the higher retention time and drug stability [93].

These vaginal dosage forms are square shaped with 5 to 10 cm of side measurement. To be inserted intravaginally, films can be folded and do not require an applicator [112]. The excipients used in the preparation of vaginal films are water soluble polymers (polyacrylates, polyethylene glycol, polyvinyl alcohol, and cellulose derivates), plasticizers (like glycerine, polyethylene glycol), disintegrated agents (like veegum, croscarmellose sodium and cross-linked PVP), fillers and dyestuffs [90]. The polymeric compound and its molecular weight affect the characteristics of the films, such as mechanical strength and disintegration time. The plasticizers are responsible for the flexibility and texture, and the disintegration agents for the increase of dissolution [112].

Therefore, this dosage form shows a high stability to be produced in a large scale and turns the drugs more stable at extreme conditions of temperature and humidity [77, 113].

Vaginal films have been used as contraceptive, but they proved to be less effective than hormonal methods, condoms and intrauterine devices [112]. Vaginal films are under investigation for different purposes, however contraceptives and microbicides are the most studied [10, 113]. Vaginal films are available in the market with different applications from Apothecus Pharmaceutical: a contraceptive film (VCF®) which contains the spermicide Nonoxynol-9, a deodorant (VCF® Dissolving Feminine Deodorant Film) and a lubrificant (VCFR® Dissolving Vaginal Lubricant Film) [90, 112].

Tampons

Tampons have been investigated to maintain vaginal pH through the delivery of lactic acid, citric acid or probiotics. Brzezinski and coworkers [114] tested tampons that release lactic acid and citric acid during menstruation. In this randomized, double bind, placebo-controlled study, 14 healthy women used normal tampons and other 14 women used the novel tampons during two consecutive menstrual cycles. The tampons with lactic and citric acid revealed an ability to reduce the high pH during menstruation, which could decrease the risk of BV.

There are tampons available in the market with a mixture of freeze-dried *Lactobacillus gasseri* LN40, *Lactobacillus fermentum* LN99, *Lactobacillus casei* subsp. *rhamnosus* LN113 and *Pediococcus acidilactici* LN23 (Ellen®, Ellen AB) with the goal to restore the normal microbiota and balance vaginal pH levels during menstruation [115].

Advantages and Limitations of Vaginal Dosage Forms

The choice of a suitable dosage form depends on several variables, such as the drug properties, the clinical requirements and the women acceptability [11]. The main advantages and limitations of each vaginal dosage form are summarized in Table **2**.

Table 2. Advantages and limitations of different vaginal dosage forms.

Dosage Form	Advantages	Disadvantages
Solutions		-very short residence time
Gels and creams	-bioavailability -low cost -easy to manufacture -acceptance (familiarity of gel concept for vaginal delivery) -lubrication and hydration effects	-messy to apply -uncomfortable -leakage -non-uniform distribution -not supply a precise dose
Tablets	-portability -precise dosing -ease of storage, handling and administration -feasibility of large scale productions -low cost -after administration, its presence is not noticed by women -improve stability of drugs -release the drug over prolonged period of time	- distribution and coverage of vaginal tissue is lower comparing with solutions and gels
Vaginal rings	-sustained/controlled drug delivery system -not interfere with sexual intercourse -not require daily administration -enables a continuous delivery of the drug	

Table 2: contd…

Vaginal films	-avoid the leakage and messiness	
	-low cost	
	-easy storage	
	-easy application	
	-high retention time and drug stability	

Improvement of Pharmaceutics by Delivery Systems

The typical vaginal formulations present weaknesses such as low contact time in the vagina, repeated administration, extended duration of therapy and low bioavailability [116].

The poor bioavailability could be overcome by novel drug delivery systems which become available with the advancement in the technology. Encapsulation of pharmaceutical ingredients is a recent concept widely used. The particles encapsulated can supply a sustained release of drugs that is important to maintain drug concentrations between administration and target site [117]. The development of adequate nanoparticles can be a challenging process because the particles can offer a high drug distribution enhancing its efficacy, however care should be taken because the nanoparticle-based drug delivery system must preserve the healthy microbiota [117].

Nanoparticles are solid colloidal particles with sizes below 1000 nm, in which pharmaceutical agents are entrapped, encapsulated or chemically attached to the surface. These systems are recognized by an excellent stability, high capability to incorporate several kinds of drugs and by the skill to modulate the pharmacokinetics of the agents used [118]. Nanoparticles can deliver different pharmaceutical agents, like small molecule drugs, peptides, proteins, nucleotides and genes. The nanoscale drug delivery systems include liposomes, micelles, dendrimers, quantum dots, nanoshells, nanocrystals, gold nanoparticles, paramagnetic nanoparticles, and carbon nanotubes [119]. The methods used to produce these particles are emulsion crosslinking, polyelectrolyte complexation, precipitation, phase separation, *in situ* polymerization, spray drying, emulsion-droplet coalescence, ionic gelation and reverse micellation techniques [18]. Vaginal nanoparticle drug delivery systems are often produced by emulsification techniques that comprise of mixing, homogenization, ultrasonication, solvent diffusion and at last, evaporation [18]. Table **3** summarizes some studies of nano/microparticles that were developed for drug delivery for the treatment of vaginal infections.

Conventional vaginal formulations have limited efficacy due to the low residence time on vaginal cavity, occuring a self-cleansing activity of vagina. This situation causes an administration more frequent of dosage forms, which is problematic and undesirable for the patient. This problem can be addressed with the use of mucoadhesives, since allow to prolong the contact to mucosal tissues due to their strong binding ability [116, 125]. There are several polymers that contain mucoadhesive properties and permit to achieve the encapsulation goal. Mucoadhesive nanopharmaceuticals have been studied with the intent of improving drug delivery in mucosal tissues. There are a variety of mucoadhesive including chitosan, alginate, pectin, carrageenan cellulose derivative, thiolated polymers, polymacrylate and carbomer [18].

The mucoadhesiveness is related with the diffusion coefficient, the solubility of the materials at the mucus and the contact time [18]. The polymeric properties that affect the retention and target sites *via* mucoadhesive bonds are the hydrophilicity, negative charge potential and the hydrogen bond forming groups [126]. Polymers that adhere to mucin-epithelial surface are classified into three categories: (i) that become sticky when placed in aqueous media, being their bioadhesion due to stickiness, (ii) that adhere through non-specific, non-covalent interactions that are electrostatic in nature and (iii) that bind to specific receptor on cell surfaces [127]. The chosen polymers should be biocompatible, have flexibility to pass the mucus, should not exhibit toxicity, should not decompose during the shelf-life of the dosage form and should be economic [126].

Table 3. Studies of nano/microparticles developed for vaginal drug delivery.

Therapeutic Agent	Method of Encapsulation	Major Findings	Reference
Clotrimazole	Liposomes were prepared by solvent evaporation, forming a thin film	-*In vitro* release studies showed a prolonged release of clotrimazole from liposomes -Liposomes guaranteed a high tissue retention of clotrimazole	[120]
Clotrimazole	Nanostructured lipid carriers with clotrimazole were prepared by stirring and ultrasonication method	Nanoparticles demonstrated more active against *C. albicans* comparing with pure drug	[121]
Itraconazole	Nanoemulsion of itraconazole was prepared using tea tree oil	It was observed a synergism of itraconazole and tea tree oil, that produced an effective antifungal thermosensitive gel	[122]

Table 3: contd...

Lactic acid	Poly (ethylene glycol)-lactic acid nanocarriers were prepared by covalently attaching lactic acid to 8-arm PEG-SH *via* cleavable thioester bonds	Nanoparticles supplied a controlled release of lactic acid for various hours, however a maximum release of only 10-14% of lactic acid was achieved	[69]
Nystatin	Microparticles containing nystatin were prepared by emulsification/internal gelation method, using alginate, chitosan and poloxamer 407 polymers	-Excellent mucoadhesive properties of microparticles were exhibited. -Nystatin encapsulated presented an antifungal effect against *C. albicans* without toxic systemic absorption.	[123]
Tenofovir	Microspheres developed by spray drying	-Microspheres were noncytotoxic to vaginal cells and to *Lactobacillus crispatus* -It has not shown an increase of inflammatory cytokines -Microspheres had a good mucoadhesion	[124]

Regulatory Requirements

Vaginal products should have normalized patterns including appearance, identity, uniform content, homogeneity assurance and composition of the drug substance. Depending on the dosage form, other assays should be performed such as viscosity, particle size, release and dissolution/disintegration rates and microbial limits [128]. The stability of the drug products should be analyzed under storage conditions, through analytical methods that detect physical and chemical modifications. Initially, drug stability must be ensured during the time of clinical trials and later, assays should be accomplished to define an expiration date for the commercial product [129].

There is lack of guidelines and regulations for vaginal products, nonetheless FDA has guidelines on the design of vaginal contraceptives and antimicrobial drugs used in treatment of gonorrhea, BV and VVC. Non clinical, pharmacological and toxicological requirements should have been submitted along with an Investigational New Drug Application, according to FDA. Before clinical trials and Investigational New Drug Application submission, reproduction studies are mandatory [16].

In the development of a vaginal drug product the most important step is the delivery of a therapeutic ingredient in a safe, effective and consistent way.

Additionally, the vaginal product should have functional features that contribute to the product utility and patient compliance [128].

Several products for treating different vaginal infections are already available on the market. Table **4** shows some of these products that are available in different dosage forms.

Table 4. Examples of marketed vaginal products.

Product	Drug	Dosage Form	Application	Company	Reference
Canesten®	Clotrimazole	Cream Tablet	Vulvovaginal candidiasis	Bayer HealthCare	[130]
Cleocin®	Clindamycin	Cream, but also available in ovules	Bacterial vaginosis	Pharmacia Upjohn	[131]
Infa VT®	Tinidazole and Clotrimazole in calcium lactate buffer base	Ointment	Vaginal infections	Lark Laboratories Ltd.	[132]
	Tinidazole Clotrimazol *Lactobacillus* spp.	Tablet	Vaginal infections		
	Metronidazole Clotrimazole *Lactobacillus* spp.	Tablet	Vaginal infections		
Lactacyd®	Lactoserum Lactic acid	Douche	Bacterial vaginosis	GlaxoSmithKline (Europe) Sanofi-aventis (outside Europe)	[133]
Metrogel-Vaginal®	Metronidazole	Gel	Bacterial vaginosis	3M Pharmaceuticals	[72]
Mycostatin®	Nystatin	Cream	Vulvovaginal candidiasis	Bristol-Myers Squibb	[134]
Vagistat-1®	Tioconazole	Ointment	Vulvovaginal candidiasis	Bristol-Myers Squibb	[135]

CONCLUSION

Vaginal cavity is an appropriate delivery site for drugs acting locally or systematically due to the rich blood supply and large surface area. Various factors are important in the development of a vaginal drug delivery system, such as safety, efficacy, physical and chemical stability of the drug in a suitable dosage form as well as the patient acceptability. Conventional vaginal drug delivery systems include douches, gels, creams, tablets or ovules. However, with the advances of technology, other dosage forms have also been developed, such as rings and vaginal films. The use of mucoadhesive polymers and encapsulation techniques permitted the design of dosage forms for controlled and/or sustained delivery of therapeutic agents, overcoming some of the limitations of traditional vaginal products. These novel dosage forms enable a prolonged residence time and an improvement of bioavailability of drugs. The research on optimization of the vaginal products is crucial for a successful treatment of vaginal infections, such as BV, VVC and trichomoniasis.

CONFLICT OF INTEREST

The authors confirm that this chapter contents have no conflict of interest.

ACKNOWLEDGEMENTS

This work was supported by the National Funds from FCT – Fundação para a Ciência e a Tecnologia through project PEst-OE/EQB/LA0016/2013. The financial support for author J. Barbosa was provided by the PhD fellowship, SFRH/BD/48894/2008 (FCT).

REFERENCES

[1]   Boris S, Barbés C. Role played by lactobacilli in controlling the population of vaginal pathogens. Microbes Infect 2000; 2(5): 543-6.
[2]   Farage MA, Miller KW, Sobel JD. Dynamics of the vaginal ecosystem-hormonal influences. Infect Dis Res Treat 2010; 3: 1-15.
[3]   Barrons R, Tassone D. Use of *Lactobacillus* probiotics for bacterial genitourinary infections in women: a review. Clin Ther 2008; 30(3): 453-68.
[4]   Bolton M, Van Der Straten A, Cohen C. Probiotics: potential to prevent HIV and sexually transmitted infections in women. Sex Transm Dis 2008; 35(3): 214-25.
[5]   Vitali B, Pugliese C, Biagi E, *et al*. Dynamics of vaginal bacterial communities in women developing bacterial vaginosis, candidiasis, or no infection, analyzed by PCR-denaturing gradient gel electrophoresis and realtime PCR. Appl Environ Microbiol 2007; 73(18): 5731-41.
[6]   de Araújo Pereira RR, Bruschi ML. Vaginal mucoadhesive drug delivery systems. Drug Dev Ind Pharm 2012; 38(6): 643-52.
[7]   Singh VK, Anis A, Banerjee I, Pramanik K, Bhattacharya MK, Pal K. Preparation and characterization of novel carbopol based bigels for topical delivery of metronidazole for the treatment of bacterial vaginosis. Mat Sci Eng C 2014; 44: 151-58.
[8]   Sekhavat L, Tabatabaii A, Tezerjani FZ. Oral fluconazole 150mg single dose *versus* intra-vaginal clotrimazole treatment of acute vulvovaginal candidiasis. J Infect Public Health 2011; 4(4): 195-9.
[9]   Sobel JD, Nyirjesy P, Brown W. Tinidazole therapy for metronidazole-resistant vaginal trichomoniasis. Clin Infect Dis 2001; 33(8):1341-6.

[10]   Grammen C, den Mooter GV, Appeltans B, *et al*. Development and characterization of a solid dispersion film for the vaginal application of the anti-HIV microbicide UAMC01398. Int J Pharm 2014; 475(1-2): 238-44.

[11]   Ferguson LM, Rohan LC. The importance of the vaginal delivery route for antiretrovirals in HIV prevention. Ther Deliv 2011; 2(12): 1535-50.

[12]   Hussain A, Ahsan F. The vagina as a route for systemic drug delivery. J Control Release 2005; 103(2): 301-13.

[13]   Kale VV, Ubgade A. Vaginal mucosa – a promising site for drug therapy. Br J Pharm Res 2013; 3(4): 983-1000.

[14]   Garg S, Tambwekar KR, Vermani K, Garg A, Kaul CL, Zaneveld LJD. Compendium of pharmaceutical excipients for vaginal formulations. Pharm Technol (Drug Delivery) 2001; 25: 14-24.

[15]   Sahoo CK, Nayak PK, Sarangi DK, Sahoo TK. Intra vaginal drug delivery system: an overview. Am J Adv Drug Deliv 2013; 1(1): 43-55.

[16]   Vermani K, Garg S. The scope and potential of vaginal drug delivery. Pharm Sci Technol Today 2000; 3(10): 359-64.

[17]   Valenta C. The use of mucoadhesive polymers in vaginal delivery. Adv Drug Deliv Rev 2005; 57(11): 1692-712.

[18]   Wong TW, Dhanawat M, Rathbone MJ. Vaginal drug delivery: strategies and concerns in polymeric nanoparticle development. Expert Opin Drug Deliv 2014; 11(9): 1419-34.

[19]   Acartürk F. Mucoadhesive vaginal drug delivery systems. Rec Pat Drug Deliv Formul 2009; 3(3): 193-205.

[20]   Thirawong N, Thongborisute J, Takeuchi H, Sriamornsak P. Improved intestinal absorption of calcitonin by mucoadhesive delivery of novel pectin–liposome nanocomplexes. J Control Release 2008; 125(3): 236-45.

[21]   Baloglu E, Senyigit ZA, Karavana SY, Bernkop-Schnürch A. Strategies to prolong the intravaginal residence time of drug delivery systems. J Pharm Pharm Sci 2009; 12(3): 312-36.

[22]   Owen DH, Katz DF. A vaginal fluid simulant. Contraception 1999; 59(2): 91-5.

[23]   Zegels G, Van Raemdonck GA, Coen EP, Tjalma WA, Van Ostade XW. Comprehensive proteomic analysis of human cervical-vaginal fluid using colposcopy samples. Proteome Sci 2009; 7: 17.

[24]   Donati L, Di Vico A, Nucci M, *et al*. Vaginal microbial flora and outcome of pregnancy. Arch Gynecol Obstet 2010; 281: 589-600.

[25]   Charlier C, Cretenet M, Even S, Le Loir Y. Interactions between *Staphylococcus aureus* and lactic acid bacteria: an old story with new perspectives. Int J Food Microbiol 2009; 131(1): 30-9.

[26]   Boskey ER, Telsch KM, Whaley KJ, Moench TR, Cone RA. Acid production by vaginal flora *in vitro* is consistent with the rate and extent of vaginal acidification. Infect Immun 1999; 67(10): 5170-5.

[27]   Donders GGG, Caeyers T, Tydhof P, Riphagen I, van den Bosch T, Bellen G. Comparison of two types of dipsticks to measure vaginal pH in clinical practice. Eur J Obstet Gynaecol Reprod Biol 2007; 134(2): 220-4.

[28]   Garcia-Closas M, Herrero R, Bratti C, *et al*. Epidemiologic determinants of vaginal pH. Am J Obstet Gynecol 1999; 180(5): 1060-6.

[29]   Simhan HN, Caritis SN, Krohn MA, Hillier SL. Elevated vaginal pH and neutrophils are associated strongly with early spontaneous preterm birth. Am J Obstet Gynecol 2003; 189(4): 1150-4.

[30]   Tevi-Bénissan C, Bélec L, Lévy M, *et al*. *In vivo* semen-associated pH neutralization of cervicovaginal secretions. Clin Diagn Lab Immunol 1997; 4(3): 367-74.

[31]   Caillouette JC, Sharp CF, Zimmerman GJ, Roy S. Vaginal pH as a marker for bacterial pathogens and menopausal status. Am J Obstet Gynecol 1997; 176(6): 1270-7.

[32]   Pavletic AJ, Hawes SE, Geske JA, Bringe K, Polack SH. Experience with routine vaginal pH testing in a family practice setting. Infect Dis Obstet Gynecol 2004; 12(2): 63-8.

[33]   Kenyon C, Colebunders R, Crucitti T. The global epidemiology of bacterial vaginosis: a systematic review. Am J Obstet Gynecol 2013; 209(6): 505-23.

[34]   Foxman B, Muraglia R, Dietz JP, Sobel JD, Wagner J. Prevalence of recurrent vulvovaginal candidiasis in 5 European countries and the United States: results from an internet panel survey. J Low Genit Tract Dis 2013; 17(3): 340-5.

[35]   Biggs WS, Williams RM. Common gynecologic infections. Prim Care Clin Office Pract 2009; 36(1): 33-51.

[36]   Kent HZ. Epidemiology of vaginitis. Am J Obstet Gynecol 1991; 165(4 Pt 2): 1168-76.

[37]   Muzny CA, Schwebke JR. Vaginal Infections. Women and health. Elsevier 2013; pp. 473-83.

[38]   Hay P. Bacterial vaginosis. Medicine, 2014; 42(7 Pt 2): 359-63.

[39]   Nugent RP, Krohn MA, Hillier SL. Reliability of diagnosing bacterial vaginosis is improved by a standardized method of gram stain interpretation. J Clin Microbiol 1991; 29(2): 297-301.

[40]   Cribby S, Taylor M, Reid G. Vaginal microbiota and the use of probiotics. Interdiscip Perspect Infect Dis 2008; 2008: 256490.

[41]   Falagas ME, Betsi GI, Athanasiou S. Probiotics for the treatment of women with bacterial vaginosis. Clin Microbiol Infect 2007; 13(7): 657-64.

[42]   Swidsinski A, Mendling W, Loening-Baucke V, *et al.* Adherent biofilms in bacterial vaginosis. Obstet Gynecol 2005; 106(5 Pt 1): 1013-23.

[43]   Dover SE, Aroutcheva AA, Faro S, Chikindas ML. Natural antimicrobials and their role in vaginal health: a short review. Int J Probiot Prebiot 2008; 3(4): 219-30.

[44]   Sobel JD. Genital candidiasis. Medicine, 2014; 42(7 Pt 2): 364-8.

[45]   Hawser SP, Douglas LJ. Resistance of *Candida albicans* biofilms to antifungal agents *in-vitro*. Antimicrob Agents Chemother 1995; 39(9): 2128-31.

[46]   Watson CJ, Fairley CK, Grando D, Garland SM, Myers SP, Pirotta M. Associations with asymptomatic colonization with candida in women reporting past vaginal candidiasis: an observational study. Eur J Obstet Gynaecol Reprod Biol 2013; 169(2): 376-9.

[47]   Eckert LO, Hawes SE, Stevens CE, Koutsy LA, Eschenbach DA, Holmes KK. Vulvovaginal candidiasis: clinical manifestations, risk factors, management algorithm. Obstet Gynecol 1998; 92(5): 757-65.

[48]   Harp DF, Chowdhury I. Trichomoniasis: evaluation to execution. Eur J Obstet Gynaecol Reprod Biol 2011; 157(1): 3-9.

[49]   Hirt RP. *Trichomonas vaginalis* virulence factors: an integrative overview. Sex Transm Infect 2013; 89(6): 439-43.

[50]   World Health Organization (WHO). Global incidence and prevalence of selectable curable sexually transmitted infections - 2008. Geneva 2012.

[51]   Saurina GR, McCormack WM. Trichomoniasis in pregnancy. Sex Transm Dis 1997; 24(6): 361-2.

[52]   Figueroa-Angulo EE, Rendón-Gandarilla FJ, Puente-Rivera J, *et al.* The effects of environmental factors on the virulence of *Trichomonas vaginalis*. Microbes Infect 2012; 14(15): 1411-27.

[53]   Lewis D. Genital candidiasis. Medicine, 2014; 42(7 Pt 2): 369-71.

[54]   Smith J, Garber GE. Current status and prospects for development of a vaccine against *Trichomonas vaginalis* infections. Vaccine 2014; 32(14): 1588-94.

[55]   Wiese W, Patel ST, Patel SC, *et al.* A meta-analysis of the Papanicolaou smear and wet mount for the diagnosis of vaginal trichomoniasis. Am J Med 2000; 108(4): 301-8.

[56]   Dey SK, Zahan N, Afrose S, *et al.* Molecular epidemiology of HIV in Asia. HIV AIDS Rev 2012; 13(2): 33-9.

[57]   Ramana LN, Anand AR, Sethuraman S, Krishnan UM. Targeting strategies for delivery of anti-HIV drugs. J Control Release 2014; 192: 271-83.

[58]   de Silva TI, Cotten M, Rowland-Jones SL. HIV-2: the forgotten AIDS virus. Trends Microbiol 2008; 16(12): 588-95.

[59]   Thomson MM, Najera R. Molecular epidemiology of HIV-1 variants in the global AIDS pandemic: an update. AIDS Rev 2005; 7: 210-24.

[60]   World Health Organization (WHO). Epidemic update and health sector progress towards universal access WHO, UNICEF, UNAIDS. Progress report 2011: Global HIV/AIDS response. Geneva 2011.

[61]   Sankoh O, Arthur SS, Nyide B, Weston M. The history and impact of HIV&AIDS. A decade of INDEPTH research. HIV AIDS Rev 2014; 13(3): 78-84.

[62]   Spence D, Melville C. Vaginal discharge. BMJ 2007; 335(7630): 1147-51.

[63]   Wilson JD, Shann SM, Brady SK, Mammen-Tobin AG, Evans AL, Lee RA. Recurrent bacterial vaginosis: the use of maintenance acidic vaginal gel following treatment. Int J STD AIDS 2005; 16(11): 736-8.

[64]   Lossick J. Treatment of sexually transmitted diseases. Rev Inf Dis 1990; 12(Suppl 6): S665-81.

[65]   Fields S, Song B, Rasoul B, *et al.* New candidate biomarkers in the female genital tract to evaluate microbicide toxicity. PLoS ONE 2014; 9(10): e110980.

[66] Van Damme L, Chandeying V, Ramjee G, *et al.* Safety of multiple daily applications of COL-1492, a nonoxynol-9 vaginal gel, among female sex workers. COL-1492 Phase II Study Group. AIDS 2000; 14(1): 85-8.

[67] Van Damme L, Govinden R, Mirembe FM, *et al.* Lack of effectiveness of cellulose sulfate gel for the prevention of vaginal HIV transmission. N Engl J Med 2008; 359(5): 463-72.

[68] Kekki M, Kurki T, Pelkonen J, Kurkinen-Räty M, Cacciatore B, Paavonen J. Vaginal clindamycin in preventing preterm birth and peripartal infections in asymptomatic women with bacterial vaginosis: a randomized, controlled trial. Obstet Gynecol 2001; 97(5): 643-8.

[69] Rajan SS, Turovskiy Y, Singh Y, Chikindas ML, Sinko PJ. Poly(ethylene glycol) (PEG)-lactic acid nanocarrier-based degradable hydrogels for restoring the vaginal microenvironment. J Control Release 2014; 194: 301-9.

[70] Voorspoels J, Casteels M, Remon JP, Temmerman M. Local treatment of bacterial vaginosis with a bioadhesive metronidazole tablet. Eur J Obstet Gynaecol Reprod Biol 2002; 105(1): 64-6.

[71] Peixoto F, Camargos A, Duarte G, Linhares I, Bahamondes L, Petracco A. Efficacy and tolerance of metronidazole and miconazole nitrate in treatment of vaginitis. Int J Gynecol Obstet 2008; 102(3): 287-92.

[72] Sanchez S, Garcia PJ, Thomas KK, Catlin M, Holmes KK. Intravaginal metronidazole gel *versus* metronidazole plus nystatin ovules for bacterial vaginosis: a randomized controlled trial. Am J Obstet Gynecol 2004; 191(6): 1898-906.

[73] Levy G, Pontonnier G, Taurelle R, Vitse M. Three-day treatment of patients with vulvovaginal candidiasis: a comparison of butoconazole inserts with econazole ovules. Curr Ther Res 1992; 52(5): 729-40.

[74] Boag FC, Houang ET, Westrom R, McCormack SM, Lawrence AG. Comparison of vaginal flora after treatment with a clotrimazole 500mg vaginal pessary or a fluconazole 150mg capsule for vaginal candidosis. Genitourin Med 1991; 67(3): 232-4.

[75] Osser S, Haglund A, Westrom L. Treatment of candidal vaginitis: a prospective randomized investigator-blind multicenter study comparing topically applied econazole with oral fluconazole. Acta Obstet Gynaecol Scand 1991; 70(1): 73-8.

[76] Dellenbach P, Thomas J-L, Guerin V, Ochsenbein E, Contet-Audonneau N. Topical treatment of vaginal candidosis with sertaconazole and econazole sustained-release suppositories. Int J Gynecol Obstet 2000; 71(Suppl 1): S47-52.

[77] Dobaria NB, Badhan AC, Mashru RC. A novel itraconazole bioadhesive film for vaginal delivery: design, optimization, and physicodynamic characterization. AAPS Pharm-SciTech 2009; 10(3): 951-9.

[78] Fan SR, Liu XP. *In vitro* miconazole susceptibility and clinical outcome in vulvovaginal candidiasis. Int J Gynecol Obstet 2007; 97(3): 207-8.

[79] Martins HPR, da Silva MC, Paiva LCF, Svidzinski TIE, Consolaro MEL. Efficacy of fluconazole and nystatin in the treatment of vaginal *Candida* species. Acta Derm Venereol 2012; 92(1): 78-82.

[80] Slavin M, Benrubi G, Parker R, Griffin C, Magee M. Single dose oral fluconazole *vs* intravaginal terconazole in treatment of candida vaginitis. J Florida Med Assoc 1992; 79(10): 693-6.

[81] Gorlero F, Macchiavello S, Pellegatta L, *et al.* Evaluation of the efficacy and tolerability of two different dosages of fenticonazole vaginal ovules (600 mg and 1000 mg) in patients with vaginal Trichomoniasis: a controlled, double-blind, randomized clinical trial *versus* placebo. Curr Ther Res 1994; 55(5): 510-8.

[82] Devlin B, Nuttall J, Wilder S, Woodsong C, Rosenberg Z. Development of dapivirine vaginal ring for HIV prevention. Antiviral Res 2013; 100(Suppl): S3-8.

[83] Karim QA, Karim SSA, Frohlich JA, *et al.* Effectiveness and safety of tenofovir gel, an antiretroviral microbicide, for the prevention of HIV infection in women. Science 2010; 329(5996): 1168-74.

[84] Reid G, Burton J, Hammond J, Bruce AW. Nucleic acid-based diagnosis of bacterial vaginosis and improved management using probiotic lactobacilli. J Med Food 2004; 7(2): 223-8.

[85] Ehrström S, Daroczy K, Rylander E, *et al.* Lactic acid bacteria colonization and clinical outcome after probiotic supplementation in conventionally treated bacterial vaginosis and vulvovaginal candidiasis. Microbes Infect 2010; 12(10): 691-9.

[86]   Marcone V, Rocca G, Lichtner M, Calzolari E. Long-term vaginal administration of *Lactobacillus rhamnosus* as a complementary approach to management of bacterial vaginosis. Int J Gynaecol Obstet 2010; 110(3): 223-6.
[87]   Reid G. Probiotics and prebiotics – progress and challenges. Int Dairy J 2008; 18(10-11): 969-75.
[88]   Borges S, Silva J, Teixeira P. The role of lactobacilli and probiotics in maintaining vaginal health. Arch Gynecol Obstet 2014; 289(3): 479-89.
[89]   Dobaria N, Mashru R, Vadia NH. Vaginal drug delivery systems: a review of current status. East Cent Afr J Pharm Sci 2007; 10(1): 3-13.
[90]   Garg S, Goldman D, Krumme M, Rohan LC, Smoot S, Friend DR. Advances in development, scale-up and manufacturing of microbicide gels, films, and tablets. Antiviral Res 2010; 88(Suppl): S19-29.
[91]   Li B, Zaveri T, Ziegler GR, Hayes JE. Shape of vaginal suppositories affects willingness-to-try and preference. Antiviral Res 2013; 97(3): 280-4.
[92]   Fetherston SM, Boyd P, McCoy CF, *et al*. A silicone elastomer vaginal ring for HIV prevention containing two microbicides with different mechanisms of action. Eur J Pharma Sci 2013; 48(3): 406-15.
[93]   Rohan LC, Sassi AB. Vaginal drug delivery systems for HIV prevention. AAPS J 2009; 11(1): 78-87.
[94]   Whitson GE, Ellis FA. Vaginal douches. SDJ MedPharmacol 1948; 1(6): 217-26.
[95]   Toedt J, Koza D, Van Cleef-Toedt K. Chemical composition of everyday products. Greenwood Publishing Group 2005; p. 98.
[96]   Nicoletti A. Perspectives on pediatric and adolescent gynecology from the allied health professional: to douche or not to douche. J Pediatr Adolesc Gynecol 2006; 19: 353-54.
[97]   Karnaky KJ. Normal physiologic vaginal douches. Am J Surg 1961; 101(4): 456-62.
[98]   Justin-Temu M, Damian F, Kinget R, Van Den Mooter G. Intravaginal gels as drug delivery systems. J Womens Health (Larchmt) 2004; 13(7): 834-44.
[99]   Gupta P, Vermani K, Garg S. Hydrogels: from controlled release to pH-responsive drug delivery. Drug Discov Today 2002; 7(10): 569-79.
[100]   Peppas NA, Bures P, Leobandung W, Ichikawa H. Hydrogels in pharmaceutical formulations. Eur J Pharm Biopharm 2000; 50(1): 27-46.
[101]   Lachman L, Lieberman HA, Kanig JL. Teoria e Prática na Indústria Farmacêutica, vol. 2. In: Fundação Calouste Gulbenkian. Lisbon: 2001; p. 907.
[102]   Mandal TK. Swelling-controlled release system for the vaginal delivery of miconazole. Eur J Pharm Biopharm 2000; 50(3): 337-43.
[103]   McNeill ME, Graham NB. Vaginal pessaries from crystalline/rubbery hydrogels for the delivery of prostaglandin E2. J Control Release 1984; 1(2): 99-117.
[104]   Sobel JD, Ferris D, Schwebke J, *et al*. Suppressive antibacterial therapy with 0.75% metronidazole vaginal gel to prevent recurrent bacterial vaginosis. Am J Obstet Gynecol 2006; 194(5): 1283-9.
[105]   Livengood CH, McGregor JA, Soper DE, Newton E, Thomason JL. Bacterial vaginosis: Efficacy and safety of intravaginal metronidazole treatment. Am j Obstet Gynecol 1994; 170(3): 759-64.
[106]   Lamont RF, Jones BM, Mandal D, Hay PE, Sheehan M. The efficacy of vaginal clindamycin for the treatment of abnormal genital tract flora in pregnancy. Infect Dis Obstet Gynecol 2003; 11(4): 181-9.
[107]   Jian-wei Z, Fang L, Ning Z, Qian M, Yan-he L. Clinical observation on treatment of 50 Patients with candidal vaginitis by Chinese herbal medicine combined with Canesten. Chin J Integr Med 2003; 9(2): 139-41.
[108]   Upmalis DH, Cone FL, Lamia CA, *et al*. Single-dose miconazole nitrate vaginal ovule in the treatment of vulvovaginal candidiasis: two single-blind, controlled studies *versus* miconazole nitrate 100 mg cream for 7 days. J Womens Health Gend Based Med 2000; 9(4): 421-9.
[109]   Duncan GW. Medicated devices and methods. US Patent 3545439, 1970.
[110]   Malcolm RK, Edwards K, Kiser P, Romano J, Smith TJ. Advances in microbicide vaginal rings. Antiviral Res 2010; 88(Suppl 1): S30-9.
[111]   Roumen FJME, Dieben TOM. Clinical acceptability of an ethylene-vinyl-acetate nonmedicated vaginal ring. Contraception 1999; 59(1): 59-62.
[112]   Machado RM, Palmeira-de-Oliveira A, Martinez-de-Oliveira J, Palmeira-de-Oliveira R. Vaginal films for drug delivery. J Pharm Sci 2013; 102(7): 2069-81.

[113] Garg S, Vermani K, Garg A, Anderson RA, Rencher WB, Zaneveld LJ. Development and characterization of bioadhesive vaginal films of sodium polystyrene sulfonate (PSS), a novel contraceptive antimicrobial agent. Pharm Res 2005; 22(4): 584-95.

[114] Brzezinski A, Stern T, Arbel R, Rahav G, Benita S. Efficacy of a novel pH-buffering tampon in preserving the acidic vaginal pH during menstruation. Int J Gynecol Obstet 2004; 85(3): 298-300.

[115] Ellen AB [homepage on the Internet]. Available from: http://www.ellenab.se/en/ [cited: 10th Nov 2014].

[116] Johal HS, Garg T, Rath G, Goyal AK. Advanced topical drug delivery system for the management of vaginal candidiasis. Drug Deliv 2014; 24: 1-14.

[117] Ensign LM, Cone R, Hanes J. Nanoparticle-based drug delivery to the vagina: a review. J Control Release 2014; 190: 500-14.

[118] Vanić Ž, Škalko-Basnet N. Nanopharmaceuticals for improved topical vaginal therapy: Can they deliver? Eur J Pharma Sci 2013; 50(1): 29-41.

[119] Desai, N. Challenges in development of nanoparticle-based therapeutics. AAPS J 2012; 14: 282-95.

[120] Jøraholmen MW, Vanić Ž, Tho I, Škalko-Basnet N. Chitosan-coated liposomes for topical vaginal therapy: assuring localized drug effect. Int J Pharm 2014; 472(1-2): 94-101.

[121] Esposito E, Ravani L, Contado C, *et al.* Clotrimazole nanoparticle gel for mucosal administration. Mat Sci Eng C 2013; 33(1): 411-8.

[122] Mirza MA, Ahmad S, Mallick MN, Manzoor N, Talegaonkar S, Iqbal Z. Development of a novel synergistic thermosensitive gel for vaginal candidiasis: an *in vitro*, *in vivo* evaluation. Colloid Surface B 2013; 103: 275-82.

[123] Martín-Villena MJ, Fernández-Campos F, Calpena-Campmany AC, Bozal-de Febrer N, Ruiz-Martínez MA, Clares-Naveros B. Novel microparticulate systems for the vaginal delivery of nystatin: Development and characterization. Carbohyd Polym 2013; 94(1): 1-11.

[124] Zhang T, Zhang C, Agrahari V, Murowchick JB, Oyler NA, Youan BC. Spray drying tenofovir loaded mucoadhesive and pH-sensitive microspheres intended for HIV prevention. Antiviral Res 2013; 97(3): 334-46.

[125] Kataria K, Garg T, Goyal AK, Rath G. Novel technology to improve drug loading in polymeric nanofibers. Drug Deliv Lett 2014; 4(1): 79-86.

[126] Andrews GP, Laverty TP, Jones DS. Mucoadhesive polymeric platforms for controlled drug delivery. Eur J Pharm Biopharm 2009; 71(3): 505-18.

[127] Park K, Robinson JR. Bioadhesive polymers as platforms for oral-controlled drug delivery: method to study bioadhesion. Int J Pharm 1984; 19(2): 107-27.

[128] Lard-Whiteford SL, Matecka D, O'Rear JJ, Yuen IS, Litterst C, Reichelderfer P. Recommendations for the nonclinical development of topical microbicides for prevention of HIV transmission: an update. J Acquir Immune Defic Syndr 2004; 36(1): 541-52.

[129] International Conference on Harmonization-Q1A (R2). Guidance for Industry. Stability testing of new drug substances and products. 2003.

[130] Canesten [homepage on the Internet]. Available from: http://www.canesten.com/en/index.php [cited: 10th Nov 2014].

[131] Milani M, Barcellona E, Agnello A. Efficacy of the combination of 2 g oral tinidazole and acidic buffering vaginal gel in comparison with vaginal clindamycin alone in bacterial vaginosis: a randomized, investigator-blinded, controlled trial. Eur J Obstet Gynaecol Reprod Biol 2003; 109(1): 67-71.

[132] Lark Laboratories [homepage on the Internet]. Available from: http://www.larklab.com/content.php?parent_id=3&page_id=35 [cited: 10th Nov 2014].

[133] Lactacyd [homepage on the Internet]. Available from: http://www.lactacyd-info.com/lal/cp/en/index.jsp [cited: 10th Nov 2014].

[134] Home Intekom [homepage on the Internet]. Available from: http://home.intekom.com/pharm/bm_squib/mstatvag.html [cited: 10th Nov 2014].

[135] Jones RN, Bale MJ, Hoban D, Erwin ME. *In vitro* antimicrobial activity of tioconazole and its concentrations in vaginal fluids following topical (Vagistat-1 6.5%) application. Diagn Microbiol Infect Dis 1993; 17(1): 45-51.

Subject Index

A

Atta-ur-Rahman (Ed.)
All rights reserved-© 2016 Bentham Science Publishers

www.ingramcontent.com/pod-product-compliance
Lightning Source LLC
Chambersburg PA
CBHW050818220326
41598CB00006B/251

* 9 7 8 1 6 8 1 0 8 1 6 0 1 *